PREMENSTRUAL SYNDROME

Ethical and Legal Implications in a Biomedical Perspective

PREMENSTRUAL SYNDROME

Ethical and Legal Implications in a Biomedical Perspective

Edited by

Benson E. Ginsburg

Biobehavioral Sciences Graduate Program
University of Connecticut
Storrs, Connecticut

and

Bonnie Frank Carter

Department of Psychiatry
Albert Einstein Medical Center
Northern Division
Philadelphia, Pennsylvania

PLENUM PRESS • NEW YORK AND LONDON

Library of Congress Cataloging in Publication Data

Conference on Legal and Ethical Implications of the Behavioral Sciences: the Premenstrual Syndrome (1984: Philadelphia, Pa.)
Premenstrual syndrome.

"Based on the Conference on Ethical Issues for Research on Biological Factors Affecting the Capacity for Responsible Behavior, held September 17–21, 1984, in Philadelphia, Pennsylvania"–T.p. verso.
Includes bibliographies and index.
1. Premenstrual syndrome–Moral and ethical aspects–Congresses. 2. Premenstrual syndrome–Law and legislation–Congresses. I. Ginsburg, Benson E. II. Carter, Bonnie Frank. III. Title. [DNLM: 1. Ethics, Medical–congresses. 2. Jurisprudence–Congresses. 3. Premenstrual Syndrome–congresses. WP 560 C748p]
RG165.C66 1984 174′.2 86-30562
ISBN-13: 978-1-4684-5277-8 e-ISBN-13: 978-1-4684-5275-4
DOI: 10.1007/978-1-4684-5275-4

Based on a Conference on Ethical Issues for Research on Biological Factors Affecting the Capacity for Responsible Behavior, held September 17–21, 1984, in Philadelphia, Pennsylvania

Softcover reprint of the hardcover 1st edition 1987
A Division of Plenum Publishing Corporation
233 Spring Street, New York, N.Y. 10013

For Judy,
whose questions launched this book,

and

For Pearl and Michael,
whose patience and encouragement sustained us in our efforts

ACKNOWLEDGMENTS

We gratefully acknowledge permissions to reprint the following materials:

Page 41, Figure 2: Courtesy of Museum of Fine Arts, Boston, MA. Honoré Daumier. Charivari, September 22, 1858. Second state, lithograph. Bequest of William P. Babcock. B4184.

Pages 52 and 53, Figures 1 and 2: From D. R. Rubinow, P. P. Roy-Byrne, M. C. Hoban, G. N. Grover, N. Stambler, and R. M. Post, in press. Premenstrual mood changes: Characteristic patterns in women with and without premenstrual syndrome. *Journal of Affective Disorders*. Reprinted by permission of *Journal of Affective Disorders*.

Page 321, Figure 1: From K. Muse, N. Cetel, L. Futterman, and I. S. Yen, 1984, The premenstrual syndrome: effects of 'medical ovariectomy,' *New England Journal of Medicine*, vol. 311, pp. 1345-1349. Reprinted by permission of the *New England Journal of Medicine*.

Page 322, Figure 2: From M. Munday, 1977, Progesterone levels in premenstrual syndrome, *Current Medical Research and Opinion*, vol. 4, pp. 16-22. Reprinted by permission of M. Munday and *Current Medical Research and Opinion*.

Page 322, Figure 3: From T. Backstrom, D. Sanders, R. Leask, D. Davison, P. Warner, and J. Bancroft, 1983, Mood, sexuality, hormones, and the menstrual cycle: Hormone levels and their relationship to the premenstrual syndrome, *Psychosomatic Medicine*, vol. 45, pp. 503-507. Reprinted by permission of T. Backstrom and Elsevier Science Publishing Co., Inc. Copyright 1983 by The American Psychosomatic Society, Inc.

Page 323, Figure 4: From W. R. Butt, J. F. Watts, and G. Holder, 1983, The biochemical background to the premenstrual syndrome. In: R. W. Taylor (Ed.), *Premenstrual Syndrome*, Medical New Tribune Ltd., London, pp. 16-24. Reprinted by permission of W. R. Butt and The Medical Tribune Group.

Pages 331, 336, and 337, Figures 1, 3, and 4: From R. L. Reid and S.S.C. Yen, 1983, Premenstrual syndrome, *Clinical Obstetrics and Gynaecology*, vol. 26, pp. 710-718. Reprinted by permission of Lippincott/Harper & Row.

Page 334, Figure 2: From G. A. MacGregor, J. E. Roulston, N. D. Karkandu, H. E. de Wardener, and J. C. Jones, 1979, Is "idiopathic" edema idiopathic? *The Lancet*, vol. 1, pp. 397-400. Reprinted by permission of G. A. MacGregor and *The Lancet*.

Page 339, Figure 5: From R. L. Reid, 1985, Premenstrual syndrome. *Current Problems in Obstetrics, Gynecology and Fertility,* J. M. Leventhal et al. (eds.), vol. 8, pp. 1-57. Copyright 1985 by Year Book Medical Publishers, Inc., Chicago.

Page 341, Figure 6: From M. Steiner, R. F. Haskett, and B. J. Carroll, 1980, Premenstrual tension syndrome: The development of research diagnostic criteria and new rating scales, *Acta Psychiatrica Scandinavica,* vol. 62, pp. 177-190. Reprinted by permission of Munksgaard International Publishers, Ltd., Copenhagen, copyright 1980.

Page 359, Figure 3: From U. Halbreich, J. Endicott, and J. Lesser, 1985, The clinical diagnosis and classification of premenstrual changes, *Canadian Journal of Psychiatry,* vol. 30, pp. 489-497. Reprinted by permission of *Canadian Journal of Psychiatry.*

Page 360, Table 4: From U. Halbreich, J. Endicott, and J. Nee, 1983, Premenstrual depressive changes: Value of differentiation, *Archives of General Psychiatry,* vol. 40, pp. 535-542. Reprinted by permission of *Archives of General Psychiatry,* copyright 1983, American Medical Association.

Pages 361 and 362, Figures 4 and 5: From U. Halbreich, J. Endicott, and J. Nee, 1982, The diversity of premenstrual changes as reflected in the Premenstrual Assessment Form, *Acta Psychiatric Scandinavica,* vol. 65, pp. 46-65. Reprinted by permission of Munksgaard International Publishers Ltd., Copenhagen, copyright 1982.

FOREWORD

As the work on a revised edition of the *Diagnostic and Statistical Manual* (DSM-IIIR) progressed, a great controversy grew over the inclusion of a new diagnostic category, "Premenstrual Phase Dysphoric Disorder." Some nosologists and scientists who study premenstrual syndrome (PMS) felt that, while a specific psychiatric disorder does exist, it occurs relatively rarely. The disorder can be characterized by recurrent periods of dysphoria on a monthly basis, in synchrony with the menstrual period. "PMS" already exists as a diagnosis in ICD 9, the international medical nomenclature. The category for DSM-IIIR was to be a specific psychiatric disorder concentrating on the dysphoric reaction, and not including all of the physical and mental symptoms that people have ascribed to this condition.

Much of the controversy that ensued had little to do with the diagnostic category or the condition itself. Rather, it concerned feelings voiced by feminist groups that the new diagnostic category would be misleading, that it would inappropriately label women as mentally ill, and that it would be affixed not only to the dysphoric disorder, but everything else that happens psychiatrically to women. We were very careful to include the caution that this diagnosis should not be made unless the person has been proven not to have a number of other conditions. We felt that this was sufficient to accommodate inclusion of the diagnostic category. However, it became clear after some time and much discussion that there was no absolute unanimity of opinion. Antagonism to the diagnosis derived from the fact that it was not a scientifically proven category. The Board of Trustees of the American Psychiatric Association determined that a special section of the DSM-IIIR, Appendix A, would list this and other tentative diagnoses which merit attention. We hoped this would encourage research and, over the next few years, provide evidence either for or against full inclusion of these diagnoses in the psychiatric nomenclature.

The following has been suggested as the diagnostic description of Periluteal Phase Dysphoric Disorder:

Associated features. Some studies suggest that there may be a higher prevalence of Depression Disorder in women with Periluteal Phase Dysphoric Disorder. Psychotic symptoms occurring exclusively in the later part of the luteal phase of the menstrual cycle have been described in rare cases.

Age at onset. The age at onset may be any time after menarche. However, women seeking treatment for the disorder are usually over the age of 30.

Natural history. The natural history of the disorder is unknown, but women seeking treatment generally report that the condition has worsened with age.

Impairment. Although subthreshold forms of this condition may be characterized only by subjective distress, the disorder as defined here requires that the symptoms seriously interfere with social or occupational functioning.

Complications. Suicidal behavior may be a complication of the disorder.

Predisposing factors. No information.

Prevalence. Although studies have indicated that mild psychological symptoms during the latter part of the luteal phase are common, the prevalence of Periluteal Phase Dysphoric Disorder is unknown, although studies of the prevalence of the syndrome in women over 18 in the community with prospective ratings are currently being conducted.

Familial pattern. No information.

Differential diagnosis. Dysmenorrhea (painful menses) is characterized by symptoms that occur with menses, whereas in Periluteal Phase Dysphoric Disorder, the onset of the symptoms is premenstrual. The diagnosis of Periluteal Phase Dysphoric Disorder should not be made if the symptoms prior to the menses are limited to pain and physical discomfort. Other disorders that are symptomatically similar to Periluteal Phase Dysphoric Disorder, such as Depressive Disorders and Panic Disorder, do not remit regularly with the onset of menses. The diagnosis of Periluteal Phase Dysphoric Disorder should not be made in an individual who is experiencing only a premenstrual exacerbation of one of these disorders. However, a diagnosis of Periluteal Phase Dysphoric Disorder may be made in addition to one of these other diagnoses if the individual experiences characteristic Periluteal Phase Dysphoric Disorder symptoms that are markedly different from those that they experience as part of the co-existing disorder.

The diagnostic criteria of Periluteal Phase Dysphoric Disorder are as follows:

A. For most menstrual cycles during the past year, symptoms in B occurred during the last week of the luteal phase and remitted within a few days after the onset of the follicular phase. In menstruating women, this corresponds to the week prior to menses, and a few days after the onset of menses. (In non-menstruating women who have had a hysterectomy, the timing of luteal and follicular phases may require the measurement of circulating reproductive hormones.)

B. At least five of the following symptoms were present for most of the time during each symptomatic periluteal phase; at least one of the symptoms was either (1), (2), (3), or (4):

   (1) marked affective lability; e.g., suddenly sad, tearful, irritable, or angry

   (2) persistent and marked anger or irritability

   (3) feeling extremely anxious, tense, keyed up, or on edge

   (4) markedly depressed mood, marked pessimism, or self-deprecating thoughts

(5) decreased interest in usual activities; e.g., work, friends, hobbies

(6) easily tired or lack of energy

(7) subjective sense of difficulty concentrating

(8) marked change in appetite, overeating, or specific food cravings

(9) hypersomnia or insomnia

(10) other physical symptoms, such as breast tenderness or swelling, headaches, joint or muscle pain, sensation of "bloating," weight gain

C. The disturbance seriously interferes with work or with usual social activities or relationships with others.

D. The disturbance is not merely an exacerbation of the symptoms of another disorder, such as Major Depression, Panic Disorder, Dysthymic Disorder or a Personality Disorder (although it may be superimposed in any of these disorders).

E. Criteria A, B, C, and D are confirmed by prospective daily self-ratings of at least two symptomatic cycles. (The diagnosis may be made provisionally prior to this confirmation.)

Some believe there is a need to separate a psychiatric condition around the menstrual period from a physiological condition. Such is the intention of proposing "Periluteal Phase Dysphoric Disorder" as a diagnostic category for DSM-IIIR. Additional research and clinical work will shed light on the validity of this distinction, as well as providing evidence about etiology.

Whether or not we ultimately find a single etiologic cause, it is important that we explore further the inter-relations among the functional and organic aspects of premenstrual syndrome. By addressing many of the difficult issues involved in understanding and treating perimenstrual dysfunction (whatever the label), the present volume is congruent with the intentions of the DSM-IIIR Task Force, and with the needs of affected women and concerned professionals.

Paul J. Fink, M.D.

Chairman
Department of Psychiatry
Albert Einstein Medical Center
Northern Division
Philadelphia, PA; and
Vice President
American Psychiatric Association

PREFACE

In an era when so many life-threatening ailments continue to pose scientifically and medically unresolved problems, our attention to the comparatively less urgent condition of "Premenstrual Syndrome" may seem misplaced. Yet, this entity, with its blurred boundaries, constitutes an interface between biomedical research, clinical practice, social, legal, and psychological concerns, and divergent ethical viewpoints. Furthermore, it exemplifies the methods and premises of these interconnected fields in relation to the objectives of each. These desiderata, so clearly illustrated in the example of premenstrual syndrome (PMS), apply as well to many other areas. In that sense, the issues addressed in the present volume go far beyond the particular syndrome with which it deals.

Premenstrual syndrome itself is far from trivial for that portion of the population clinically affected, and for those who have to address its consequences in a social, legal, psychological, medical, and/or ethical context. For these reasons, we felt it should serve as a focus for an international, multidisciplinary think-tank whose results would merit wider dissemination. The product is this volume. We are grateful to the section on Ethics and Values in Science and Technology (EVIST) of the National Science Foundation and to the Humanities, Science and Technology (HST) program of the National Endowment for the Humanities for their support of the Conference and the derivative activities leading to this publication (Grant RII-8409835 entitled "Conference on Ethical Issues for Research on Biological Factors Affecting the Capacity for Responsible Behavior"). We are also grateful for the helpful advice we received from Dr. Rachelle Hollander, EVIST Program Director, and from the National Science Foundation reviewers regarding the recruitment of qualified participants and suggestions for procedures to maximize the interactions which we sought.

Participants were chosen to represent the diversity of relevant fields — ethicists, legal scholars, clinicians, biomedical researchers, sociologists, psychologists, psychiatrists, feminists, and criminologists. All submitted papers in advance of the Conference, which were presented and discussed in an intensive 5-day encounter. The final sessions were divided into topic groups that attempted to distill and summarize the sense of the discussions. These evaluative summaries are recapitulated in the appendix. The chapters themselves were re-written later by the participants to reflect their own views in the light of the discussions. The volume also includes contributions from several invitees who were unable to attend, but who sent their papers for discussion and feedback.

As editors as well as participants, it was our responsibility to ensure that the final products were carefully reviewed in their various professional contexts, as well as in the light of the transcripts of the discussions, and to intrude our editorial judgments on matters of style and organization. We are grateful to our colleagues for sharing their expertise, for their careful reviews of their papers to reflect the interactions at the Conference, and for their final drafts, which generally involved modifications based on further review, all of which enabled this volume to be more than a mere collation of disparate contributions. Our collaboration was necessarily intermittent due to the demands of our regular duties and to our geographic separation that could not be effectively bridged by the use of the mails and the telephone. It required, in addition, numerous weekends, evenings, and other "free" times at professional meetings, as well as budgeting "vacation" periods for this purpose. Particular thanks are due to Kathy Moriarty, who acted as liaison, copy editor, and lay reader, and whose skill and esthetic sense in the preparation of camera-ready copy are responsible for the pleasing and readable format of this volume.

We also would like to thank Dea Silbertrust for review of the law literature when we were first developing the Conference proposal; Stephen Stelzer, Paul J. Fink, and Susan Bernini for their efforts in facilitating the move of the Conference to Philadelphia; Barbara Mattleman for smoothing many of the details involved in that move; Susan Moushegian for assistance above and beyond the call of any duty in preparing materials for the conferees; and Elizabeth Epstein for her assistance in preparing the subject index. We further gratefully acknowledge the help that we received from Plenum Press in various technical areas, and from our home institutions in providing time and encouragement to permit us to work together.

With respect to our own contributions to the planning and execution of the Conference and of this publication, they are so interdigitated that neither of us should be seen as primary editor. In a very real sense, each of us has been both of us in a shared working experience in which we were able to achieve a synthesis while preserving our separate contributions.

Bonnie Frank Carter
Benson E. Ginsburg

August, 1986

CONTENTS

INTRODUCTION

ETHICAL ISSUES

LEGAL ISSUES

SOCIAL ISSUES

PSYCHOLOGICAL ISSUES

BIOMEDICAL ISSUES

CONCLUSIONS

INTRODUCTION

PREMENSTRUAL SYNDROME:

STUDIES IN INTERDISCIPLINARY PROBLEM-SOLVING

Bonnie Frank Carter, Ph.D.

Department of Psychiatry
Albert Einstein Medical Center
Northern Division
Philadelphia, Pennsylvania

INTRODUCTION

On September 17, 1984, 22 professionals from the United States, Canada, and Great Britain convened at the Albert Greenfield Center at SugarLoaf in Philadelphia, Pennsylvania, for five days of intensive discussion. The disciplinary composition of the full group is schematically presented in Figure 1. This group included lawyers, but their subject would not be limited to the law; it included physicians and biomedical researchers, but their contributions would not be limited to medical concerns; the group included professors, but their discussions would not be constrained to the academic area. Among the latter were philosophers, sociologists, psychologists, ethicists, criminologists, and feminists, whose contributions, like those of the physicians and lawyers, would not be limited to their parochial concerns. Moreover, what made this gathering truly unique was the participants' mutual purpose of reciprocal education and the subsequent mutual goal of working together as a problem-solving team on the basis of shared interdisciplinary information. Their focus would be on the premenstrual syndrome as an example of a bio-psycho-social behavioral complex about which considerable uncertainty remains, and yet regarding which numerous demands for specific concrete responses are made upon the biomedical, legal, and social science disciplines.

Premenstrual syndrome (PMS) can be defined as the occurrence of mildly-to-severely disruptive physical and/or psychological symptoms, recurrent in association with the premenstrual phase of the menstrual cycle. Further delineating features include: extent of functional disruption created by the symptoms; degree of freedom from symptoms during the postmenstrual baseline period; and the degree of responsiveness to specific etiologically-inferred ameliorative measures. These additional factors characterizing the syndrome vary substantially in the importance assigned them by various investigators, and are the basis of enormous controversy.

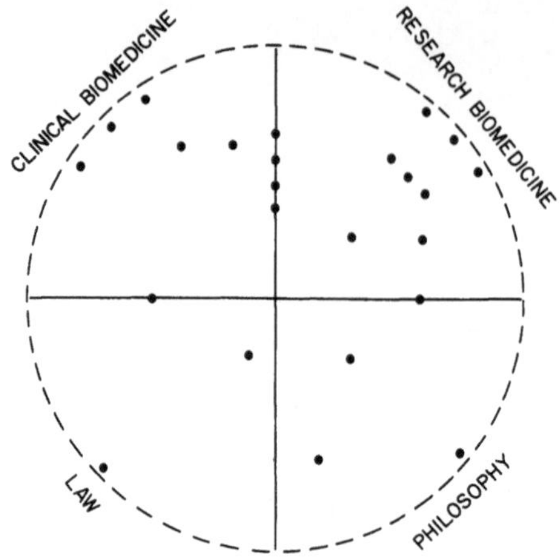

Fig. 1. Conference participants' disciplinary affiliations: A schematic representation.

TOWARD AN INTEGRATED APPROACH

Everyone has heard of the story of the six blind men and the elephant. This book represents just such an endeavor to create the whole out of the sum of its seemingly unrelated parts.

Presented here are the various views required to "see" the phenomenon of premenstrual syndrome in its entirety. Some readers will be constrained by limitations of time or interest to focus on a portion of the total picture, but our purpose in this volume is to provide the opportunity for conceptualizing the whole. As in the story of the blind men and the elephant, recognition of the total entity (and therefore, the ability to formulate meaningful conclusions about it) can only be accomplished by an *integration* of the various facts derived from the disparate disciplines concerned with the phenomenon.

As expert as we each may be in our own field, even if this expertise extends to multiple related fields, we remain ignorant in other relevant areas. Ignorant, that is, but not stupid. A competent professional certainly has the intellectual capacity to understand the intricacies of another specialized area. Although such knowledge is not beyond the grasp of our mental faculties, its acquisition may push us beyond the limits of available time, and further, beyond the limits of our humility. Few among us could afford a return to the intense investment of time and self, coupled with the ever-present risk of exposure to criticism, required by resuming the status of full-time student.

The 1984 Conference was designed to meet these difficulties in communication across professions. All participants were required to be present throughout the five days, as papers were read, issues discussed, and statements formulated. In this way, each person was exposed to the same information base as everyone else. Physicians, for example, learned definitions of legal constructs; scientists confronted principles of ethics and the multiple meanings of "normalcy;"

philosophers grappled with the immediacy of clinical needs. And in the end, everyone was involved in drafting summary statements which epitomized the current status in each of three areas: social science research and public policy; biomedical issues; and legal ethics (see appendix to this book). The Conference ended with everyone more knowledgeable than at the outset and acutely aware of further questions and the ongoing need to find answers.

Following the Conference, all participants submitted revised papers, integrating what they brought with what they got. These papers constitute the present volume, which has been constructed to reflect this same ongoing evolution of information. It is not a self-help manual nor a treatment compendium. Such books are already available, including several written by contributors to the present volume (e.g., Dalton, 1984, 1985; Harrison, 1984; Lauersen & Stukane, 1985; Norris & Sullivan, 1983). Rather, this book is for those who want to understand the full picture of premenstrual syndrome based on current and inclusive knowledge. It is intended for researchers attempting to identify the etiological bases of PMS; for clinicians trying to compassionately and effectively treat the symptoms and the patterns of behavior experienced as disruptive by some of their patients; for attorneys whose first priority is (and must be) providing the best possible legal defense for their clients; for social scientists, feminists, and ethicists concerned with protecting the rights of women while affording them the benefits of medical and legal support; and for the interested lay public whose right to know is well served by the kind of comprehensive synthesis provided here.

THE SEARCH FOR SIMPLE ANSWERS

All efforts at full explication of the complexities of human behavior must confront and surmount the common human predilection for simple and quick answers. This is no less true for premenstrual syndrome than for other behavioral occurrences. Our attention to PMS must, therefore, begin by analyzing sources of the "search for simple answers," so that we may avoid these pitfalls in our later discussions.

Current Western society seems to be dominated by a quest for simple and concrete explanations. Fast food establishments are omnipresent with their promise of instant gratification for a basic need. The 30-minute format remains the staple of televised entertainment and continues to reinforce the premise that life situations not only can be presented and understood within a few minutes, but can even reach resolution within that limited time frame. Television commercials continue in the rapid-fire visual and auditory mode adopted and intensified by the music video industry, and both imply that a more deliberate consideration of facts is somehow outdated and unnecessary. Almost everywhere we turn, there are examples of the request to get to "the bottom line." The attorney's carefully constructed defense is lost in the news report announcing the verdict. Detailed medical care involving the coordination of multiple specialties is forgotten in the resulting statements of diagnosis and prognosis. Years, even decades, of carefully constructed experimental design are lost in the media proclamation of a scientific "breakthrough." Even presentations of new findings to colleagues at scientific meetings are typically compressed into a 15- or 20-minute time frame. And yet, the word "complex" remains the most accurate descriptor of human behavior, and because of its complexity, our knowledge is always tentative and uncertain.

Difficulties in tolerating uncertainty are well documented in the medical and mental health professions. In the practice of clinical genetics, problems are reported in patients' comprehension and recall of probabilistic statements (Lippman-Hand, 1982; Lippman-Hand & Fraser, 1979), while in communications about prognosis for terminal illness, the problem with uncertainty is sometimes experienced as occurring within the physician (Katz, 1984; Seaman, 1985). As "politicians and others would like simple answers to complex questions" (Edsall, 1981, p. 13), it becomes increasingly necessary to eliminate the counterproductive search for simple answers. Otherwise, the most careful and complete scholarship is in danger of being overly distilled and thereby underutilized. Therefore, what follows is a discussion of some of the psychological reasons that simple answers are so appealing and that complex uncertain situations are so poorly tolerated. By understanding the dynamics of the problem, we are better able to deal with it in order that the interactions among us should be maximally productive. Our premises in conducting the Conference derived from these dynamics.

THE DYNAMICS OF REDUCTIONISM

All human beings have the capacity (and, to a greater or lesser degree, the tendency) to "split" our thinking into exaggerated and mutually exclusive categories. This cognitive process of polarizing people or events as into all "good" or all "bad" has its roots in the initial childhood recognition of the "other" (typically the mother) as separate from self (Mahler, Pine, & Bergman, 1975). As the infant begins to know herself or himself as distinct from the nurturing and therefore powerful parent, the possibility of loss of that other becomes conscious as well. Prior to the stage where "good" (or desired) actions can be integrated with "bad" (or rejected) events, the infant conceptualizes only one extreme at a time. Hence, the parent is perceived alternately as good or bad prior to being recognized as both simultaneously. The latter integration may seem so logically congruent with the earlier perceptions as to be simply inevitable, but its development can very easily be disrupted. Evidence of this is the increasing prevalence of adults presenting to the mental health profession as struggling with problems attributable to Borderline Personality Disorder. This psychiatric designation specifies a personality structure so markedly characterized by "splitting" that this is a hallmark criterion for diagnosis [*Diagnostic and Statistics Manual of Mental Disorders*, Edition 3 (DSM-III), 1980; see Gunderson & Singer (1975) and Kernberg (1975) for further discussion].

In normal development, integration of the divergent aspects of "good" and "bad" is based on repeated presentations of small frustrations followed by re-establishment of the nurturant connection, all against a background of reliable consistency, or what is known as "good enough mothering" (Winnicott, 1965). At the present time in our society, this necessary pattern is frequently disrupted by such realities as decreased availability of helpers for the primary caretaker, increased isolation of the nuclear family, decreased parental availability due to increasing divorce rates and two-wage-earner families; and the existence of parents who are themselves narcissistically deprived, depressed, or otherwise emotionally disturbed (Miller, 1981). This last factor is both a result and a self-perpetuating cause of inadequate parenting. Furthermore, these individual, familial, and societal factors are cited as causal to other problems of life in the late 20th century, including teenage suicide, teenage pregnancy, and drug and alcohol abuse. There are many obvious and obscure interrelationships among these factors, but a full discussion of these is beyond the present purpose. Here, the point is this: Continued reliance on dichotomous thinking into adulthood appears to be increasingly prevalent in this culture, and is one source of our identifiable preference for simple answers and our general inability to tolerate "gray" uncertainty, ambiguity, and profound complexity.

The limit that exists in our intellectual capabilities is another source of the preference for simple answers and the related intolerance of ambiguity.[1] When the phenomenon we wish to study has components in excess of our attentional capacity, empirically demonstrated as limited to seven items (± 2) (Miller, 1956), we must analyze our object of study into smaller, more manageable components. We then can consider the full complexity of the subject matter only by integrating several partially overlapping pieces. In taking these steps, we are confronted with our inherent mental limitations. Such limitations in an aspect of behavior that comprises an essential basis for sense of self-esteem can even be perceived as defect (Kohut, 1972, p. 146):

> "We take our thought processes as belonging to the core of our self and we refuse to admit that we may not be in control of them. . . The loss of limb can. . . be mourned, like the loss of a love object (Tolstoy's description of Anatole Kuragin's farewell to his amputated leg is a deeply moving illustration of this process; 1866, Book 10, Chapter 7, pp. 907-908); a defect in the realm of our mental functions, however, is experienced as loss of self."

The usual response to a "loss of self," including being confronted with one's intellectual limits, is anger. More precisely, we experience narcissistic rage in response to what is perceived as damage to one's self or a narcissistic injury. The fact that intense affect such as narcissistic rage further hinders cognitive capacity increases the pressure to avoid circumstances of greater complexity than what we can quickly assimilate; i.e., feelings of narcissistic injury resulting from recognition of our cognitive limitations increase our tendencies to avoid ambiguity and to demand simple answers.

We all endeavor to maintain a feeling of intellectual competence and a sense of an integrated self. Nevertheless, "Narcissistic blows are unavoidable and the propensity to respond to them with rage is ubiquitous" (Kohut, 1985a, p. 63). Although these two facts are easily acknowledged as theoretically valid, a third fact interferes with our accepting them as personally (as well as professionally) veridical; and with our understanding the connection between perceived narcissistic injury and an intolerance of ambiguity. The third fact is that normal anger (normal meaning healthy, as well as normal meaning ubiquitous) is often repressed during development by raising children in ways which "refuse to let them express their anger and suffering except at the risk of losing their parents' love and affection" (Miller, 1983, p. 106). In order to circumvent this problem, and thereby to clarify the connection between narcissism and intellectual closed-mindedness, the following illustration is cited as a more easily recognized example of narcissistic rage. This example involves (Kohut, 1972, p. 147; see also Kohut, 1985a, b):

> ". . . the emotional reaction of children to slight injuries. When a child has stubbed his toe or pinched his finger, his

---

[1] My thanks to Henry Beck, Ph.D., for directing my attention to this point.

response expresses a number of feelings. . . The child gives voice not only to his physical pain and fear, but also to his wounded narcissism. 'How can it be? How can it happen?' his outraged cries seem to ask."

And as it is that a child with a stubbed toe seeks to avoid repeating the experience of the self-offensive pain, so too does the adult confronted with intellectual limitations seek to avoid repetition of that psychological affront, as is done by seeking or erroneously creating simple answers.

Individual narcissism and splitting converge in the phenomenon of "we/they" thinking. Dividing people into categories or groups is a means of decreasing uncertainty or ambiguity in a complex situation. If the criteria for inclusion are specified in sufficient detail, it is simply a matter of processing the details to reach a clear decision about group membership. Such categorizations further serve narcissistic needs because whatever the "we" group is — be it defined as different from the "they" group according to criteria of sex, race, social class, functional status, or occupational group — "we" are always represented as "better" than "they" are. Thus, the we/they split fulfills the narcissistic need for enhancement of self through identification with a valued, even idealized, group.

Increased acceptance of individual differences would be facilitated by emphasizing the reality that any group comparison is more accurately reflected by a continuum than by a dichotomy, but this is resisted precisely because it clouds identification of group membership. A focus on the needs of the self can provide not only an understanding of what is occurring in such splits, but also suggests a means of alleviating this destructive way of thinking. In a discussion of work with actively delusional patients, Kohut (1985b, p. 250) stated, "Insofar as you can build a bridge of empathy to a person, to that extent he is not psychotic." While the designation of psychosis is not particularly relevant to PMS (see chapter by Sadoff, this volume, for further discussion of a continuum of normal to psychotic thought processes), the possibility of bridging a gap in comprehension through empathy is critical. The particular group distinctions relevant to PMS are in regard to sex: across gender (males versus females) and among women (those with PMS versus those without it). Here again, it is necessary to emphasize the necessity of acknowledging and assimilating events and feelings which we might prefer to repress, and again reference to childhood occurrences provides an excellent illustration (Miller, 1983, p. 177):

> "To empathize with what a child is feeling when he or she is defenseless, hurt, or humiliated is like suddenly seeing in a mirror the suffering of one's own childhood, something many people must ward off out of fear while others can accept it with mourning. People who have mourned in this way understand. . . the dynamics of the psyche. . ."

While each of us may not experience "PMS" *per se*, we have all experienced, in other contexts and to varying degrees, the feelings of a PMS sufferer. We will be best able to improve our research and treatment efforts if we utilize these available empathic connections (see chapters by Ginsburg and by Vergare, this volume, for further elaboration).

PREMENSTRUAL SYNDROME AS A MULTIFACETED COMPLEX ENTITY

The psychological parameters discussed here as pressures toward erroneously simplified answers are particularly relevant to PMS. Etiology, or the cause of behavioral events, is a major area where the expectation of simple answers creates spurious conflict. In other words, is PMS caused by biological factors, or is it caused by psycho-social factors? Although it is generally not recognized, it seems inevitable that the truth encompasses both domains, and that all of the following will be found to exist:

1. Some women will have premenstrual disruptions of usual function resulting directly from biological changes.

2. Others will have such disruptions resulting directly from psychological factors. For some women, this will occur in addition to biologically-caused changes, in which cases:

   (a) psychological problems may derive from the biological occurrences; or

   (b) psychological problems and contributing biological factors may arise from independent sources.

3. For still other women, premenstrual dysfunction will arise solely from psychological factors, which may, in turn, lead to biological changes.

4. Contextual dynamics provide a further source for premenstrual symptomatology; e.g., past and present family circumstances, social and cultural attitudes, religious and political beliefs. As with biological and psychological factors, social parameters will be of major import for some women and of lesser relevance for others.

To adequately consider premenstrual syndrome as an inclusive entity with varying manifestations, and to attempt to achieve an understanding encompassing its definition, its causes, and its effects, we must recognize the possibility that all of the above situations exist. In fact, given the ways in which human behavior develops and occurs, it should be expected that all of the above do exist. We must especially remind ourselves that the identification of any one causal mechanism in a complex behavior should not be misconstrued as meaning that others do not exist, nor should the label PMS be misconstrued as implying a unitary syndrome rather than one based on complicated and possibly diverse interacting components converging on a common range of definable endpoints; hence, a syndrome.

No finding of one etiological factor is likely to translate into a single treatment and thereby eliminate the myriad concerns involved in the experience and study of PMS. This book stands as a specific example of the kind of broad-based interdisciplinary and integrative discussion essential to improvements for the existence of humankind; not simple. . . not quick. . . not easy. . . but essential.

USING THIS VOLUME

As an addition to the above emphasis on the importance of viewing the present volume as an integrated whole, the following discussion highlights the areas of uncertainty and controversy regarding PMS. In keeping with the apprentice tradition of teaching by example, it is presented in the form of questions with explanatory comments. These are drawn from the initial questions from which the Conference structure and content were developed, and therefore will include references to those chapters in which relevant issues are discussed and answers suggested. Consequently, this listing is appropriate as a study guide.

What is the name of this phenomenon we are discussing? The field includes the following designations: Premenstrual Tension Syndrome (PMTS) (e.g., Frank, 1931); Premenstrual Distress (e.g., Freed, 1945); Premenstrual Syndrome (PMS) (e.g., Dalton & Greene, 1953); Premenstrual Dysphoria (e.g., Steiner & Carroll, 1977); Premenstrual Changes (PMC) (e.g., Endicott, Halbreich, Schacht, & Nee, 1981); Premenstrual Stress Syndrome (PMSS) (e.g., Press, 1983); and Premenstrual Dysphoric Disorder (PDD) (e.g., revisions suggested to the *Diagnostic and Statistics Manual of Mental Disorders, Edition 3* (DSM-III) (Fisher, 1986). Most recently, a diagnosis of Periluteal Phase Dysphoric Disorder is being considered in reference to the DSM-IIIR (see Foreword by P.J. Fink, this volume). While each of these labels was created to emphasize particular symptoms and/or etiology, all have general referents in common, and should be recognized as having more overlap than differentiation.

Does PMS really exist? What is it? How should it be defined? Certainly, premenstrual "changes" occur (see chapters by Ericksen and by Halbreich & Endicott), but the manifestations can affect almost every internal and external human system (see chapters by O'Brien; Rubinow) with differing degrees of severity or impact. The timing of symptoms (i.e., the consistency of cyclic occurrence) is questioned by some (chapters by Blechman & Clay; Rubinow; Sampson), while seen by others (chapter by Dalton) as the essential minimum criterion for diagnosis. Even the possibility of a symptom-free postmenstruum may be doubted, as interpersonal conflicts can easily continue once started (see, for example, chapter by Reid). The author(s) of each chapter was requested either to provide a definition of PMS or to specify the reasons a definition could not be stated. Accordingly, this book contains many "definitions" of PMS. Given the continuing uncertainties, including but not limited to those listed below, this absence of a single definition is as it should be. It is left to the reader to draw his or her own conclusions.

Is premenstrual syndrome a unitary condition or does use of this label erroneously imply a singular entity? Beyond the fact that few human behavioral conditions are so simple in either their causes or their effects, there is evidence of substantial heterogeneity (of causal pathways), as well as a multiplicity (of causal systems) for PMS (see chapters by Ginsburg; Rubinow; Steiner & Haskett). Singular approaches generate more error than information (see chapters by Bell; Bird; Ginsburg).

How many women are affected by this phenomenon? Any designation of the percentage of women who have PMS depends upon the definition being employed, and particularly on the severity of "symptoms" and the method by which their presence is assessed. Accordingly, prevalence remains an open question (see chapter by Ericksen), with a wide range of percentages cited across investigators (see chapters by O'Brien; Reid; Rubinow). The prevalence question has significant implications for public perception and media representation (see chapter by Parlee), as people are wont to believe "*if one* woman is unable to function fully, or commits an aggressive act premenstrually, *then all* women. . ."

Do the changes that occur during the premenstrual phase warrant the label "syndrome"? What are the implications of such labeling? These questions bring in such philosophical and social issues as normalcy, stigmatization, right of the individual *vis-à-vis* the group, the roles of the media, cultural and familial training, and consumer advocacy (see chapters by Bell; Cassara; Ericksen; Macklin; Norris; Parlee; Ruble & Brooks-Gunn). Although medical designations are generally intended to be neutral, these designations are frequently, even typically, given value connotations. For example, it has been questioned whether inclusion as a psychiatric diagnosis promotes understanding or blame (Goleman, 1985). It is important for us to recognize the interpretations inferred from our words and actions, and to attempt prevention of predictable errors whenever possible.

Is (or are) PMS something which warrants treatment? This again relates to the question, "What is normal?" But even if warranted, *what kind of treatment would be appropriate?* Should PMS be addressed through a medical model (chapter by Bell), and viewed endocrinologically (chapters by Dalton; Reid; Sampson) or psychiatrically (chapter by Vergare); or perhaps through a behavioral (chapter by Blechman & Clay) or socio-cultural framework (chapter by Ericksen)? [We remind you to recognize that these "examples" are stated by way of emphases, as the overwhelmingly predominant view in this book is that a multidisciplinary approach is essential, both for research and for treatment of PMS.]

Some awareness of the impending onset of menses is the most common occurrence for women. In fact, total lack of any such awareness is not only extremely rare, but may itself be associated with certain potentially problematic emotional constellations (Foresti, Ferraro, Reithaar, Berlanda, Volpi, Drago, & Cerutti, 1981). When premenstrual changes create no disruption or only minor disruption of usual activities, it may be sufficient for the woman to simply take note of the time in her cycle, be aware and accepting of the bodily functions involved, and go on about her business, be it in the home, the work place, or whatever. If subjectively-defined major disruption results from the noted changes (perhaps thereby more appropriate to be labeled "symptoms," or as part of a "syndrome"), then treatment is likely to be sought.

Does PMS exist exclusive of other medical, psychological, or social conditions? Again, this would appear unlikely on the basis of the usual complexity of the human condition, and here also, there is specific research addressing areas of overlap and their significance (chapters by Halbreich & Endicott; Steiner & Haskett; Vergare). It is particularly important to remember that an over-emphasis on PMS as "the cause" of particular situations can lead to inappropriately ignoring other sources, be they intra-psychic or interpersonal (see chapter by Vergare), or cultural or political (see chapter by Bell).

Where does PMS fit into the legal arena? Within the context of the meaning of "responsibility," does PMS have any impact on legal responsibility (chapters by Boorse; Houlgate)? Does it (ever) constitute a diminution of capacity in the legal sense so that it warrants some mitigation of legal culpability (chapters by Boorse; Dalton; Jeffery; Sadoff)? Directly related to these questions are the issues raised by criminologists and philosophers: Rehabilitation versus retribution; biological and/or psycho-social causation of crime; and acceptability of internment versus the unacceptability of treatment (chapters by Jeffery; Macklin).

What do we do now? While it is clear that more data are needed to fully answer the above questions, many situations exist currently which cannot responsibly be evaded pending further research. Such situations exist in the clinical domain, where self-identified PMS sufferers are seeking help from gynecologists (chapter by Reid), psychologists (chapter by Blechman & Clay), psychiatrists (chapters by Sampson; Steiner & Haskett; and Vergare), as well as peer (chapter by Cassara) and professional (chapter by Norris) self-help groups. Progesterone therapy is more fully discussed in the present volume than other treatments due to its prominence in the field and the resulting need for considering the issues its use raises.

Circumstances requiring direct and immediate attention have also arisen in the legal arena, as in the 1982 case where Attorney Stephanie Benson, while not introducing PMS as a defense *per se*, introduced PMS as a relevant factor in the criminal ajudication of Shirley Santos in the matter of child abuse (Clausen, 1982). Although the relevance of PMS was not fully decided because the case was settled in a pretrial hearing when Judge Donald Jacoby recommended discharge conditional on the defendant seeking adequate treatment for her symptoms, the Judge did state the following (Certified Court Record, April 29, 1982, pp. 29-30):

> "As to the issue of premenstrual syndrome, a good deal of public discussion has surfaced recently here and abroad about it. Apparently, if this case proceeds to trial the issue of viability of such a defense would be tested. Notwithstanding that, this Court wishes to make this observation. . . Inasmuch as eruptions of the mind are admissible evidence at criminal trials, why then should proof of physiological eruptions of the body likewise not be admitted? A rhetorical question at this moment but perhaps that will be grappled with at another time."

This statement is open to some contradictory interpretations [e.g., Holtzman (1984) versus Benson (personal communication, September 20, 1984)]; and as such, summarizes the still tentative situation of PMS in relation to diminished capacity in the United States. This is in contrast to the situation in Great Britain, where PMS is sometimes accepted as the basis for mitigated punishment [*Regina v. Craddock*, *Regina v. English* in Dalton (1984); versus *Regina v. Smith (Sandie)* reported by Caryl-Thomas (1982)], although it continues to arouse substantial debate (e.g., Brahams, 1981). [See chapters by Boorse and by Sadoff for further discussion of the legal issues involved, and by Bell regarding the socio-cultural context.]

Even while such situations demand immediate action, regardless of extant knowledge, attention must also be directed to long-term consequences. In addition to guidelines provided by the Federal Government (chapter by Rubinow), facts and frameworks taken from history and sociology (chapter by Bell), from biomedical ethics and philosophy (chapters by Boorse; Houlgate; and Macklin), and from critical evaluations of research (chapters by Halbreich & Endicott; Rubinow; and Steiner & Haskett) provide essential cautions.

CONCLUSIONS

As noted in the Introduction to this chapter, decisions about actions to take are in part directed by the ethics of one's particular professional discipline (Goldman, 1980). There may be differences of opinion among colleagues. For example, "Scientists can honestly disagree as to what inferences can be legitimately drawn from the facts"

(Edsall, 1981, p. 12). Nevertheless, general agreement about the priorities and purposes of a profession provide significant guidance for decision-making: ". . . above all. . . the passion for getting at the truth should be the dominant passion for scientific workers when they are trying to act as responsible scientists" (Edsall, 1981, p. 14). Interdisciplinary efforts force us into the difficult task of working across divergent professional priorities (Cassell, 1985), but the resulting geometric increase in available problem-solving capability justifies the effort. Contributions from many academic and applied disciplines were involved in creating this book. We, the editors and the contributors, present it as our contribution to furthering the understanding of premenstrual syndrome, as an example of a human behavioral complexity by professionals and the general public alike.

ACKNOWLEDGMENTS

The author is appreciative of comments and suggestions on a preliminary draft from the following members of the Study Group in Self Psychology and Object Relations of the Philadelphia Society for Psychoanalytic Psychology: Kathleen Arcuri, Ph.D.; Nicholas Kirsch, M.A.; and Bonnie Randolph, Psy.D.

REFERENCES

Brahams, D., 1981. Premenstrual syndrome: A disease of the mind? *The Lancet 2:* 1238-1240.

Caryl-Thomas, E., 1982. Pre-menstrual syndrome — whether a defence. *Criminal Law Review*, August, pp. 531-532.

Cassell, E. J., 1985. *The Place of the Humanities in Medicine.* The Hastings Center, Hastings-on-Hudson, NY.

Clausen, P., 1982. Not guilty because of PMS? *Newsweek,* November 8, p. 111.

Dalton, K., 1984. *Premenstrual Syndrome and Progesterone Therapy* (second edition). Year Book Publishers, Chicago, IL; and William Heineman Medical Books, London.

Dalton, K., 1985. *Once A Month: A Complete Guide to the Symptoms, Effects and Treatment of Premenstrual Syndrome* (second edition). Hunter House, Claremont, CA.

Dalton, K. and R. Greene, 1953. The premenstrual syndrome. *British Medical Journal 1:* 1007.

Edsall, J. T., 1981. Two aspects of scientific responsibility. *Science 212:* 11-14.

Endicott, J., U. Halbreich, S. Schacht, and J. Nee, 1981. Premenstrual changes and affective disorders. *Psychosomatic Medicine 3:* 514-517.

Fisher, K., 1986. DSM-III-R: Amendment process frustrates non-MDs. *American Psychiatric Monitor,* February, pp. 17, 18, 24.

Foresti, G., M. Ferraro, P. Reithaar, C. Berlanda, M. Volpi, D. Drago, and R. Cerutti, 1981. Premenstrual syndrome and personality traits: A study on 110 pregnant patients. *Psychotherapy & Psychosomatics 36:* 37-42.

Frank, R. T., 1931. The hormonal causes of premenstrual tension. *Archives of Neurology and Psychiatry (Chicago) 26:* 1053-1057.

Freed, S., 1945. The treatment of premenstrual distress with special consideration of the androgens. *Journal of the American Medical Association 127:* 377-379.

Goldman, A. H., 1980. *The Moral Foundations of Professional Ethics.* Rowena and Littlefield, Totowa, NJ.

Goleman, D., 1985. New psychiatric syndromes spur protest. *The New York Times,* November 19, Section C, pp. 1 and 16.

Gunderson, J. G. and M. T. Singer, 1975. Defining borderline patients: An overview. *American Journal of Psychiatry 132:* 1-10.

Harrison, M., 1984. *Self Help for Premenstrual Syndrome.* Random House, New York, NY.

Holtzman, E., 1984. Premenstrual syndrome: The indefensible defense. *Harvard Women's Law Journal 7:* 1-3.

Katz, J., 1984. Why doctors don't disclose uncertainty. *Hastings Center Report,* February, pp. 35-44.

Kernberg, O., 1975. *Borderline Conditions and Pathological Narcissism.* Jason Aronson, New York, NY.

Kohut, H., 1972. Thoughts on narcissism and narcissistic rage. *The Psychoanalytic Study of the Child 27:* 360-400. [Reprinted in: C. B. Strozier (Ed.), 1985. *Self Psychology and the Humanities: Reflections on a New Psychoanalytic Approach.* W. W. Norton, New York, NY, pp. 124-160.]

Kohut, H., 1985a. On leadership. In: C. B. Strozier (Ed.), *Self Psychology and the Humanities: Reflections on a New Psychoanalytic Approach.* W. W. Norton, New York, NY, pp. 51-72.

Kohut, H., 1985b. One needs a twinkle of human as a protection against craziness. In: C. B. Strozier (Ed.), *Self Psychology and the Humanities: Reflections on a New Psychoanalytic Approach.* W. W. Norton, New York, NY, pp. 244-253.

Lauersen, N. H. and E. Stukane, 1983. *PMS: Premenstrual Syndrome and You.* Simon & Schuster, New York, NY.

Lippman-Hand, A., 1982. communication and decision making in genetic counseling. In: *Human Genetics, Part B: Medical Aspects.* Allan R. Liss, New York, NY, pp. 511-519.

Lippman-Hand, A. and F. C. Fraser, 1979. Genetic counseling: Parents' responses to uncertainty. *Birth Defects: Original Article Series, 15 (5C):* 325-339.

Mahler, M. S., F. Pine, and A. Bergman, 1975. *The Psychological Birth of the Human Infant.* Basic Books, New York, NY.

Miller, A., 1981. *Prisoners of Childhood.* (Translated by R. Ward.) Basic Books, New York, NY. [Published in paperback in 1983 as *The Drama of the Gifted Child.* Basic Books, New York, NY.]

Miller, A., 1983. *For Your Own Good: Hidden Cruelty in Child-rearing and the Roots of Violence.* (Translated by H. and H. Hannum.) Farrar Strauss Giroux, New York, NY.

Miller, G. A., 1956. The magical number seven plus or minus two: Some limits on our capacity for processing information. *Psychological Review 63:* 81-97.

Norris, R. V. and C. Sullivan, 1983. *PMS: Premenstrual Syndrome.* Rawson Associates, New York, NY.

Press, M. P., 1983. Premenstrual stress syndrome as a defense in criminal cases. *Duke Law Journal 1:* 176-195.

Seaman, B., 1985. Coping with uncertainty. *Hastings Center Report,* February, p. 47.

Steiner, M. and B. J. Carroll, 1977. The psychobiology of premenstrual dysphoria: Review of theories and treatments. *Psychoneuroendocrinology 2:* 321-335.

Winnicott, D. W., 1965. *Maturational Processes and the Facilitating Environments: Studies in the Theory of Emotional Development.* New York International Universities Press, New York, NY.

ETHICAL ISSUES

THE PREMENSTRUAL SYNDROME (PMS) LABEL: BENEFIT OR BURDEN?

Ruth Macklin, Ph.D.

Department of Epidemiology and Social Medicine
Albert Einstein College of Medicine
Bronx, New York

INTRODUCTION: THE PREMENSTRUAL SYNDROME PHENOMENON

Inquiry into the premenstrual syndrome (PMS) phenomenon raises a cluster of questions involving conceptual, scientific, moral, social, and legal concerns. The moral concerns might at first seem to be the only ones that directly raise ethical questions, but a closer look reveals that the conceptual, social, scientific, and legal issues also have ethical dimensions. It is by now a well accepted fact that science is not a value-free enterprise. Research into PMS and the proposed medical and social treatment of sufferers provides an illustrative case study of the ways in which value considerations pervade the domain of biomedical science, in both research and treatment.

The following characteristics of PMS give rise to that cluster of questions: its uncertain status as a disease entity or as deviant behavior; the unknown etiology of PMS (in particular, whether there is a neurobiological substrate); whether a diagnosis of PMS should be allowed as a mitigating or exculpating factor for criminal offenses, and if so, whether it should be allowed only if PMS qualifies as a disease; the difficulty of comparing the benefits with the burdens of labeling individuals as sufferers from a disease; and the potential for discrimination against women as a consequence of their being possible candidates for the PMS label.

In seeking to understand the value dimensions of the PMS phenomenon, it is necessary first to sketch a conceptual map of the territory. Philosophers have called this "exploring the logical geography" of a concept. In the present context, the territory includes the concepts of normal and abnormal, disease and illness, proper and improper functioning, and related notions. In order to understand what sort of phenomenon PMS is (or is thought to be), and what are the implications of labeling women believed to suffer from the premenstrual syndrome, we must first map out the conceptual territory. That will pave the way for examining the implications of construing PMS as a medical, a social, or a moral phenomenon.

The way in which a deviation from a social or behavioral norm is conceptualized has implications for individuals who deviate from that norm and, as a result, are given a label to reflect their aberrancy. Assigning a medical condition to a person whose behavior is socially deviant has different consequences from ascribing a label that confers moral praise or blame. And although it may be possible to devise a term for socially deviant behavior that is purely descriptive, social conduct is so often subject to approval or disapproval that labels initially designed to be value-free are unlikely to remain neutral.

Recreational drug use in our society provides an illustration of how the same behavior pattern can be variously labeled as a medical or psychiatric disorder, as a moral failing, and as criminal conduct (Gaylin, Murray, & Macklin, 1984). Narcotic and cocaine addicts are said to suffer from a psychiatric disorder by virtue of their addictive behavior, and they are typically disapproved of morally as well. Because the criminal law defines possession and use of these substances as felonies, users of these substances are at the same time labeled criminals. A clue that moral disapproval is built into the description of individuals who use these or even less harmful substances is that the terms "abuse" and "abuser" have come to replace the neutral words "use" and "user." With legal drugs, such as alcohol and nicotine, dependence and abuse are exempt from the criminal label, but the medical label may still be applied. People who use these substances are less likely to be subject to general moral disapproval in our society (in contrast to Islamic states), although some religious groups in Western culture proscribe alcohol and tobacco on what they consider moral grounds.

It is worth recalling the changes that have come about in the past two decades regarding the conceptualization of marijuana use, changes that reflect the dramatic increase in incidence and prevalence of that behavior, especially among younger members of the population. Before the mid-1960's, the "reefer madness" conception prevailed: Marijuana was thought to be a dangerous drug on a par with opiates, a drug whose use was believed to result in uncontrolled and often criminal behavior. Its widespread use in the late 1960's and early 1970's by college students and others who were not "drop-outs" from society led to a changed social perception, even among those who continued to disapprove of recreational use of marijuana. The culmination of this changed perception was the decriminalization of state laws, making the use and possession of marijuana a misdemeanor.

The reverse holds true for cocaine, a substance that was not only legally available in the 19th and early 20th centuries, but was used by such notable figures as Sigmund Freud, Ulysses S. Grant, Pope Leo XIII, and Thomas Edison (Grinspoon & Bakalar, 1976). There was little or no stigma attached to cocaine use, perhaps because the drug was employed as a "performance enhancer," enabling its users to work long hours and require less sleep. The original formula for Coca-Cola[R] contained a small amount of cocaine, but this ingredient was removed as the substance became disapproved and eventually illegal. Despite the considerable increase in the past decade in the recreational use of cocaine, especially among middle-class people, there are few signs that it will be decriminalized or demedicalized, as has largely occurred with marijuana. The difference in the social, medical, and legal attitudes toward these two drugs is, in part, a function of the empirical evidence available after years of experience. Unlike marijuana, cocaine has been shown to have genuinely addicting properties, as well as serious physical and psychological effects from heavy use.

This illustration is suggestive for PMS in a number of ways. It shows the complexity of any effort to conceptualize social and behavioral deviations from the norm, since such deviations are often accompanied by social attitudes of disapproval, and those attitudes may change from one historical era to another. Furthermore, the illustration demonstrates the overlapping categories into which the same piece of deviant behavior can fall: drug abuse is considered at one and the same time a psychiatric disorder, a moral failing, and illegal conduct. The uncertainty surrounding the classification of PMS and the proper way to view sufferers from this condition are functions of factors in addition to those that can be answered by scientific inquiry.

It may seem a more straightforward task to label deviations from a biological norm than departures from a behavioral or social norm, but the apparent simplicity evaporates on closer scrutiny. Not every deviation from biological norm qualifies as a disease or disorder. Consider height, for example. Very short or very tall persons are not thought of as suffering from a disease or disorder, unless their abnormal height is attributed to a metabolic disturbance or other physiologic malfunction. In such cases, other signs of the presence of disease can be detected clinically or by means of diagnostic tests. It would be far too broad a definition of "disease" to allow any deviation from a statistical norm, considered by itself, to be sufficient for labeling an abnormality as a "disease."

What else is required before the deviation can correctly be characterized as a disease or disorder? The answer is not obvious, and controversies have arisen about the proper classification of a number of statistically aberrant behavior patterns. Examples include hyperactive behavior in childhood, also called hyperkinesis and Minimal Brain Dysfunction (MBD); homosexuality, a category that has undergone a striking history of changes in nomenclature in the psychiatric profession over the past decade; the genotypic XYY male; and now, PMS. Understanding what these examples have in common should provide some clue to why both scientific and moral controversies continue over their proper classification. Controversy has surrounded the labeling of children as suffering from MBD, given the absence of an established biological basis for assigning the label despite undeniable evidence that children identified as hyperkinetic respond to treatment with certain drugs. Homosexuality used to be considered a psychiatric disease, but is now construed as a choice of lifestyle in homosexuals who accept their own sexual orientation, a conceptual change that did not come about as a result of new scientific evidence, but instead from changed social perceptions and from political activism. And studies of XYY males raised controversy in the scientific community not only about the validity of some of the scientific methods employed in the research, but also over the ideological premises of behavior genetics. In all these examples, as in that of PMS, the question of whether the label is accurately applied is not one to which science alone can provide the answer. But even when the application of a label is scientifically sound, these examples raise the issue of the potential harm such labels can confer on their bearers.

The shortcomings of using statistical deviation from a biological or behavioral norm as a criterion for the presence of disease have been widely discussed and generally acknowledged. But that agreement has not ended the scientific and moral debate. Failure of agreement has led to efforts to arrive at a more precise definition, one that places boundaries around the proper candidates and rules out inadmissible ones. One suggestion is to begin with the statistical deviation, but only call it a disease if the biological or behavioral aberrancy results from a failure of proper functioning of the organ system or physiologic mechanism. Another proposal is to take a reduced ability to function on the part of the entire organism as an additional necessary condition. Other candidates have been proposed (Caplan, Englehardt, & McCartney, 1981). Leading recent attempts to define "disease" typically entail some reference to the notion of function and what it is for the organism to function properly (Boorse, 1981; Margolis, 1981).

All this suggests that at least two different meanings of the term "abnormal" are in regular use. First, "abnormal" sometimes means, simply, deviation from a statistical norm. Taken by itself, that deviation implies nothing about the causes of the abnormality, nor does it say anything about how society reacts or how the individual who exhibits the deviation feels or behaves as a result of it.

A second meaning of "abnormal" denotes a departure from "proper" structure or function. The term "proper" is itself ambiguous, sometimes conveying moral value, and at other times simply the value inherent in working according to design. Both meanings are normative, or value-laden. However, the former meaning reflects societal values, expressed in the idea of "proper conduct" referring merely to etiquette, perhaps, or to the more important psychiatric and moral judgments that a person is behaving "inappropriately" in social circumstances. The second meaning of "proper functioning" captures the norm from which departures are to be construed as disorders, diseases, or dysfunctions.

To call a physical or behavioral state abnormal in this sense presupposes an underlying scientific theory that explains the phenomenon, even if that theory is not yet fully developed. This appears to be the current state of research regarding PMS. Several contributors to this volume have developed hypotheses based on their own scientific research and that of others. Although disagreement persists among the proponents of these hypotheses, it is likely that continued research will lead to a resolution of the scientific aspects of the dispute. However, unless a promising explanatory theory is advanced — a theory that enables an understanding of behavioral deviance based on a scientifically validated knowledge of structure and function — a deviation can only be characterized as abnormal in the first sense; that is, as statistically deviant.

In the domain of human behavior, the quest for a well-confirmed, explanatory theory continues, with little resolution in sight for long-standing controversies. The situation regarding these different meanings of "normal" and "abnormal" has been summarized as follows (Livermore, Malmquist, & Meehl, 1968, pp. 78-79):

> "From a biological viewpoint, it is not inconsistent to assert that a sizable proportion — conceivably a majority — of persons in a given population are abnormal or aberrant. Thus if an epidemiologist found that 60% of the persons in a society were afflicted with plague or avitaminosis, he would (quite correctly) reject an argument that 'since most of them have it, they are okay, i.e. not pathological and not in need of treatment.' It is admittedly easier to defend this nonstatistical, biological-fitness approach in the domain of physical disease, but its application in the domain of behavior is fraught with difficulties."

Among the difficulties these authors probably have in mind are the cross-cultural variations in norms of conduct that make application of the biological fitness approach to behavior questionable. Even within our our own society, subcultural variations in the behavior of different ethnic groups and varying norms of success contribute to the problem of determining which of conflicting modes of social behavior are well adapted, and which are manifestations of pathology of some sort. To the extent that scientific research into PMS uncovers the underlying mechanisms, these difficulties may become resolved.

There is still another meaning of "abnormal," a meaning that contains a built-in moral judgment. Typically, this meaning is reserved for human conduct, and is not applied to physiological functioning of organisms, to animal behavior, or, of course, to machines. To call human conduct "abnormal" in this third sense is to make a value judgment, implicitly or explicitly. When certain forms of sexual conduct are deemed "abnormal," it is not clear without further explication whether "abnormal" is meant in the statistical sense, a sense that is value-neutral; or in the sense of "improper," in which a negative value judgment is part of the meaning of the term. The functional meaning of "abnormal" might also apply to the example of sexual conduct for those who see humans as the products of design by a creator who intended sexual practices only for the purpose of procreation. Those who maintain such beliefs hold that the purpose of sexual conduct is propagation of the species, and any deviation from that purpose constitutes abnormal behavior in the normative rather than the statistical sense. A version of this view is apparent in the Roman Catholic dogma asserting that masturbation is an "intrinsically and seriously disordered act" (Vatican Congregation for the Doctrine of the Faith, 1976).

ABNORMALITY, DISEASE, AND ILLNESS

There are, then, three distinct meanings of the term "abnormal": statistical deviance; deviation from design or correct functioning; and socially or ethically unacceptable conduct. The applications of these three meanings are not always clear and distinct, and their uses are especially likely to overlap when statistical deviance is accompanied by moral disapproval (as used to be the case with divorce), or when conduct is believed to deviate from proper functioning and is also considered morally unacceptable (as with any recreational sexual activity for those who approve of sex only for procreative purposes). Only in the case of the second meaning — deviation from design or correct functioning — is there a basis for ascribing the concept of *disease* to the deviant behavior or functioning.

This already complex conceptual picture is further complicated by the notion of *illness*. The concepts of disease and illness have been explored and debated at length, and although controversy still exists over the proper way to understand these related yet distinct notions, there is general agreement that the concept of disease is an objective one, to be applied on the basis of scientific criteria, while illness contains a subjective element, referring essentially to the sufferer's discomfort, pain, or feelings of distress stemming from the condition. According to this distinction, disease may be found in an individual on the basis of objective evidence; yet if the person is not (perhaps, not yet) suffering from that condition, the concept of illness does not apply. Examples include a variety of conditions typically called "presymptomatic" or "asymptomatic," and perhaps also certain "subclinical" phenomena. The person in whom these physiological deviations are found may not experience subjective feelings of discomfort or distress. Yet the condition might even be a life-threatening disease, as in the case of hypertension diagnosed by means of tests.

Boorse (1981, p. 555) characterizes the relationship between disease and illness as follows:

"A disease is an *illness* only if it is serious enough to be incapacitating, and therefore is (i) undesirable for its bearer; (ii) a title to special treatment; and (iii) a valid excuse for normally criticizable behavior."

According to this account, disease is a concept that is largely or purely descriptive, while illness is a concept that is normative and makes essential reference to social interactions and to the moral accountability of the person. But the author of this passage, in a note appended to a reprinting of his original article, makes the following disclaimer (Boorse, 1981, p. 560):

". . . the view that illness is disease laden with values. . . now seems a mistaken concession to normativism. Illness is better analyzed simply as systematically incapacitating disease, hence as no more normative than disease itself."

Still further disagreement exists over whether the concept of disease may itself be value-laden, or whether it must be construed as a "purely descriptive" notion. According to one view (Margolis, 1981, p. 566):

"It is clear why the concept of disease, though not entirely isomorphic with the concept of illness, makes no sense without reference to appropriate norms. A diseased state. . . is a morbid or abnormal state of some sort. . . Illness is simply a diseased state manifest to an agent through that agent's symptoms. . ."

Some of this confusion can be cleared up by noting that not all values are moral values. Therefore, the norms of proper functioning usually taken to be implicit in the definition of disease are not to be construed as moral norms. Although wide agreement exists in support of social norms that place high value on the ability to work productively and to adapt to social and occupational roles, departure from those accepted roles need not be a moral failing. Some individuals adhere to subjective values that permit departures from social norms, departures that do not result in harm to others but may result in failure on the part of these individuals to comply with conventional measures of success and adaptation. Women exhibiting symptoms of PMS may suffer disapproval at the hands of their employers or husbands because of failure to live up to accepted norms of behavior in their occupational or marital roles. But falling short of those norms is not inherently immoral, nor should it qualify such women for the disease label. If, however, a correlation between specific neurobiological states and the emotions and behavior of PMS women is verified, that would provide evidence for the existence of disease. It still would not count as illness, though, unless the additional conditions are met that warrant calling a disease an illness.

LABELING AND ITS IMPLICATIONS

The social consequences of pinning a label on people for some purpose or another are well known. We have only to reflect on how labels stick even when they are later withdrawn, or how a particular label may create or alter a self-image, whether or not the label is correctly applied. The best known examples are probably in the area of mental retardation. A designation applied early in life can endure, even if the grounds for applying the label are later discovered to be mistaken. The undesirable social consequences of labeling persons as mentally retarded, and the stigma the label carries even when correctly applied, has led some advocates of the mentally retarded to disavow the use of labels altogether. These advocates of the mentally retarded go further than simply denying the ascription of a stigmatizing label, however. Their advocacy extends to social and educational efforts as well: "mainstreaming" in schools and attempts to "normalize" the life of mentally retarded persons as much as possible. In addition to deinstitutionalization, these efforts have included placement in residential communities and finding employment for those retarded persons capable of holding unskilled jobs in the mainstream of society (Macklin & Gaylin, 1981).

The consequences of other sorts of labeling are perhaps more instructive for an analysis of the PMS phenomenon. The controversy a decade ago over a research program involving efforts to identify infants with the XYY chromosomal abnormality provides a good case study (Gaylin, Macklin, & Powledge, 1981), with some striking analogies to PMS. Both are situations in which a biological phenomenon with presumed implications for socially deviant behavior is subjected to scientific investigation. In both instances, it is suggested that finding a biological cause of antisocial or aggressive behavior can mitigate the individual's moral responsibility for that behavior, and might even contribute to a legal defense of "diminished capacity" for violent criminal acts. Both cases have raised questions about the ethics of research design. A major concern is that the very identification of persons with these conditions is likely to lead to a "self-fulfilling prophecy" regarding aggressive or antisocial conduct (Gaylin et al., 1981, pp. 98-119). In both cases, worries have also been voiced about the social consequences of labeling persons as XYY or PMS. Will individuals so labeled be ostracized? Might mandatory screening programs be established or made a condition of employment? A similar conceptual question arises about both instances of abnormality: How should males having that chromosomal anomaly be characterized, and how should women exhibiting deviations from the norm in their conduct and feeling during the premenstrual period be characterized?

At another level, an ideological conflict continues to rage: Some critics have opposed on moral grounds research that seeks to identify biological determinants of human behavior. They argue that almost all human behavior is a product of numerous and complex interacting causes, and genetic determinism is a pernicious idea that will lead to discrimination, ostracism, and perhaps even forced interventions into the lives of those found to be "genetically programmed" to act in certain ways (Powledge, 1981). Their ideological opponents claim that only by identifying the root causes of antisocial or other deviant forms of behavior can we fashion appropriate responses: punishment, therapy, or rehabilitation in the case of criminal offenders, and medical intervention in cases where individuals are found to have chemical imbalances or deficiencies believed to cause their aberrant behavior (Jeffery, this volume).

This ideological debate reveals both the risks and benefits of labeling a condition as a disease. It also forces us to distinguish between an opposition to research based on possible applications of research findings, and criticism of research based either on direct harms to research subjects or ways in which research subjects may be wronged in the conduct of the investigation; for example, by being deceived or by having significant information about the research withheld from them (Scanlon, 1981). Both criticisms were leveled against research projects designed to study XYY, with replies in defense of the research offered by the investigators and their supporters (Gaylin et al., 1981).

DISEASE LABELING: BENEFIT OR HARM?

A great deal has been written about the negative consequences of labeling. Much less attention has been paid to the benefits to an individual or a class of persons as a result of labeling them as bearers of a disease or disability. In the wake of legislative efforts and judicial decisions over the past several decades, disabled and handicapped persons are now entitled to numerous social benefits. Whether the benefits are in the form of direct monetary payments, job entitlements, special education or other services, parking spaces, ramps, and other requirements for public buildings, persons with all sorts of physical and mental disabilities can enjoy those benefits only by accepting the label denoting their status.

Yet whether it is a benefit or a harm to label people as bearers of disease or disability remains controversial. As noted earlier, advocates for the mentally retarded stand on both sides of this debate, with some arguing that the retarded benefit most by not being labeled, but rather by "normalizing" and "mainstreaming" them into society. Opponents claim that labeling permits the retarded to qualify for special education and other services that will benefit them more in the long run by increasing their level of functioning and by enabling them to achieve greater independence (Macklin & Gaylin, 1981). Analogous benefits can be postulated for PMS: Women labeled as sufferers might be motivated to seek psychiatric or other professional help; the anxiety sufferers experience might be alleviated by their knowledge that they have an identifiable condition afflicting other women as well; and the label may result in greater tolerance by others of the behavior of PMS women during the premenstrual period. But unlike mentally retarded children and probably most adults who cannot assess for themselves whether a label is more of a benefit or a burden, women who are candidates for the PMS label are the ones most appropriate to judge the risks and benefits of a label applied to them.

A different yet related version of this controversy is the long-standing debate over the concept of mental illness, and the implications of labeling persons diagnosed as having a psychiatric disorder. One of the foremost critics of the concept of mental illness, the polemical psychiatrist Thomas Szasz, has waged war against institutional psychiatry on many fronts. His arguments against the very concept of mental illness are complex and varied, but one point is pertinent to the emerging situation regarding PMS. On the question of whether a disease label is beneficial to the sufferer or not, he is somewhat equivocal. At one point, while reviewing the history of psychiatric theory and practice, Szasz (1961, p. 221) writes:

> "From the standpoint of our present analysis, the entire change in renaming certain illnesslike forms of behavior from 'malingering' to 'hysteria' (and 'mental illness') can be understood as nothing but a linguistic change employed for the purpose of achieving a new type of action-orientedness in the listener. The verbal change. . . served to command those charged with dealing with 'hysterics' to abandon their moral-condemnatory attitude toward them and to adopt instead a solicitous and benevolent attitude, such as befitted the physician *vis-a-vis* his patient."

Elsewhere in the same work, Szasz comments on the tendency in this century to reclassify various forms of behavior and social practices as illnesses (Szasz, 1961, p. 43):

> "During [the past 60 or 70 years] a vast number of occurrences were reclassified as 'illnesses.' We have thus come to regard phobias, delinquencies, divorce, homicide, addiction, and so on almost without limit as psychiatric illnesses."

Szasz contends that this is "a colossal and costly mistake," and claims that one of its consequences has been that although "some members of suffering humanity were promoted. . . to higher social rank, this was attained at the cost of obscuring the logical character of the observed phenomena" (p. 295). One need not concur fully with Szasz's general conclusions about mental illness to raise similar questions about PMS: Is its classification as an illness likely to promote sufferers to higher social rank? And even if it would have that consequence, would it do so at the cost of obscuring the logical character of the PMS phenomenon?

The answer to the question, Is it a favor to people to assign a label of disease, disorder, or disability? is far from clear. On the one hand, labels can be misapplied, stigmatizing, and hard to shake even when the conditions for applying the label in the first place are no longer present. On the other hand, to designate someone as diseased or disabled may entitle that person to monetary, social, educational, and medical benefits not otherwise available. Also, if Szasz is correct, in at least some cases, people are "elevated to higher social rank" once classified as sick rather than as evil, malingering, or some other socially undesirable category. Being entitled to receive medical treatment seems like an unqualified benefit of being labeled. But it is a mixed blessing when a presumably pathological condition or "disease syndrome" such as PMS is still under investigation. Whatever "treatment" can be offered is at best highly experimental, with unknown risks and benefits. The same may be said, of course, for many other conditions undergoing clinical investigation at any given time. Even if the presence of disease is incontrovertible, therapeutic benefits are uncertain, and some treatments may even prove harmful in the long run. An additional concern in the case of PMS, as noted throughout this essay, is that the risks and benefits of the very act of labeling sufferers are as unclear as the risks and benefits of experimental treatment.

To identify a behavioral pattern as the product of an underlying disease can at the same time stigmatize the individual and also serve to mitigate responsibility for harmful or irresponsible actions. We have only to think of epilepsy, and the way in which sufferers have fared throughout history. It is hard to deny that a stigma continues to haunt epileptics, despite the facts that the condition is not contagious and those who suffer from it can in no way be held responsible for its presence. On the other hand, certain benefits surely accrue to epileptics as a result of the present medical understanding and treatment of the disease, in contrast to earlier eras when moral condemnation and religious opprobrium were the rule. Epileptics cannot be held morally responsible for their behavior during a seizure, but they are properly held accountable for failure to take necessary precautions in undertaking activities such as operating an automobile or other machinery when they are aware that the onset of a seizure may lead to harming themselves or others. When there is a strong probability that harm to others is likely to occur, intervention can be ethically justified according to the "harm principle" — the moral principle that permits interference with an individual's liberty in order to protect innocent persons from harm. If relevant similarities exist between PMS and epilepsy, and possibly other biological deviations such as the XYY chromosomal anomaly, it is fair to assume that appending the label to afflicted individuals will be a mixed blessing to them and hold promise for providing added protections to society.

MEDICAL AND LEGAL PATERNALISM

"Paternalism" can be defined as coercing people or otherwise manipulating them for their own good. The good in question can be the life or health of those coerced, as in the case of suicide prevention and in successful efforts to override patients' refusal of medical treatments. Involuntary commitment on any grounds besides "dangerousness to others" is paternalistic, as are laws preventing the manufacture and sale of laetrile, and laws making users of narcotics and stimulant drugs subject to criminal penalties. When paternalism occurs through the use of laws or government regulations, it is usually termed "legal paternalism." But there is a great deal of individual paternalism practiced by professionals in many fields, by family members towards one another, and in various other situations in which people interact. A common example of individual paternalism is withholding information from people "for their own good."

The classic instance of paternalism, and the circumstance that gives rise to the name of the concept, is that of protective behavior of parents toward their minor children. Most people agree that paternalism regarding young children is entirely justifiable, if not morally obligatory. Controversy arises over the age at which it is no longer justifiable to coerce youth for their own good, with some "child liberationists" seeking an early age of liberation from parental domination, while others take the legal age of majority or conditions of emancipation as the appropriate dividing line.

It is not only minor children, however, who have been viewed as appropriate subjects for paternalistic behavior by caretakers or society. Mentally retarded persons, those afflicted with severe mental disorders, and other adults believed to suffer from diminished capacity of one kind or another have also been deemed candidates for justifiable paternalism. Although the very concept of paternalism has had a bad press in recent years, there are few thoughtful people who are unwilling to allow any instances whatever of paternalism toward adults as ethically acceptable. The key lies in specifying the conditions under which paternalism on the part of individuals toward one another, or on the part of the government through its statutes, courts, and regulations, is justifiable.

Psychiatry plays a key role in this picture. The idea of diminished capacity, although fundamentally a common-sense notion, has acquired a status that requires psychiatric experts to apply it properly. If people have to be evaluated as suffering from diminished capacity, it suggests that some sort of expertise is necessary for making that evaluation. It is surely true that psychiatrists are expert at diagnosing mental disorders and emotional dysfunctions, based on their theoretical knowledge and clinical experience, but the concept of diminished capacity is not such a disorder or dysfunction. The judgment that a person suffers from diminished capacity might rest on a psychiatric evaluation, but the judgment itself has a social and moral component. The social component provides the background context against which to judge whether a society member's behavior does, in fact, exhibit diminished capacity. The moral component absolves the person from full responsibility as a moral agent, thus mitigating moral blame or criminal culpability. Whatever the areas in which psychiatric expertise exists — and they are many and varied — that expertise does not encompass the moral domain. A judgment of "diminished capacity" has to be the conclusion of a moral argument, not a professional evaluation based on diagnostic expertise. If the judgment that a person suffers diminished capacity as a result of a medical or psychiatric condition is to be used as an excusing condition for moral agency, it requires more than a medical or psychiatric diagnosis to draw that conclusion. There is general agreement (with a few notable exceptions, such as Thomas Szasz) that if paternalism can be justified at all beyond the application to children, it is permissible in the case of adults whose cognitive or affective capacities are severely impaired. The determination of when those conditions exist is a complex matter, requiring the expertise of psychiatrists, but not limited to the role that professional group can play.

The same conclusion obviously holds for other medical professionals. A finding that there is a genetic predisposition to PMS or any other biological or behavioral syndrome is not by itself sufficient for drawing a moral conclusion of diminished responsibility for actions; nor is it a license for professional intervention on behalf of a patient or research subject. If PMS is "medicalized" by the use of psychiatric diagnostic criteria and through an identification of a biological substrate and genetic predispositions, it becomes a fertile breeding ground for a form of medical paternalism that probably cannot be morally justified. Even if scientific research leads to eventual confirmation of the existence and nature of a premenstrual syndrome, the decision of whether to seek professional help properly belongs with the sufferer. Some people who suffer from chronic pain prefer to endure the pain rather than risk the side effects of medication. Many women choose to undergo the discomforts of menopause and take the risks associated with osteoporosis, instead of being subject to the potential hazards of prolonged hormonal therapy. It is unacceptably paternalistic for professionals to exert undue influence on patients into accepting treatment "for their own good." To make a competent, scientifically-based diagnosis of PMS is not paternalistic. But to insist that medical or psychiatric treatment is the only reasonable option is to engage in medical paternalism.

ETHICAL, SOCIAL, AND LEGAL IMPLICATIONS OF PREMENSTRUAL SYNDROME LABELING

The most important factors of moral relevance to PMS are whether treatment is mandatory or voluntary, and whether the recommended therapy is still in its research phase or has become accepted treatment. It is by now well established in the biomedical and behavioral fields that for research to be conducted in an ethical manner, subjects must freely grant their informed consent. That ethical requirement includes disclosure of at least the following elements: the purpose of the research; what procedures will be done; the risks of those procedures, including psychological and social risks, as well as risks of physical harm; the expected benefits of the research to the subject and to others; and alternatives the subject may choose (Department of Health and Human Services Regulations, 1981).

The moral requirement of freely granted, fully informed consent to research involving human subjects rules out any mandatory experimental treatment programs, such as those that existed in a number of prisons in the early 1970's (Gaylin et al., 1981). Whether alternatives to incarceration should also be ruled out on ethical grounds is a question that must be examined on a case-by-case basis. Moral debate has surrounded cases of surgical castration offered to repeated sex offenders as an alternative to life imprisonment; and a program of anti-androgen therapy (so-called "chemical castration") as a condition for release from prison has also been controversial (Macklin, 1982). In these cases, those who sought to give sex offenders an alternative to prison have been accused of making a coercive offer, one that a prisoner with a life sentence "could not refuse." The most controversial aspects of these experimental programs, however, revolved around their likelihood of success. The unproven nature of these interventions allowed the distinct possibility that an offender could submit to surgical or chemical castration, thus earning his freedom, and return to society only to perpetrate more acts of sexual violence. In that situation, there would be no benefits from the research, either to the subject or to others — and both the offender and his innocent victims would end up being harmed.

It is also widely agreed, in the United States at least, that a patient's consent for treatment must be as fully informed and as freely granted as is true in the research setting. Additional elements proposed as ethically required for informed consent to treatment are the costs, if any, to the patient, and the uncertainty concerning the likelihood of benefit (President's Commission, 1982). But what about screening, as opposed to treatment, for a condition like PMS or XYY? Could mandatory screening of any sort be morally permissible? One argument that it could not rests on the absence of any existing treatment or cure for these particular conditions, in contrast to PKU, for instance, for which mandatory newborn screening has met with little opposition. Recall again the furor that ensued some years ago concerning the research program involving newborn screening for XYY (Gaylin et al., 1981), in which consent was sought on a voluntary basis from women in labor. According to a woman who was the admitting aide at Boston Hospital for Women, where the controversial research was conducted, she "handed the consent forms to women in labor, and they had to be signed as quickly as possible; there was no time to read the lengthy explanation, and no one on hand qualified to answer questions" (Gaylin et al., 1981, p. 105).

Another instructive analogy is that of screening for sickle cell disease, which met with considerable opposition as a potentially racist policy following its introduction as a mandatory procedure in several states. Those who proposed mandatory screening for sickle cell carriers maintained that their motive was solely to help blacks by providing information enabling them to make informed choices regarding marital partners and reproductive decisions. Similarly, mandatory screening for PMS might be defended as an aid to women generally, enabling those at risk to become aware of their potential for depression or uncontrolled aggressive behavior. Yet, it takes little imagination to conceive of the uses to which such information could be put by employers, by insurance companies, or by a law-and-order government policy using prevention of crime as a rationale for coercive intrusions into the privacy of its citizens.

Although there can be no paternalistic justification for putting mandatory therapeutic or screening programs for PMS in place, the question of a nonpaternalistic rationale can still be raised. The ethical principle that might be used to justify such interventions is the "harm principle" mentioned earlier — the moral principle that permits interference with an individual's liberty in order to protect innocent persons from harm. The harm principle serves as a justification for involuntary commitment of individuals believed to be "dangerous to others," a practice civil libertarians fault as being nothing other than preventive detention, a concept traditionally proscribed by our criminal justice system.

Here is another instance in which the power and authority of the psychiatric profession are evident. In the absence of mechanisms within the criminal justice system enabling preventive detention of persons believed dangerous to others, psychiatric testimony in civil proceedings can accomplish the same end: incarceration of persons who have not (yet) committed a criminal offense. However, the potential for abuse of information gained through genetic or other screening programs is not limited to involuntarily obtained data. Medical professionals in possession of information about patients or research subjects could be faced with a subpoena requiring that they disclose information for the purpose of judicial proceedings. It is hard to predict whether such legal developments will occur with any frequency as a result of further research into PMS, and it is impossible to judge at this stage whether disclosure of confidential information about patients would be morally permissible. But, it is best to contemplate the consequences for afflicted women and for society well in advance of the need to make pressing policy decisions.

CONCLUSIONS

In order to draw sound conclusions about the ethical, social, and legal consequences of PMS labeling, on the assumption that PMS is recognized as a genuine psychobiological phenomenon, it must be determined whether the syndrome should be accepted as a moral (and legal) excusing condition. Does it diminish an individual's responsibility for action? This question is not a scientific one; it cannot be answered by the biological or the social sciences alone, although data provided by scientific research are surely relevant. It is not a matter for scientific discovery, but rather a matter for social and moral decision. How the issue is decided depends on what theory of moral responsibility for action is most reasonable, and in particular, whether a discovery that conduct is at least partially caused by biological predispositions makes any difference in ascribing responsibility to the individual. Learned behavior may be just as difficult to change, and a person is as much a product of acquired tendencies to act as of innate propensities. Both values and ideological presuppositions underlie the positions people are likely to take on these matters. Continued interdisciplinary inquiry and debate are essential to understanding the problems and fashioning an acceptable approach to the issues raised by the PMS phenomenon.

REFERENCES

Boorse, C., 1981. On the distinction between disease and illness. In: A. L. Caplan, H. T. Engelhardt, Jr., and J. J. McCartney (Eds.), *Concepts of Health and Disease*. Addison-Wesley Publishing Company, Reading, MA, pp. 545-560.

Caplan, A. L., H. T. Engelhardt, Jr., and J. J. McCartney (Eds.), 1981. *Concepts of Health and Disease*. Addison-Wesley Publishing Company, Reading, MA.

Department of Health and Human Services Regulations on Protection of Human Subjects, 1981. 45 CRF 46.

Gaylin, W., R. Macklin, and T. M. Powledge (Eds.), 1981. *Violence and the Politics of Research*. Plenum Press, New York, NY.

Gaylin, W., T. H. Murray, and R. Macklin (Eds.), 1984. *Feeling Good and Doing Better: Ethics and Nontherapeutic Drug Use*. Humana Press, Clifton, NJ.

Grinspoon, L. and J. B. Bakalar, 1976. *Cocaine*. Basic Books, New York, NY.

Livermore, J. M., C. P. Malmquist, and P. E. Meehl, 1968. On the justifications for civil commitment. *University of Pennsylvania Law Review 117:* 75-96.

Macklin, R., 1982. *Man, Mind, and Morality: The Ethics of Behavior Control*. Prentice-Hall, Englewood Cliffs, NJ.

Macklin, R. and W. Gaylin, 1981. *Mental Retardation and Sterilization: A Problem of Competency and Paternalism*. Plenum Press, New York, NY.

Margolis, J., 1981. The concept of disease. In: A. L. Caplan, H. T. Engelhardt, Jr., and J. J. McCartney (Eds.), *Concepts of Health and Disease.* Addison-Wesley Publishing Company, Reading, MA, pp. 561-577.

Powledge, T. M., 1981. How not to study violence. In: W. Gaylin, R. Macklin, and T. M. Powledge (Eds.), *Violence and the Politics of Research.* Plenum Press, New York, NY, pp. 49-140.

President's Commission for the Study of Ethical Problems in Medicine and Biomedical and Behavioral Research, 1982. *Making Health Care Decisions.* U.S. Government Printing Office, Washington, D.C.

Scanlon, T. M., 1981. Ethics and the control of research. In: W. Gaylin, R. Macklin, and T. M. Powledge (Eds.), *Violence and the Politics of Research.* Plenum Press, New York, NY, pp. 225-246.

Szasz, T., 1961. *The Myth of Mental Illness.* Hoeber-Harper, New York, NY.

Vatican Congregation for the Doctrine of the Faith, 1976. Declaration on sexual ethics. *New York Times,* January 16, 1976.

NEUROSCIENCE RESEARCH AND PREMENSTRUAL SYNDROME: SCIENTIFIC AND ETHICAL CONCERNS

Stephanie J. Bird, Ph.D.

Science, Technology, and Society Program; and
The Center for Technology, Policy and Industrial Development
Massachusetts Institute of Technology
Cambridge, Massachusetts

INTRODUCTION

A very small percentage of women experience severe, incapacitating, and disabling symptoms, suggestive of underlying physiological dysfunction, which is increasingly being referred to as premenstrual syndrome (PMS). Other women experience symptoms which are troubling, but which do not severely limit their ability to function socially or professionally. Many women experience detectable changes premenstrually which are not sufficiently severe to be considered a syndrome, either objectively or subjectively. Some women detect changes premenstrually, such as increased energy, creativity, or sexual drive, which they consider positive. A relatively few women detect no changes at all. Discussion of the widespread occurrence of PMS based upon including all women who detect any changes premenstrually as experiencing at least mild PMS has focused professional and public attention on the topic. This has the potential advantage of increased funding for research. However, it also has the effect of labeling all women of reproductive age as likely PMS sufferers. Such a label may have a negative, stigmatizing effect. This is an example of the ethical implications of behavior linked to biology.

PMS is a phenomenon with characteristics intriguing and challenging to neuroscience research. Its symptoms and expression suggest a role of endogenous compounds in brain function that is only beginning to be explored by neuroscience researchers. Yet research in this area has broad implications in need of consideration. The neurosciences focus on various aspects of biology, but there are two major factors which are both outcomes of and contributors to that biology. These are self-perception and behavior, both of which are strongly influenced by social factors. In addition, social issues both influence, and are influenced by, science. These relationships raise scientific and ethical concerns that merit examination.

NEUROSCIENCE RESEARCH

Neuroscience can be defined as that body of research directed toward understanding the molecular, cellular, and intercellular processes in the central nervous system (CNS) and the way in which those processes are integrated in functional control systems, with an emphasis on research which ultimately relates CNS function to behavior. The neurosciences address all levels of structural and functional capacity: ions and molecules, gene expression and other aspects of neurochemistry; neuroanatomy, including both the fine structure of individual neurons and other cells of the nervous system, and the pathways and interconnections of various brain regions in higher organisms; neurophysiology of cells, of cell groups, and of the brain as a whole; neuropharmacology, including the cellular and intercellular effects and interactions of endogenous substances, as well as exogenous naturally-occurring and synthetic compounds; and behavior, including simple behaviors like the startle reflex, and more complex behaviors such as learning, language, and other higher brain functions. Although the brain is generally considered a single organ and the nervous system an anatomical and physiological system like the circulatory system or the digestive system, the brain and the nervous system are more complex, interconnected and interactive than the whole rest of the body. The CNS contains a remarkable number of different cell types, and groups of cells, called nuclei, which are connected and interact through the more obvious connections and also through mechanisms of neuromodulation and regulation so subtle that they are only beginning to be perceived (Kretzinger, 1981; Schmitt, 1984). Indicative of the extraordinary complexity of this single organ is the fact that there are more genes expressed uniquely and specifically in brain tissue than in the whole rest of the body taken together (Hahn, Van Ness, & Chaudhari, 1982). At the same time, the brain is intimately involved in and affected by all other bodily systems.

There has recently been an increased understanding of the role of hormones in brain function, at both the cellular and the molecular levels (Krieger & Hughes, 1980; McEwen, 1980; Nock & Feder, 1981). With respect to PMS, the hormones associated with reproductive functions are of particular interest, although it is not likely that they are the only endogenous substances involved in the expression or experience of this malady (Abraham, 1980; Muse, Cetel, Futterman, & Yen, 1984; Reid & Yen, 1981). Not only do hormones regulate their own concentrations in the bloodstream via a sophisticated feedback system, usually involving the hypothalamus (Krieger, 1980), but they also affect a variety of other areas of the brain, many of which do not seem to have any obvious role in reproductive behavior (McEwen, Davis, Parsons, & Pfaff, 1979). Receptors for estrogen and progesterone have been shown to influence gene expression and the sensitivity of neurons to other neuroactive substances (McEwen, 1982). In addition, steroid hormones are likely to have a physiological effect on neurons in several brain regions which do not have any obvious role in reproductive function (e.g., areas of the cortex, brainstem, spinal cord, and cranial nerve nuclei) (Pfaff & Keiner, 1973; Sar & Stumpf, 1973; Stumpf & Jennes, 1984; Yu & McGinnis, 1984). For example, receptors for testosterone have been found in the hypoglossal nucleus, a brain region which controls movement of the tongue (Yu & McGinnis, 1984). Besides the hormones themselves, hypothalamic releasing factors, which are simple peptides, have been shown to have functions outside the strict confines of their role in regulation of trophic hormone release from the pituitary (Koranyi, Whitmoyer, & Sawyer, 1977; Riskind & Moss, 1979; Sakuma & Pfaff, 1980; Sirinathsinghji, Whittington, Audsley, & Fraser, 1983; Valentino, Foote, & Aston-Jones, 1983). In addition, pituitary hormones that regulate the function of target glands and their synthesis and release of hormones have been shown to have roles in brain areas that are not directly involved in regulation of hormone levels (de Weid, 1980; Harlan, Shivers, & Pfaff, 1983; Sodersten, Henning, Melin, & Ludin, 1983). Thus, for example, the pituitary hormone, vasopressin, which is primarily responsible for water retention by the kidney and thereby the maintenance of normal blood volume, has also been shown to affect both sexual behavior (Sodersten et al., 1983) and memory (de Weid, 1980). Adrenocorticotrophic hormone is a trophic pituitary hormone primarily responsible for stimulating the synthesis and release of the adrenal hormone cortisol. However, it, too, acts directly on a number of brain regions to affect learning, memory, and other behaviors (de Weid, 1980). These and other studies have resulted in a growing appreciation of both the demonstrated and potential roles of endogenous compounds long associated with the reproductive system in functions not considered to be directly or solely involved in reproductive function or behavior.

There are also a number of neurotransmitters (compounds used for communication between nerve cells) that influence the neurobiology of reproductive function and the reproductive system, as well as having other functions. Because the hypothalamus is interconnected with most, if not all, of the other parts of the brain, a given releasing factor may be regulated by several neurotransmitters (Krieger, 1980). Neurotransmitters exert an influence all along the hypothalamic-pituitary-gonadal axis. In particular, the transmitter norepinephrine is associated with gonadotropin releasing factor secretion in the hypothalamus, and another transmitter, dopamine, further stimulates trophic hormone release from the pituitary (Frohman, 1980). Neurotransmitters also affect the action of reproductive hormones by specifically modifying the sensitivity of brain cells to the hormones (Nock & Feder, 1981). Throughout the CNS, there is great overlap of different transmitter systems, anatomically, physiologically, and pharmacologically, and no doubt there is comparable overlap of behaviors related to them.

INTERACTIONS OF PHYSIOLOGY, PSYCHOLOGY, AND BEHAVIOR

In general, the neurosciences focus on the physical basis of mental activity, on how it is that the brain generates thoughts and feelings. Mental activity has diverse physiological effects. Nightmares can produce a cold sweat and a pounding heart; the memory of an argument or a frightening experience can increase heart rate and blood pressure and redden the face. These are expressions of the physiological impact of mental activity on other bodily systems. Within the brain itself, mental activity is another side of the coin of physiological activity (Bloom, Lazerson, & Hofstadter, 1985). External events also have an impact on brain function, both physiologically and psychologically. Initial sensory perception (for example, visual perception) arises from alterations in the conformation of molecules in cells in the eye that induce electrical changes in the cells themselves (Brobeck, 1973). The electrical signal is carried along a distinct, diverging and converging pathway, to various specific brain regions, inducing a variety of physiological changes at each stage, some of which have yet to be identified. These physiological changes are due to the sensory input itself. In addition, there may be a psychological impact of the same external event. For example, the death of a loved one can clearly have a significant psychological impact, producing grief, anxiety, anger and stress. The emotions associated with such an event affect behavior. The psychological experience of anxiety and stress induces physiological changes in the balance and activity of a number of hormones (Kopin, 1980; Sachar, 1980). These, in turn, influence behavior in a complex and intricate fashion. Anxiety and stress may lead to sleeplessness, lack of appetite, and weight loss. They may also have a further psychological impact and result in a sense of helplessness and depression. Sadness may be expressed through tears, although how emotions are expressed may often depend upon cultural prescriptions, standards, and values. Some individuals in some cultures express grief through tears, wailing, or even self-mutilation; others repress the feelings; still others do not consider behavioral expressions of grief as options, consciously or unconsciously identifying them as inappropriate. In addition to behavioral expressions of grief, the self-perception of emotions is likely to be influenced by both the social context of the event and internalized social perceptions. The presence or absence of supportive family and friends may mitigate or exacerbate emotional responses. Personal philosophy and religious beliefs, both strongly influenced by social values and perceptions, can affect one's evaluation of the significance of death in the cycle of life. Biology, psychology, and social factors combine and interact to affect the experience and behavior associated with the loss of a loved one.

PREMENSTRUAL SYNDROME: A DYNAMIC INTERACTION IN A SOCIAL CONTEXT

The experience and expression of PMS can be seen as a dynamic interaction of neurobiological, psychological, and social elements (Fig. 1), similar to that of grief, with one major difference: the experience of grief is associated with an external event, while PMS is closely linked to the internal biology of the individual. The majority of the symptoms that have come to be recognized as extreme premenstrual changes associated with PMS have major neurological or psychological components, or both (Table 1). The physiological changes that underlie PMS may have a direct psychological effect; that is, there may be a psychological experience that is "the other side" of the neurophysiological changes that are taking place. Yet, there are additional psychological factors, intimately intertwined with the direct psychological effects of the physiological changes and occurring simultaneously in a given individual. They may be evoked by the biological changes of PMS; they may have nothing to do with PMS; they may be due to external circumstances. Because they occur in the same individual, the perceptions and experiences overlap and interact, and, indeed, may not be distinct from each other. Other psychological events may potentiate or mitigate the psychological and physiological effects of PMS. As an example, consider that many people lack the time and energy to fulfill all their personal and professional obligations, as well as those things they feel they ought to do, never mind all the things they would like to do. This is likely to result in a sense of tension, aggravation, or frustration,

Table 1. Some of the Symptoms Associated with PMS.

Abdominal bloating	Depression	Migraine
Abdominal cramping	Edema	Mood swings
Acne	Fainting	Nausea
Aggression	Fatigue	Palpitations
Alcohol intolerance	Food cravings	Seizures
Anxiety	Headache	Sex drive changes
Asthma	Hemorrhoids	Sinus problems
Back pain	Herpes	Sore throat
Breast swelling and tenderness	Hives	Styes
	Insomnia	Suicidal thoughts
Bruising	Irritability	Urinary difficulties
Clumsiness	Joint swelling and pain	Weight gain
Confusion	Lethargy	Withdrawal from others

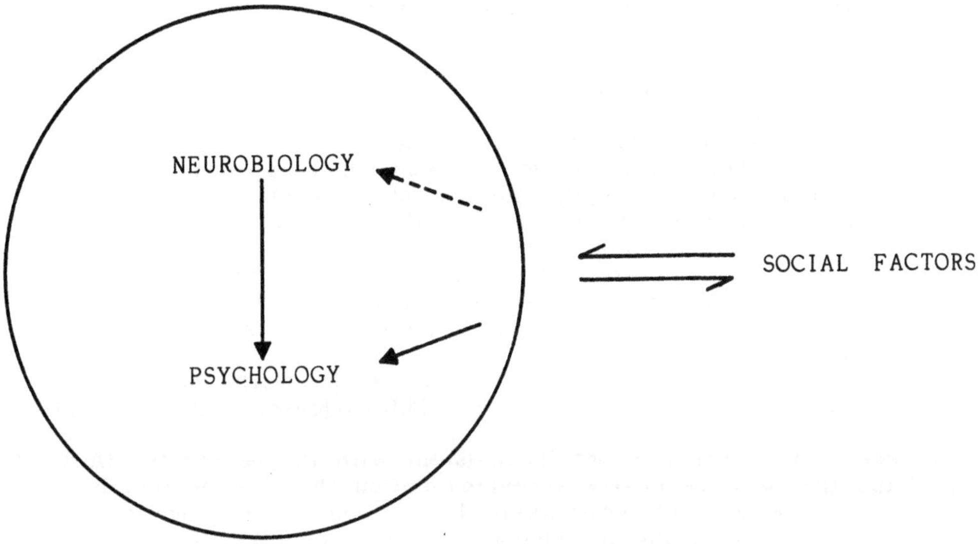

Fig. 1. The dynamic interaction between neurobiology, psychology, and social factors determine both the way in which PMS is expressed and how it is experienced and perceived by the individual. Biology in the form of hormones, gonadotropins, and other endogenous compounds, and psychological factors, such as self-confidence and anxiety, interact to determine perception and behavior. These are both profoundly influenced in subtle and obvious ways by social factors in the form of societal perceptions of appropriate behavior, duties, and responsibilities of women, and of the fundamental nature of women. These societal views affect the individual both because they are expressed in interpersonal relationships with others, and because they are internalized by the individual and thereby affect her perception and evaluation of herself. Verbal and non-verbal behaviors affect the way in which the individual is viewed (and potentially the group she is perceived as representing) and thus, in turn, influence social perceptions.

at least occasionally. Tension may be exacerbated by PMS (Harrison, 1982), either indirectly or perhaps directly. For a particular individual, symptoms may include fatigue. This may add to the frustration of not having enough time or energy to accomplish all the tasks that need to be done. In addition, one of the neurobiological changes associated with PMS may be stimulation of a hypothetical neurological center primarily responsible for the perception and expression of irritability. Psychological elements both related and unrelated to PMS may be acting at the same brain center through different transmitters or through the same transmitters, a final common pathway, producing a specific behavior or perception.

Social factors, in the form of popular opinion, "common knowledge," and common sense, can influence an individual's perception of herself and of her environment, as well as the perceptions of others and of society at-large. They affect a woman's expectations of herself and her evaluation of the feasibility of her goals, as well as of her own ability to affect her world. Social perceptions of the nature of women and of their role in society are deeply embedded in the social fabric.

In the 6th century B.C., Semonides wrote:

> "One day she smiles and is happy; a stranger who sees her in the house will praise her, and say, 'There is no woman better than this among all mankind, nor more beautiful.' But on another day she is unbearable to look at or come near to; then she raves so that you can't approach her, like a bitch over her pups, and she shows herself ungentle and contrary to enemies and friends alike. Just so the sea often stands without a tremor, harmless, a great delight to sailors, in the summer season; but often it raves, tossed about by thundering waves. It is the sea that such a woman most resembles in her temper; like the ocean, she has a changeful nature."
>
> — Semonides, 6th century B.C.
> (Lloyd-Jones, 1975, p. 43)

His poetic description is not inconsistent with the generally offered (and perhaps therefore generally accepted) notion that women are, by nature, emotional, moody, and temperamental. Although now Semonides might be thought to be providing an eloquent account of PMS, to the extent that women are thought of as inherently temperamental, women with PMS who find their mood swings intolerable are trapped by the stereotype which classifies their moods as an inescapable feature of womanhood and thereby to be accepted as is.

Social factors influence both how PMS is perceived by others and how it is experienced. In the words of a man who accompanied his wife to the gynecologist where she was seeking treatment for PMS (Harrison, 1982, p. 45):

> "My wife is fine for two weeks out of the month. She's friendly and a good wife. The house is clean. Then she ovulates and suddenly she's not happy about her life. She wants a job. She wants to go back to school. Then her period comes and she is all right again."

His, and presumably her, understanding of PMS (and thus of what should be treated and cured) is, at least in part, the result of societally-determined stereotypes. The general view of a woman's duties and responsibilities, and of her role in society, may affect perceptions of PMS both for the outside observer and for the woman herself. Societal expectations of the duties of a woman, of how she ought to spend her time, are internalized and affect her perception of herself, and of her identity as a woman. To the extent that societal standards and values are in conflict with the goals and desires of the individual, they may compound the effects of PMS and other psychological factors. This reemphasizes the fact that PMS is a dynamic, psychosocial, biological phenomenon.

ETHICAL IMPLICATIONS

Any label or categorization emphasizes similarities and minimizes differences, blurring even relevant and significant distinctions. Although over 150 different symptoms have been associated with PMS, most women who have PMS experience only a few of these symptoms which recur cyclically and define PMS for them (Abraham, 1980; Endicott, Halbreich, Schacht, & Nee, 1981). No matter which symptoms a particular woman may have, it is likely that the label of PMS will carry with it the stigma associated with the most negative of these symptoms. Women whose symptoms include bloating, migraines, breast tenderness, and fatigue, and who identify themselves as having PMS, are likely to be suspected by others of having a tendency toward violence or a loss of self control, although both of the latter are very rare behaviors for women, even among women with PMS. Acknowledgment and emphasis by the medical community on the variability of PMS both in symptomatology and in severity could help to alleviate stigma associated with the PMS label.

The dynamic, interactive nature of PMS also has implications for the way in which PMS is perceived by the medical community and how it is presented to the general public. Medical community discussion of the importance of the interaction between physiological, psychological, and social elements in the experience and expression of PMS and emphasis on this dynamic relationship in the presentation of PMS to patients and their families, to the media, and to the public at large will help to counteract the two opposing, simplistic notions associated with PMS: (1) that it is "all in their heads," and (2) that "women are victims of their biology." Both of these portrayals are pejorative, and each places the locus of the condition within the individual. Neither acknowledges the significance of social factors in the experience and perception of PMS. Scientists and clinicians who have been educated and trained to understand that brain structure and function and attendant behaviors are extraordinarily complex, intricate, and subtle have the responsibility to avoid oversimplification of the role of biology in behavior, which is not only inaccurate, but perpetuates stigmatizing depictions of biobehavior.

Another result of the emphasis on biological factors in behavior, to the exclusion of psychological and social elements, is that it tends to dictate a biological solution. To the extent that behavior is believed to be rooted in biology, methods for changing that behavior will be selected for their effectiveness in altering the relevant biology. Yet biological intervention may have a variety of hidden dangers. These include the possibility of harmful side effects or long-term effects. The risks of side effects and long-term effects are an aspect of medical treatments in general. Particularly relevant examples include the physiological, psychological, and social consequences of full hysterectomy (including ovariectomy) (Morgan, 1982; Zussman, Zussman, Sunley, & Bjornson, 1981), and the changes associated with "medical oophorectomy" (Muse et al., 1984), both potential medical treatments for PMS (Muse et al., 1984; Reid, 1985). Biological approaches also inherently emphasize the necessity for change in the individual, to the exclusion of changes needed beyond the individual (Conrad & Schneider, 1980). Furthermore, for phenomena with substantial psychological and social components, a purely biological approach is likely to be ineffective. Recognition of the multifaceted nature of PMS emphasizes the importance of developing treatment programs that are not only rational and cautious with respect to potential side effects and untoward long-term effects, but are also multifaceted themselves. Although a regimen that addresses diet, exercise, peer and professional counseling, participation in support groups, and education in stress management and coping strategies primarily focuses on and requires alteration in the individual, it also acknowledges the dynamic relationship among a variety of factors, some of which are external to the individual. For some with severe symptoms, such a multifaceted approach to PMS may be insufficient. A variety of over-the-counter remedies, diet supplements, and prescription drugs have been proposed as treatments for the symptoms of PMS (Eagan, 1983). None have been demonstrated safe and effective, and all pose potential risks, some as yet unidentified. The complex nature of PMS and the absence of a safe, reliable treatment emphasizes the point that it is the individual who must assess and weigh the risks, costs, and benefits of medical intervention. This is likely to be difficult given that both risks and benefits may be uncertain or unknown, and costs may be not only financial, but also personal and social since intervention may alter life style and ultimately, perhaps, relationships.

While a purely biological approach to PMS is inappropriate, emphasis on psychological and/or social factors to the exclusion of biological ones is inaccurate. However significant psychological factors may be in the experience and expression of PMS, a number of factors emphasize the physiological basis for PMS. PMS has been observed in a variety of cultures (Janiger, Riffenburgh, & Kersh, 1972; Snowden & Christian, 1983), and a purely psychological etiology for PMS has not been demonstrated (Gannon, 1981; Golub, 1985; Goudsmit, 1983). Most significantly, premenstrual changes in feeding, social withdrawal, restlessness, and aggression have been noted in non-human primates (D. Goldfoot, personal communication; Hausfater & Skoblick, 1985; Janiger et al., 1972).

The dynamic interaction of biological, psychological, and social elements is fundamental to PMS. To approach it as any one of these alone is to lose a measure of understanding of the phenomenon.

THE INFLUENCE OF SOCIETY ON SCIENCE

Social factors are of relevance to PMS not only because of their role in the experience and perception of PMS, but also because of their influence on the work of scientists and clinicians. Before beginning their professional training, scientists and clinicians, like other professionals, spend at least 20 years living in and learning from society. Knowledge acquired in the formative, pre-school years serves as a foundation, which is later modified through formal schooling. In addition, societal standards, values, and perceptions permeate advertising, the media, and all other sources of "common knowledge." They become an inextricable part of the individual scientist's world view. These culturally-determined factors, in conjunction with general education and scientific training, affect the direction of research. All these components together determine which issues are recognized as problems and which are considered amenable to study. They influence the way in which scientific hypotheses are framed and how they are addressed. They govern the solutions that are recognized and acknowledged as reasonable. The influences of society also affect the kinds of data collected and the methods used to collect them, how the data are interpreted, and the recommendations, either stated or implied, regarding the application of research findings (i.e., applications which are endorsed or acknowledged as valid and appropriate uses of the research).

Examples of the influence of social factors in determining the directions of research, and in the scientific explanations accepted as reasonable, have been cited (Chorover, 1979; Gould, 1981; Longino & Doell, 1983). For example, in the 1850's during pre-Civil War times, the Medical Association of Louisiana formed a committee that was headed by the preeminent physician Samuel A. Cartwright and charged with investigation of the health and diseases of the American blacks of the period (i.e., the slaves). Cartwright and his committee did an extensive study and made a thorough report to the Association which was later published (Cartwright, 1851). Two of the many findings reported were physiological explanations of behaviors both well known and troubling to the citizens of the time. One was a "mental illness" suffered by certain blacks, labeled "drapetomania," which resulted in a tendency among its sufferers to run away. Cartwright and colleagues recommended an approach that could serve as a preventive: On the one hand, treatment of slaves should not be too cruel or neglectful. On the other hand, Negroes should not be treated with too much familiarity; rather awe and reverence should be exacted, as otherwise "they will despise their masters." Cartwright recognized a problem and developed a solution consistent with his world view and experience, and with his training and education. It seemed reasonable and it fit with societal perceptions and understanding, as well as the social needs of the time.

Cartwright also described a disorder associated with improper aeration of the blood that produced the behavioral problem described as "rascality" by slave owners and overseers. The appropriate home remedy for this ailment was thorough washing followed by application of oil. The oil was then slapped into the skin with a broad leather strap, and the patient put to hard work outdoors such as chopping wood or splitting rails. Although the contemporary reader recognizes this study as strongly spiced with the expectations and values of the time, and a conscious or unconscious interest and effort to maintain the political status quo, it can also be recognized as an attempt by professionals to address a commonly recognized problem from their own special perspective. Some suggest that PMS and other women's health issues function to maintain the political status quo (e.g., Ehrenreich & English, 1978). Discussion of this issue is beyond the scope of this paper. However, these examples from pre-Civil War medicine demonstrate that social values can creep into science without being recognized as such.

A continuing area of neuroscience research is the investigation of the role of sex hormones in determining behavior. A large body of work has demonstrated the importance of male and female sex hormones for gender-related anatomical, physiological, and behavioral sex characteristics (for reviews, see Bardin, 1980; Davidson, 1980; Michael, 1980; and Yen, 1980). The hormones are essential for the development and maintenance of gonads and secondary sex characteristics and of appropriate sexual behavior in laboratory animals. In addition, the absence of androgens (male sex hormones) in the developing brain of newborn rodents is necessary for the development of a female, cycling brain and for the expression of female sexual behavior in the sexually mature animal (see Gorski, 1980, for review). The presence of androgens during the critical period shortly after birth results in a "male" brain and male sexual behavior in the adult.

One group of recent studies (Ehrhardt & Meyer-Bahlburg, 1981) focuses on young women with congenital adrenocorticohyperplasia, a disorder which exposes an individual to abnormally large doses of androgens during development. One measure considered is the extent of "tomboyism" in the behavior of these young women. Tomboyism is defined operationally as a preference for active outdoor play rather than less active indoor play, as a preference for male rather than female playmates, as an emphasis on career over housewifery, and as a decreased interest in small infants and play of motherhood roles. It is unavoidable that the observer examining the behavior of these young women will have a concept of both female behavior and male behavior and of "tomboy" behavior. These concepts will inevitably be influenced by culturally-derived perceptions of feminine and masculine characteristics. Furthermore, in these studies, behavioral information was obtained from parents, teachers, and the subjects themselves, all of whom knew of the abnormal physiological condition and are likely to have had expectations regarding its impact. Social perceptions are an inherent, required component of this research — it is socialization behaviors which are under examination. Yet, it is important to recognize and acknowledge that social values are embedded in these perceptions.

Throughout the course of scientific investigation, the research question must be simplified and assumptions made (Star, 1983). The introduction of some bias is inescapable, especially in research assessing normal and abnormal behavior (Bird, 1986). In order for an outside observer to determine the nature of that bias, the simplification process should be explicitly noted and, in particular, assumptions upon which the research is based should be identified at every level of experimentation, from problem formulation to data interpretation. One example in the area of PMS research is the selection of a control population. Whether men, children, women on the pill, women without premenstrual changes, or women with PMS are selected as an experimental control, some assumptions are made regarding the validity and value of the experimental design. These assumptions need to be made clear. The bias which investigators inevitably bring to their work ought to be identified, since not to do so misrepresents the nature of the research.

MEDICALIZATION AND THE BIOLOGICAL PERSPECTIVE

Professionally, individuals consider, address, assess, and approach problems from their own particular perspective, within a specific context. Psychiatrists, endocrinologists, and neuroscientists each consider issues within a particular framework from a particular viewpoint. A neurobiologist could not avoid considering a subject like PMS from a neurobiological perspective. Training and experience provide an orientation in which a problem is evaluated and relevant aspects identified. The viewpoint that develops from professional education and training has two consequences. It not only influences how the problem is analyzed, but also governs what solutions or interventions are recognized and recommended. Financial reward, power, and control have been cited (Illich, 1976; Larson, 1977; Starr, 1982) as motives behind the medicalization of a wide range of topics, including alcoholism, child birth, dying, drug addiction, homosexuality, menopause, mental illness, suicide and violence. Indeed, financial gain and power may result from the medicalization of such subjects. However, rather than conscious or even unconscious expectations of personal or professional aggrandizement, it seems likely that the biological perspective may be largely responsible for the medicalization of these issues. In addition, professional emphasis on biology by "experts" should be viewed in the context of a growing general recognition of the role of biological factors in some aspects of behavior, and the perception of legitimization and exculpation associated with physical illness as contrasted with the social stigma and onus of blame attached to mental illness. Although it is easy to place responsibility for medicalization on the medical community or the established power structure, medicalization grows in a receptive and complex social environment (Riessman, 1983).

A second consequence of a medical or biological education is that such training can unduly and inappropriately narrow the focus of an observer's attention. If the larger context of the subject and other relevant components are not considered, scientists and other specialists may find ourselves in the same predicament as Monsieur Babinet in the etching by Honoré Daumier (Fig. 2), whose high-powered technology has limited his ability to find what he seeks. An awareness of the limitations of our tools and perspectives may permit sensitivity and receptivity to the ways in which other perspectives may complement our own.

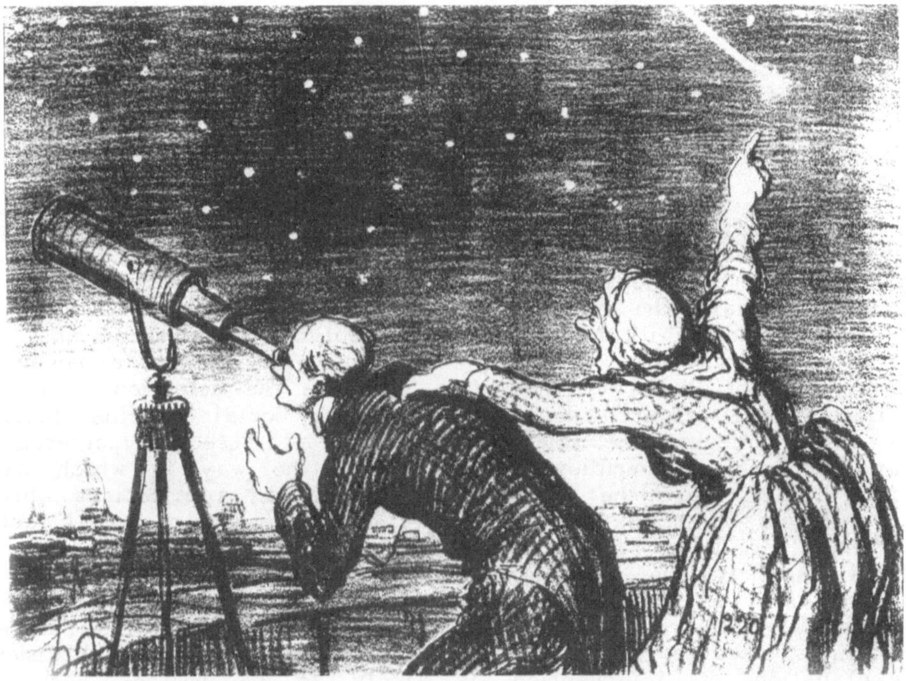

Fig. 2. This Daumier print suggests the circumstance that may arise if the neurobiological foundations and implications of PMS are emphasized to the exclusion of psychological and social factors. [Daumier's legend reads: *"M. Babinet prévenue par sa portière de la visite de la Comète."* Monsieur Babinet is informed by his housekeeper of the comet's arrival. Honoré Daumier, 1808-1879. Charivari, September 22, 1858. Second state, lithograph bequest of William P. Babcock B4184. Lithograph reproduced through the courtesy of the Museum of Fine Arts, Boston, MA.]

SOCIAL IMPACTS OF SCIENCE

Finally to be considered is the fact that while society has an impact on science, science, in turn, has an impact on society. Science is widely perceived as the search for truth, both within and beyond the scientific community. Society values science; it recognizes scientific observations and discoveries as the source of innumerable and spectacularly diverse benefits that improve life, not only through creature comforts, but through increased longevity and improved health. Scientific research is funded by various components of society with the expectation that scientists are looking for and will find "the truth." This truth will be used as the basis for the development of social and public policy. Although there is a growing awareness that science is value-laden, it is not generally recognized, and thus not acknowledged, that scientific truth is not absolute.

There is also general pressure for a truth that is simple — Is PMS a disease or isn't it? Should PMS be a mitigating factor for violent crime or shouldn't it? Simple truths facilitate the development and implementation of policy. Yet, to quote H. L. Mencken, "For every human problem, there is a solution that is simple, neat and wrong."

For a complex issue like PMS, it is vital that scientists not succumb to the pressure to provide a simple explanation and oversimply at the expense of accuracy.

CONCLUSIONS

PMS, like other complex behavioral phenomena, is an expression of the dynamic interaction of biological, psychological, and social factors. This has implications both for the medical interventions proposed to address it, and the manner in which it is presented and viewed by the biomedical community and the general public. Social perceptions, values, and standards are not only a component of the experience and expression of PMS, but they also influence the direction of science by affecting the research done by scientists. Social elements influence to a varying degree the scientific problems addressed, hypotheses posed, and methodologies employed, as well as the way in which data are interpreted and the recommendations and applications proposed. Recognition of the extent and nature of the impact of social factors on science permits a more accurate and candid representation of scientific findings. Science is widely represented as, and believed to be, a search for the truth. Acknowledgment of factors which may affect the nature of that truth makes possible a more appropriate use of research findings. Because PMS is a complex phenomenon, a simple, unidimensional explanation or intervention is likely to be neither accurate nor appropriate.

ACKNOWLEDGMENTS

This material was prepared with support from the National Science Foundation (Grant RII-8318803) and the National Endowment for the Humanities (Grant RH-20542). The views expressed are those of the author and do not necessarily reflect the views of NSF or NEH.

REFERENCES

Abraham, G. E., 1980. Premenstrual tension. *Current Problems in Obstetrics and Gynecology 3:* 1-39.

Bardin, C. W., 1980. The neuroendocrinology of male reproduction. In: D. T. Krieger and J. C. Hughes (Eds.), *Neuroendocrinology*. Sinauer Associates, Sunderland, MA, pp. 239-247.

Bird, S. J., 1986. Ethical, legal and social implications of PMS. Unpublished manuscript.

Bloom, F. E., A. Lazerson, and L. Hofstadter, 1985. *Brain, Mind, and Behavior*. Freeman and Co., New York, NY.

Brobeck, J. R. (Ed.), 1973. *Best and Taylor's Physiological Basis of Medical Practice*, 9th edition. Williams and Wilkins, Baltimore, MD.

Cartwright, S. A., 1851. Report on the diseases and physical peculiarities of the Negro race. *New Orleans Medical and Surgical Journal* (May): 691-715. [Reprinted in: A. L. Caplan, H. T. Engelhardt, Jr., and J. J. McCartney (Eds.), 1981. *Concepts of Health and Disease*. Addison-Wesley, Reading, MA, pp. 305-325.]

Chorover, S. L., 1979. *From Genesis to Genocide*. MIT Press, Cambridge, MA.

Conrad, P. and J. W. Schneider, 1980. *Deviance and Medicalization: From Badness to Sickness*. C. V. Mosby, St. Louis, MO.

Davidson, J. M., 1980. Hormones and sexual behavior in the male. In: D. T. Krieger and J. C. Hughes (Eds.), *Neuroendocrinology*. Sinauer Associates, Sunderland, MA, pp. 232-238.

de Weid, D., 1980. Hormonal influences on motivation, learning, memory, and psychosis. In: D. T. Krieger and J. C. Hughes (Eds.), *Neuroendocrinology*. Sinauer Associates, Sunderland, MA, pp. 194-204.

Eagan, A., 1983. The selling of premenstrual syndrome: Who profits from making PMS "the disease of the 80's"? *Ms.* (October): 26-32.

Ehrenreich, B. and D. English, 1978. *For Her Own Good: 150 Years of the Experts' Advice to Women.* Anchor Press/Doubleday, Garden City, NY.

Ehrhardt, A., H. Meyer-Bahlburg, 1981. Effects of prenatal sex hormones on gender-related behavior. *Science 211:* 1312-1313.

Endicott, J., U. Halbreich, S. Schacht, and J. Nee, 1981. Premenstrual changes and affective disorders. *Psychosomatic Medicine 43:* 519-529.

Frohman, L. A., 1980. Neurotransmitters as regulators of endocrine function. In: D. T. Krieger and J. C. Hughes (Eds.), *Neuroendocrinology*. Sinauer Associates, Sunderland, MA, pp. 44-57.

Gannon, L., 1981. Evidence for a psychological etiology of menstrual disorders: A critical review. *Psychological Reports 48:* 287-294.

Golub, S., 1985. Premenstrual syndrome: The developmental point of view. In: N. Kase (Ed.), *Premenstrual Syndrome: New Findings and Controversies.* In press.

Gorski, R. A., 1980. Sexual differentiation of the brain. In: D. T. Krieger and J. C. Hughes (Eds.), *Neuroendocrinology*. Sinauer Associates, Sunderland, MA, pp. 215-222.

Goudsmit, E. M., 1983. Psychological aspects of premenstrual symptoms. *Journal of Psychosomatic Obstetrics and Gynecology 2:* 20-26.

Gould, S. J., 1981. *The Mismeasure of Man.* W. W. Norton, New York, NY.

Hahn, W. E., J. Van Ness and N. Chaudhari, 1982. Overview of the molecular genetics of mouse brain. In: F. O. Schmitt, S. J. Bird, and F. E. Bloom (Eds.), *Molecular Genetic Neuroscience.* Raven Press, New York, NY, pp. 323-334.

Harlan, R. E., B. D. Shivers, and D. W. Pfaff, 1983. Midbrain microinfusions of prolactin increase in the estrogen-dependent behavior, lordosis. *Science 219:* 1451-1453.

Harrison, M., 1982. *Self-Help for Premenstrual Syndrome.* Matrix Press, Cambridge, MA.

Hausfater, G. and B. Skoblick, 1985. Perimenstrual behavior changes among female yellow baboons: Some similarities to premenstrual syndrome (PMS) in women. *American Journal of Primatology 9:* 165-172.

Illich, I., 1976. *Medical Nemesis: The Expropriation of Health.* Pantheon, New York, NY.

Janiger, O., R. Riffenburgh, and R. Kersh, 1972. Cross cultural study of premenstrual syndrome. *Psychosomatics 13:* 226-235.

Kopin, I. J., 1980. Catecholamines, adrenal hormones, and stress. In: D. T. Krieger and J. C. Hughes (Eds.), *Neuroendocrinology.* Sinauer Associates, Sunderland, MA, pp. 159-166.

Koranyi, L., D. I. Whitmoyer, and C. H. Sawyer, 1977. Effect of thyrotropin releasing hormone, luteinizing hormone releasing hormone and somatostatin on neuronal activity of brain stem reticular formation and hippocampus in the female rat. *Experimental Neurology 57:* 807-816.

Kretzinger, R. H., 1981. Mechanisms of selective signalling by calcium. *Neurosciences Research Program Bulletin 19:* 211-334.

Krieger, D. T., 1980. The hypothalamus and neuroendocrinology. In: D. T. Krieger and J. C. Hughes (Eds.), *Neuroendocrinology.* Sinauer Associates, Sunderland, MA, pp. 3-12.

Krieger, D. T. and J. C. Hughes (Eds.), 1980. *Neuroendocrinology.* Sinauer Associates, Sunderland, MA.

Larson, M. S., 1977. *The Rise of Professionalism: A Sociological Analysis.* University of California Press, Berkeley, CA.

Lloyd-Jones, H., 1975. *Females of the Species: Semonides on Women.* Noyes Press, Park Ridge, NJ.

Longino, H. and R. Doell, 1983. Body, bias and behavior: A comparative analysis of reasoning in two areas of biological science. *Signs 9:* 206-227.

McEwen, B. S., 1980. The brain as a target organ of endocrine hormones. In: D. T. Krieger and J. C. Hughes (Eds.), *Neuroendocrinology.* Sinauer Associates, Sunderland, MA, pp. 33-42.

McEwen, B., 1982. Steroid hormone action in the brain: Cellular and behavioral effects. In: F. O. Schmitt, S. J. Bird, and F. E. Bloom (Eds.), *Molecular Genetic Neuroscience.* Raven Press, New York, NY, pp. 265-275.

McEwen, B., P. G. Davis, B. Parson, and D. W. Pfaff, 1979. The brain as a target for steroid hormone action. *Annual Review of Neuroscience 2:* 65-112.

Michael, R. P., 1980. Hormones and sexual behavior in the female. In: D. T. Krieger and J. C. Hughes (Eds.), *Neuroendocrinology.* Sinauer Associates, Sunderland, MA, pp. 223-231.

Morgan, S., 1982. *Coping with Hysterectomy.* Dial, New York, NY.

Muse, K. N., N. S. Cetel, L. A. Futterman, and S.S.C. Yen, 1984. The premenstrual syndrome: Effects of "medical ovariectomy." *New England Journal of Medicine 311:* 1345-1349.

Nock, B. and H. H. Feder, 1981. Neurotransmitter modulation of steroid action in target cells that mediate reproduction and reproductive behavior. *Neuroscience and Biobehavioral Reviews 5:* 437-447.

Pfaff, D. W. and M. Keiner, 1973. Atlas of estradiol-concentrating cells in the central nervous system of the female rat. *Journal of Comparative Neurology 151:* 121-158.

Reid, R. L., 1985. Premenstrual syndrome. *Current Problems in Obstetrics, Gynecology, and Infertility 8:* 1-57.

Reid, R. L. and S.S.C. Yen, 1981. Premenstrual syndrome. *American Journal of Obstetrics and Gynecology 139:* 85-104.

Riessman, C. K., 1983. Women and medicalization: A new perspective. *Social Policy 14:* 3-18.

Riskind, P. and R. L. Moss, 1979. Midbrain central gray: LHRH infusion enhances lordotic behavior in estrogen-primed ovariectomized rats. *Brain Research Bulletin 4:* 203-205.

Sachar, E. J., 1980. Hormonal changes in stress and mental illness. In: D. T. Krieger and J. C. Hughes (Eds.), *Neuroendocrinology.* Sinauer Associates, Sunderland, MA, pp. 177-183.

Sakuma, Y. and D. W. Pfaff, 1980. LH-RH in the mesencephalic central grey can potentiate lordosis reflex of female rats. *Nature 283:* 566-567.

Sar, M. and W. E. Stumpf, 1973. Autoradiographic localization of radioactivity in the rat brain after injection of 1,2-^{3}H-testosterone. *Endocrinology 92:* 251-256.

Schmitt, F. O., 1984. Molecular regulators of brain function: A new view. *Neuroscience 13:* 991-1001.

Sirinathsinghji, D.J.S., P. E. Whittington, A. Audsley, and H. M. Fraser, 1983. β-endorphin regulates lordosis in female rats by modulating LH-RH release. *Nature 301:* 62-64.

Snowden, R. and B. Christian, 1983. *Patterns and Perceptions of Menstruation.* St. Martin's Press, New York, NY.

Sodersten, P., M. Henning, P. Melin, and S. Ludin, 1983. Vasopressin alters female sexual behaviour by acting on the brain independently of alterations in blood pressure. *Nature 301:* 608-610.

Star, S. L., 1983. Simplification in scientific work: An example from neuroscience research. *Social Studies of Science 13:* 205-228.

Starr, P., 1982. *The Social Transformation of American Medicine.* Basic Books, New York, NY.

Stumpf, W. E. and L. Jennes, 1984. The A-B-C (Allocortex-Brainstem-Core) circuitry of endocrine autonomic integration and regulation: A proposed hypothesis of the anatomical-functional relationships between estradiol sites of action and peptidergic-aminergic neuronal systems. *Peptides 5, Supplement 1* (Fayetteville): 221-226.

Valentino, R. J., S. L. Foote, and G. Aston-Jones, 1983. Corticotropin-releasing factor activates noradrenergic neurons of the locus coeruleus. *Brain Research 270:* 363-367.

Yen, S.S.C., 1980. Neuroendocrine regulation of the menstrual cycle. In: D. T. Krieger and J. C. Hughes (Eds.), *Neuroendocrinology.* Sinauer Associates, Sunderland, MA, pp. 259-272.

Yu, W.H.A. and M. Y. McGinnis, 1984. Demonstration of androgen receptors in cranial nerve motor nuclei. *Society for Neuroscience Abstracts 10:* 901.

Zussman, L., S. Zussman, R. Sunley, and E. Bjornson, 1981. Sexual response after hysterectomy-oophorectomy: Recent studies and reconsideration of psychogenesis. *American Journal of Obstetrics and Gynecology 140:* 725-729.

PRACTICAL AND ETHICAL ASPECTS OF PHARMACOTHERAPEUTIC EVALUATION

David R. Rubinow, M.D.

Psychiatry Consultation-Liaison
National Institutes of Health; and
Unit on Peptide Studies
Biological Psychiatry Branch
National Institute of Mental Health
Bethesda, MD

INTRODUCTION

Premenstrual syndrome exemplifies the convergence of science and superstition, experience and belief, political consciousness and political subjugation, inquiry and ideology. The current state of confusion surrounding this disorder impacts on the decisions made regarding its treatment. In the following paper, I will pose a series of questions about the ethical and practical principles of pharmacotherapeutic evaluation with specific reference to the premenstrual syndrome(s) (PMS).

WHAT IS THE NATURE OF THE PROCESS BY WHICH ONE MAKES ETHICAL DECISIONS? [1]

Ethical decisions or decisions of principle have as their main characteristics prescription and universalizability. Ethical or value judgments are not simply propositions, observations, or descriptive statements, but rather prescribe, command, guide choices, regulate conduct, and answer the question, "What shall I do?" Both moral and non-moral values derive from or appeal to certain generalizable principles or standards in contrast to the simple imperative which also guides choices. Ethical or moral values differ from non-moral value judgments in the type of principles that are appealed to; moral principles are principles for the conduct of human beings as human beings and cannot be accepted without influencing the way in which we conduct ourselves. These principles are universalizable, consistent, general, and broad as opposed to oriented to specific opinions of an individual. In sum, ethics describes the process of a human being's conduct as a human being; ethical principles necessarily entail and prescribe actions. Decisions of principle, then, can be seen as entailing the assent of the doer that the action prescribed is correct even if he were to become the recipient of the action, all other relevant respects being equal.

---

[1] This section was adapted from the work of R. M. Hare (1964, 1965).

WHAT PRINCIPLES GUIDE THE FOOD AND DRUG ADMINISTRATION (FDA) PHARMACOTHERAPEUTIC EVALUATION PROCESS?

The guiding principle in medicine is often conceptualized as *primum non nocere* — non-maleficence or "above all do no harm," although it is more accurately described as beneficence — "do more good than harm" (Macklin, this volume). These principles appear also to guide the decision-making process of the Food and Drug Administration (FDA). Thus, examination of FDA IND Form 1571 (Notice of Claimed Investigational Exemption for New Drug), as well as the transcripts of the Fertility and Maternal Health Drugs Advisory Committee meetings, makes clear the FDA's concern with the following: (1) drug safety (first and foremost); (2) the justification for administering a drug to a human, including demonstrations of the efficacy of the drug and the significance of a clinical trial employing the drug; and (3) provision of sufficient information to the recipient of the drug to permit assessment of the potential risks and benefits.

These concerns have been specifically applied to the question of progesterone treatment in three FDA advisory committee meetings between 1976 and 1983. In 1976, the FDA Obstetrics and Gynecology Advisory Committee reviewed the use of progesterone suppositories for the treatment of luteal phase defects; i.e., the presence of inadequate ovarian progesterone secretion in otherwise regular ovulatory cycles, a problem most commonly associated with infertility (Transcript and Answers to Questions by the Food and Drug Administration's Obstetrics and Gynecology Advisory Committee, July 15, 1976). The Committee noted that there was no evidence that progesterone administration during pregnancy was associated with birth defects and that published reports suggested the efficacy of physiologic doses of progesterone as treatment for luteal phase defects. They concluded that data from at least two random assignment prospective placebo-controlled studies were necessary in order to assess the efficacy of progesterone for these defects. The Committee also noted that their current presumption of safety was based on a dosage of progesterone not exceeding that necessary to obtain normal luteal phase serum progesterone levels.

In 1981, the Fertility and Maternal Health Drugs Advisory Committee concluded that progesterone was safe for the treatment of "reproductive disorders" and that despite the absence of randomized clinical trials, the results of studies involving "a well-defined clinical and endocrinological patient population" indicated the efficacy of progesterone for the treatment of luteal phase deficiency (Transcript and Answers to Questions by the Food and Drug Administration's Fertility and Maternal Health Drugs Advisory Committee, November 5-6, 1981). It was recommended that the label be changed to indicate that progesterone and 17-OH progesterone caproate did not appear to have significant teratogenic potential. Recommended doses of progesterone for luteal phase deficiency were 12.5 milligrams intramuscularly each day or 25-milligram suppositories twice per day. The Committee stated that "for safety sake" and in the absence of Phase One bioavailability/absorption studies, a maximum dose of 250 milligrams of intravaginal progesterone each day for 14 days should not be exceeded for the "treatment of premenstrual syndrome." (Phase One studies determine the human toxicity, metabolism, absorption, excretion, preferred route of administration, safe dose range, etc. of a drug.)

In 1983, the Fertility and Maternal Health Drugs Advisory Committee requested discussion of premenstrual syndrome and its treatment with progesterone as an agenda item (Transcript and Answers to Questions by the Food and Drug Administration's Fertility and Maternal Health Drugs Advisory Committee, February 17, 1983). The intent of the Committee was to review evidence for the safety of progesterone for the treatment of premenstrual syndrome or, in its absence, to define the studies necessary to establish the safety of progesterone for premenstrual syndrome. The Committee concluded that the safety but not the efficacy of progesterone had been demonstrated for premenstrual syndrome. Recommendations were made for double-blind, placebo-controlled, crossover studies employing up to a maximum of 200 milligrams per day by suppository. Dosages above this level were not to be employed until Phase One pharmacokinetic/absorption studies were completed. Finally, it was recommended that informed consent acknowledge the "experimental nature of the treatment and the limited knowledge of the long term effects of the higher doses regimen."

The FDA's actions appear consonant with the stated aim of ensuring safety. Nonetheless, it might be argued that the FDA's caution in evaluating progesterone treatment of premenstrual syndrome does indirectly produce harm and thus violates the principles proscribing harm-producing actions. Does the caution of the FDA result in delayed determination of the efficacy or lack of efficacy of progesterone at the doses employed in clinical practice, thereby potentially resulting in the withholding of treatment (with consequent prolongation of suffering) or in the unnecessary exposure of PMS patients to potentially dangerous elevated drug levels? Should it be the position of the FDA to expedite rather than delay those studies that might indeed answer the question of the safety and efficacy of doses of progesterone recommended by some and prescribed by many? Does the FDA caution perpetuate the disbelief of physicians about the existence of PMS and mandate the unavailability of recommended treatment? These questions address the role of the FDA as disseminator of information, molder of public policy, and regulator of clinical medical practice. However, the FDA may view its paramount role as protecting people from harm, rather than promoting their safety or symptomatic relief. Additionally, changes in clinical practice frequently precede FDA sanction, as was seen, for example, with the standard use of propranolol for the treatment of cardiac arrhythmias prior to FDA approval for this indication. Thus, the FDA might argue that clinicians will do as they please, but the FDA will not approve a medication for a clinical condition so long as doubts about its safety or efficacy exist. If at present there is no evidence of risk associated with progesterone treatment in lower doses for other indications, then perhaps the FDA's caution with respect to higher doses for premenstrual syndrome may relate as much to the concern about justification for use as it does to the concern for safety.

HOW DOES ONE EVALUATE THE JUSTIFICATION FOR AND EFFICACY OF PHARMACOTHERAPY?

A variety of practical/methodological and ethical problems complicate clinical pharmacotherapeutic research. The failure of investigators to consider basic methdologic questions prior to conducting studies of premenstrual syndrome accounts in large part for the inconsistency and ungeneralizability of data collected (Rubinow & Roy-Byrne, 1984), as well as for the all too frequent effort to transform blind spots into dogma.

(1) What disorder is the pharmacotherapy to be used for?

(2) How does one diagnose the disorder to be treated?

In clinical research as well as in clinical practice, the first question that must be posed is, "How do you define that which you wish to study (or treat)?" A preliminary definition of premenstrual syndrome is as follows: The cyclic recurrence of symptoms of sufficient severity so as to interfere with certain aspects of life and that occur with a consistent and predictable relationship to menstruation. In order to operationalize this definition, several derivative questions must be answered (Rubinow & Roy-Byrne, 1984).

(A) What are the symptoms that are experienced?

The list of symptoms that have been attributed to the premenstrual syndrome is formidable and includes practically any symptom that one might expect to encounter in a general medical practice. Perhaps the best attempt to date to deal with the diversity of symptoms is the Premenstrual Assessment Form (PAF) of Halbreich, Endicott, Schacht, and Nee (1982). These authors hope that this instrument will identify clinically meaningful symptom clusters; however, they appropriately caution that their subsyndromes are not mutually exclusive and must at present be viewed as descriptors rather than diagnoses. Thus, for the time being, the type of symptom is of little utility in the diagnosis of premenstrual syndrome.

(B) What is the intensity or severity of the symptoms experienced?

Generally, this question has been addressed in a sporadic and idiosyncratic manner. Further problems have included: The failure of investigators to measure symptom severity (Sutherland & Stewart, 1965); the attribution of clinical significance to statistically significant but clinically insubstantial changes (Taylor, 1979); and the utilization of a scale with insufficient sensitivity to differences in severity and reflecting categories rather than dimensions (Abraham, 1980), with consequent greater vulnerability to the effects of perceptual bias (Ruble & Brooks-Gunn, 1979).

(C) When do the symptoms occur in relation to menstruation?

This question is clearly crucial to the diagnosis of premenstrual syndrome, for it is the timing of the appearance and offset of symptoms in relation to menstruation that establishes them as menstrually-linked and thus distinguishes them from other non-menstrually-related symptoms. In general, definitions of "premenstrual" have varied from study to study (Dalton, 1964; Kramp, 1968; Sutherland & Stewart, 1965) with little attention devoted to the non-premenstrual portion of the cycle.

(D) What is the symptomatic baseline upon which symptoms occur?

Premenstrual symptoms must be evaluated in the context of the remainder of the menstrual cycle in order to be able to successfully distinguish among premenstrual appearance of symptoms, premenstrual exacerbation of pre-existing symptoms, and premenstrual continuation of symptoms. These distinctions are rarely addressed. Additionally, few authors have attempted to define the acceptable amount of variance in symptoms over the course of the menstrual cycle (Parlee, 1973) or to assess the relationship of symptoms to other life events.

(E) By what methods can one establish the menstrual linkage of symptoms?

It is now clear that a *history* of menstrually-linked symptoms does not predict their prospective confirmation. Despite numerous demonstrations that retrospective ratings are not generally validated by daily prospective ratings (Abplanalp, Donnelly, & Rose, 1979; McCance, Luff, & Widdowson, 1937; Sampson & Prescott, 1981) and are influenced by information processing biases (Ruble & Brooks-Gunn, 1979), most studies to date have used retrospective reports of menstrually-related symptoms as the sole entry criterion without prospectively confirming, *prior* to study entry, the existence of the relationship between symptom occurrence and menstruation. In two studies employing retrospective assessment and prospective, longitudinal daily ratings, Endicott and Halbreich (1982) confirmed the presence of premenstrual syndrome in only 59 percent of 48 women presenting with a history of PMS. We obtained similar confirmation using visual analogue scale self-ratings in only 69 out of 160 or 43 percent of putative PMS sufferers. Examples of daily rating patterns obtained in individuals and groups of women with and without confirmed premenstrual syndrome are illustrated in Figures 1 and 2. In recognition of the multitude of factors thwarting attempts to obtain diagnostic uniformity and cross-study comparability, we operationally defined a menstrually-related mood disorder as at least a 30 percent increase in mean mood symptom score for each individual during the week prior to menstruation compared with the week following menstruation in at least two out of three cycles (Rubinow, Roy-Byrne, Hoban, Gold, & Post, 1984), a definition similar to that adopted by the National Institute of Mental Health/Public Health Service (NIMH/PHS) Research Workshop in April, 1983.

(3) By what measures is therapeutic outcome assessed, and can these measures be reliably obtained?

At present, there is no generally accepted way of objectively rating a syndrome that more often consists of internally experienced symptoms than objective behavioral signs. The lack of standardized observer rating instruments sensitive to meaningful changes in mood in relation to the menstrual cycle is suggested by the observation by Haskett, Steiner, Osmun, and Carroll (1980) of a mean Hamilton Depression Scale score of only 12 (compared with a score of 16, a standard minimum required for depression studies) in a group of women with "severe premenstrual syndrome" during their symptomatic phase. Thus, at present one must use self-ratings obtained on a daily basis and employing an ordinal or interval measure of symptom severity in order to properly evaluate the magnitude and the timing of the change in symptoms.

(4) What non-specific effects of treatment complicate therapeutic evaluation?

A frequently observed phenomenon is the mitigation of symptoms experienced by women completing daily self-rating forms. Whether this change is a product of an empathic and accepting therapeutic relationship, an enhanced sense of order, predictability and self-control, or a formal validation of suffering rather than derogation or contempt, it is nonetheless a factor that may produce treatment artifact if treatment trials are initiated early in the self-rating process. Placebo response rates in patients with PMS have been reported as high as 80 percent by some investigators (J. Endicott, personal communication, April 14, 1983).

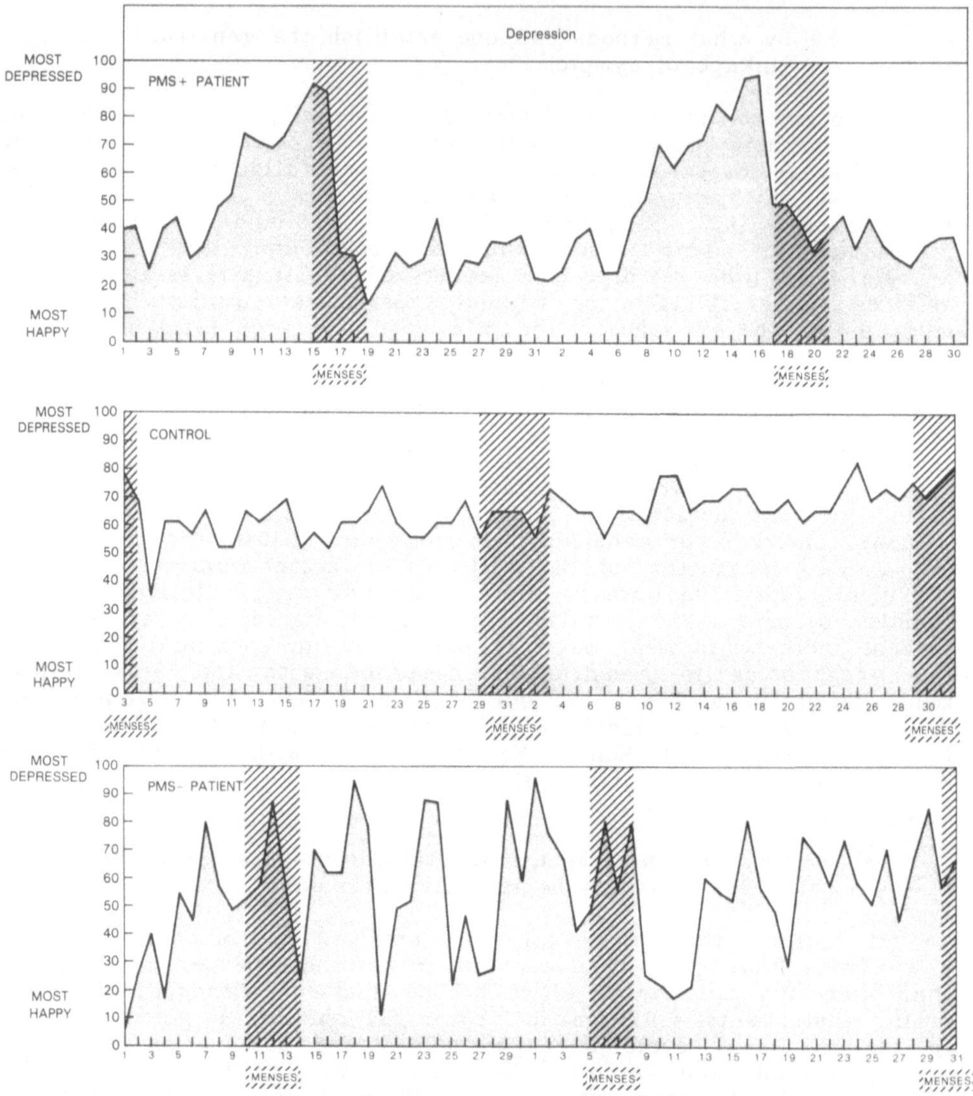

Fig. 1. Daily A.M. depression ratings of a patient with confirmed premenstrual syndrome (PMS+), a control patient with no premenstrual complaints, and a patient with premenstrual complaints but no confirmatory evidence of premenstrual syndrome (PMS-). [From: Rubinow et al., 1986. Reprinted with permission of *Journal of Affective Disorders.*] (See also Rubinow et al., 1984.)

While perhaps a reflection of inadequate diagnostic entry criteria or insufficiently long treatment cells that obscure possible time-dependent attentuation of response, placebo response rates of this magnitude make the demonstration of the therapeutic superiority of any active agent a practical impossibility. In sum, given this degree of methodologic chaos, it is not surprising that progesterone may be viewed as an unproven treatment for an ill-defined disorder of questionable consequence.

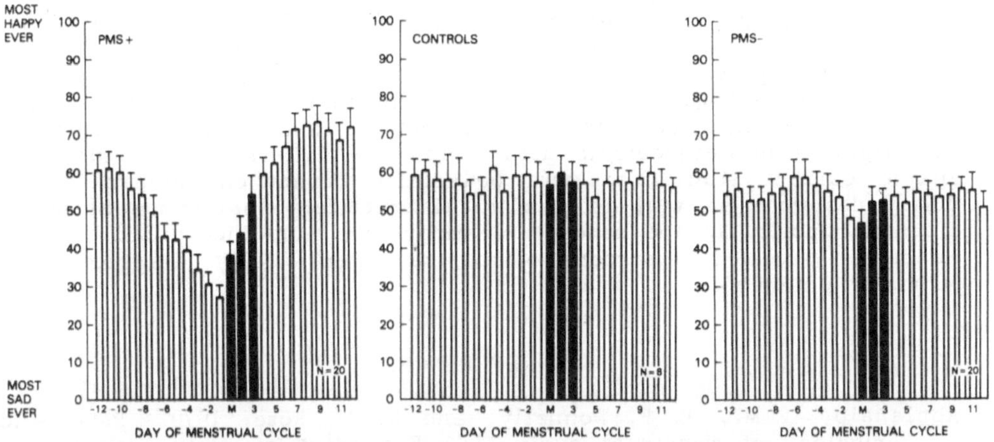

Fig. 2. Mean daily A.M. depression ratings in groups of women with (PMS+) and without (PMS-) confirmed premenstrual syndrome and controls. Menses is indicated by solid histograms. [From: Rubinow et al., 1986. Reprinted with permission of *Journal of Affective Disorders.*]

CONCLUSIONS

The ethical problems encountered in clinical research are derived from those principles guiding the conduct of the investigator as a human being and physician. Clinical research techniques may at times appear to be discordant with the guiding principle of beneficence, "do more good than harm." This principle influences decisions to withhold treatment, treat with placebo, maintain a treatment blind, and perform procedures unnecessary to the treatment of an individual patient.

Withholding treatment where no effective treatment exists is different from the situation in which effective treatment is withheld in order to test a treatment of unproven efficacy. In the case of premenstrual syndrome, withholding pharmacotherapy during the initial cycles of self-rating can be justified as necessary to permit the diagnostic assessment required for prescription of an indicated treatment or avoidance of unnecessary or non-indicated treatment. Treatment with placebo (in crossover studies where patients also receive active treatment) can also be justified in order to prevent prescription of a treatment with additional risks and no additional benefits. One is, however, on ethically more treacherous ground when the dictates of the study supersede the interests of the individual subject. If, for example, treatment cells are three months in length, should a subject be left on placebo for three months when it appears clear that symptomatic relapse or exacerbation has occurred after one month? Should a patient be exposed to pain or potential procedural risk (even slight) if the information obtained from the procedure will not directly benefit the patient? Such questions are not easily answered, for the "relevant respects" providing the context for the operation of the guiding principles are intricate and include such factors as degree of discomfort, altruistic satisfaction, and financial coercion.

The more general question, however, of the justification for and encouragement of research on PMS is more easily resolvable. In the context of the suffering or even self-perception of suffering of thousands of women, failure to actively support research designed to promote diagnostic clarity and determine therapeutic efficacy and safety is a statement of disbelief. Otherwise, one could not place oneself in the position of a person suffering intense and, at times, devastating intra- and interpersonal discomfort and yet maintain that efforts to understand and alleviate this suffering should not be supported. Attention by investigators to methodologic detail prior to initiating their studies may enable current studies to more powerfully impact on research funding policy decisions as well as on clinical practice. Inattention by molders of public policy to the conceptual importance and widespread impact of menstrually-related disorders would be scientifically disgraceful and ethically untenable.

REFERENCES

Abplanalp, J. M., A. F. Donnelly, and R. M. Rose, 1979. Psychoendocrinology of menstrual cycle, I: Enjoyment of daily activities and moods. *Psychosomatic Medicine 41:* 587-604.

Abraham, G. E., 1980. The premenstrual tension syndromes. In: L. K. McNall (Ed.), *Contemporary Obstetric and Gynecologic Nursing, Vol. 3.* Mosby Co., St. Louis, MO.

Dalton, K., 1964. *The Premenstrual Syndrome.* Charles C. Thomas, Springfield, IL.

Endicott, J. and U. Halbreich, 1982. Psychobiology of premenstrual change. *Psychopharmacology Bulletin 18:* 109-112.

Halbreich, U., J. Endicott, S. Schacht, and J. Nee, 1982. The diversity of premenstrual changes as reflected in the Premenstrual Assessment Form. *Acta Psychiatrica Scandinavica 65:* 46-65.

Hare, R. M., 1964. *The Language of Morals.* Oxford University Press, New York, NY.

Hare, R. M., 1965. *Freedom and Reason.* Oxford University Press, New York, NY.

Haskett, R. F., M. Steiner, J. N. Osmun, and B. J. Carroll, 1980. Severe premenstrual tension: Delineation of the syndrome. *Psychiatry 15:* 121-139.

Kramp, J. L., 1968. Studies of the premenstrual syndrome in relation to psychiatry. *Acta Psychiatrica Scandinavica (Suppl.) 203:* 261-267.

McCance, R. A., R. C. Luff, and E. Widdowson, 1937. Physical and emotional periodicity in women. *Journal of Hygiene (London) 37:* 571-611.

Parlee, M. B., 1973. The premenstrual syndrome. *Psychological Bulletin 80:* 454-465.

Rubinow, D. R. and P. P. Roy-Byrne, 1984. Premenstrual syndromes: Overview from a methodologic perspective. *American Journal of Psychiatry 141:* 161-172.

Rubinow, D. R., P. P. Roy-Byrne, M. C. Hoban, P. W. Gold, and R. M. Post, 1984. Prospective assessment of menstrually-related mood disorders. *American Journal of Psychiatry 141:* 684-686.

Rubinow, D. R., P. P. Roy-Byrne, M. C. Hoban, G. N. Grover, N. Stambler, and R. M. Post, 1986. Premenstrual mood changes: Characteristic patterns in women with and without premenstrual syndrome. *Journal of Affective Disorders,* in press.

Ruble, D. N. and J. Brooks-Gunn, 1979. Menstrual symptoms: A social cognition analysis. *Journal of Behavioral Medicine 2:* 171-194.

Sampson, J. A. and P. Prescott, 1981. The assessment of the symptoms of premenstrual syndrome and their response to therapy. *British Journal of Psychiatry 138:* 399-405.

Sutherland, H. and I. Stewart, 1965. A critical analysis of premenstrual syndrome. *The Lancet 1:* 1180-1183.

Taylor, J. W., 1979. The timing of menstruation-related symptoms assessed by a daily symptom rating scale. *Acta Psychiatrica Scandinavica 60:* 87-105.

APPENDIX

A.M.

Name ____________ Month/Year ____________

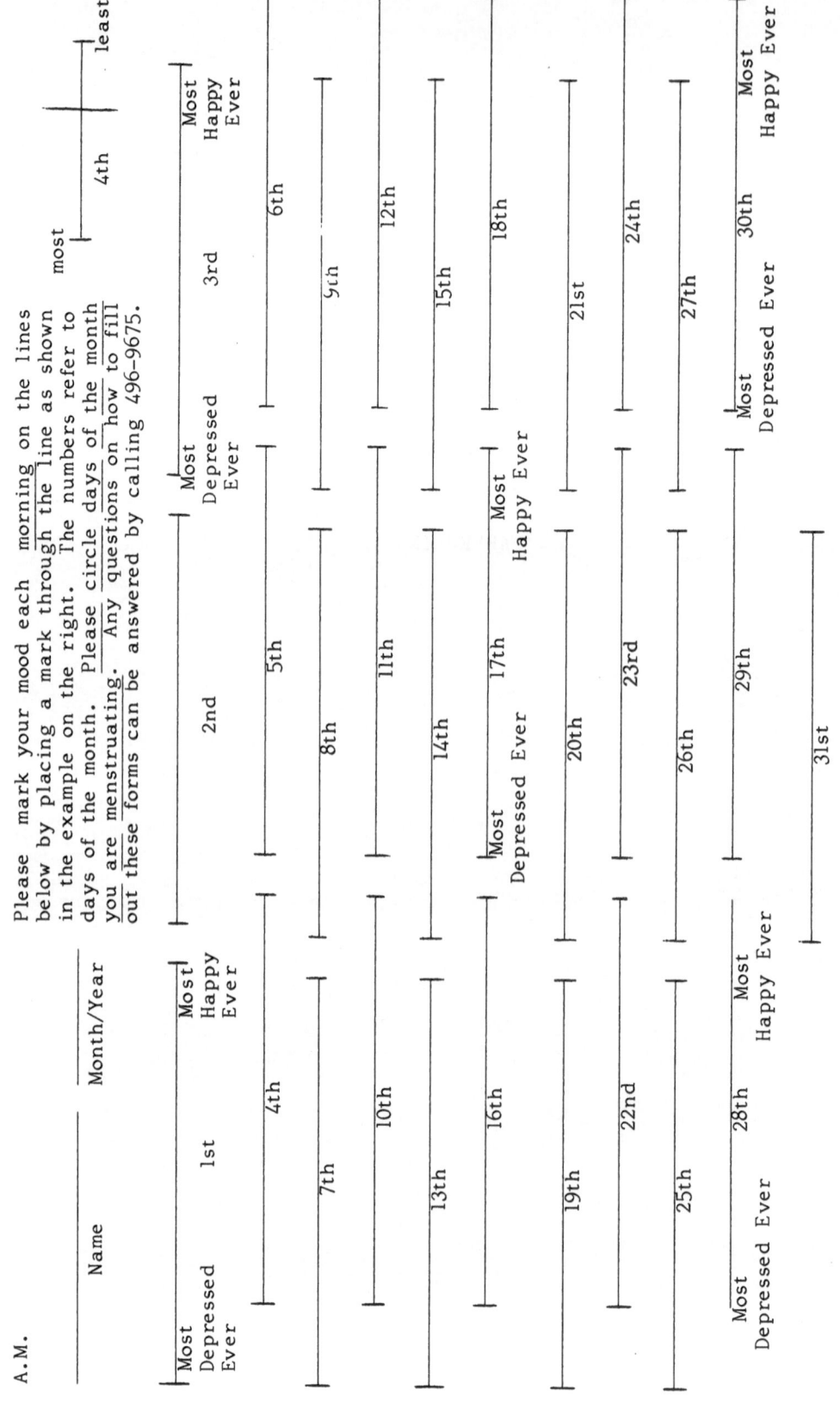

Please mark your mood each morning on the lines below by placing a mark through the line as shown in the example on the right. The numbers refer to days of the month. Please circle days of the month you are menstruating. Any questions on how to fill out these forms can be answered by calling 496-9675.

most — 4th — least

Most Depressed Ever — 1st — Most Happy Ever

2nd

Most Depressed Ever — 3rd — Most Happy Ever

4th

5th

6th

7th

8th

9th

10th

11th

12th

13th

14th

15th

16th

Most Depressed Ever — 17th — Most Happy Ever

18th

19th

20th

21st

22nd

23rd

24th

25th

26th

27th

Most Depressed Ever — 28th — Most Happy Ever

29th

Most Depressed Ever — 30th — Most Happy Ever

31st

HAMILTON PSYCHIATRIC RATING SCALE FOR DEPRESSION

Subject ____________________ Rater ____________________ Date ____________

Mark each item on left half of scoring sheet on row specified
Use marking positions 0 - 4, columns 1 - 5

1. Depressed Mood (Sadness, hopeless, helpless, worthless)
   0 = Absent
   1 = These feeling states indicated only on questioning
   2 = These feeling states spontaneously reported verbally
   3 = Communicates feeling states non-verbally — i.e., through facial expression, posture, voice, and tendency to weep
   4 = Patient reports VIRTUALLY ONLY these feeling states in his spontaneous verbal and non-verbal communication

2. Feelings of Guilt
   0 = Absent
   1 = Self reproach, feels he has let people down
   2 = Ideas of guilt or rumination over past errors or sinful deeds
   3 = Present illness is a punishment. Delusions of guilt
   4 = Hears accusatory or denunciatory voices and/or experiences threatening visual hallucinations

3. Suicide
   0 = Absent
   1 = Feels life is not worth living
   2 = Wishes he were dead or any thoughts of possible death to self
   3 = Suicide ideas or gesture
   4 = Attempts at suicide (any serious attempt rates 4)

4. Insomnia Early
   0 = No difficulty falling asleep
   1 = Complains of occasional difficulty falling asleep -- i.e., more than 1/2 hour
   2 = Complains of nightly difficulty falling asleep

5. Insomnia Middle
   0 = No difficulty
   1 = Patient complains of being restless and disturbed during the night
   2 = Waking during the night — any getting out of bed rates 2 (except for purposes of voiding)

6. Insomnia Late
   0 = No difficulty
   1 = Waking in early hours of the morning but goes back to sleep
   2 = Unable to fall asleep again if he gets out of bed

7. Work and Activities

0 = No difficulty
1 = Thoughts and feelings of incapacity, fatigue or weakness to activities; work or hobbies
2 = Loss of interest in activity; hobbies or work -- either directly reported by patient, or indirect in listlessness, indecision and vacillation (feels he has to push self to work or activities)
3 = Decreases in actual time spent in activities or decrease in productivity. In hospital, rate 3 if patient does not spend at least three hours a day in activities (hospital job or hobbies) exclusive of ward chores
4 = Stopped working because of present illness. In hospital, rate 4 if patient engages in no activities except ward chores, or if patient fails to perform ward chores unassisted

8. Retardation (Slowness of thought and speech; impaired ability to concentrate; decreased motor activity)

0 = Normal speech and thought
1 = Slight retardation at interview
2 = Obvious retardation at interview
3 = Interview difficult
4 = Complete stupor

9. Agitation

0 = None
1 = Fidgetiness
2 = Playing with hands, hair, etc.
3 = Moving about, can't sit still
4 = Hand wringing, nail biting, hair-pulling, biting of lips

10. Anxiety Psychic

0 = No difficulty
1 = Subjective tension and irritability
2 = Worrying about minor matters
3 = Apprehensive attitude apparent in face or speech
4 = Fears expressed without questioning

11. Anxiety Somatic

0 = Absent	Physiological concomitants of anxiety, such as:
1 = Mild	Gastro-intestinal — dry mouth, wind, indigestion, diarrhea, cramps, belching
2 = Moderate	
3 = Severe	
4 = Incapacitating	Cardio-vascular — palpitations, headaches
	Respiratory — hyperventilation, sighing
	Urinary frequency
	Sweating

12. Somatic Symptoms Gastrointestinal

0 = None
1 = Loss of appetite but eating without staff encouragement. Heavy feelings in abdomen
2 = Difficulty eating without staff urging. Requests or requires laxatives or medication for bowels or medication for G.I. symptoms

13. Somatic Symptoms General

0 = None
1 = Heaviness in limbs, back or head. Backaches, headaches, muscle aches. Loss of energy and fatigability
2 = Any clear cut symptom rates 2

14. Genital Symptoms

0 = Absent
1 = Mild
2 = Severe

Symptoms such as: Loss of libido
Menstrual disburbances

15. Hypochondriasis

0 = No present
1 = Self-absorption (bodily)
2 = Preoccupation with health
3 = Frequent complaints, requests for help, etc.
4 = Hypochondriacal delusions

16. Loss of Weight Rate either A or B

A. When rating by history:

0 = No weight loss
1 = Probably weight loss associated with present illness
2 = Definite (according to patient) weight loss
3 = Not assessed

B. On weekly ratings by ward psychiatrist, when actual weight changes are measured:

0 = Less than 1 lb. weight loss in week
1 = Greater than 1 lb. weight loss in week
2 = Greater than 2 lb. weight loss in week
3 = Not assessed

17. Insight

0 = Acknowledges being depressed and ill
1 = Acknowledges illness but attributes cause to bad food, climate, overwork, virus, need for rest, etc.
2 = Denies being ill at all

18. Diurnal Variation

A. Note whether symptoms are worse in morning or evening. If NO diurnal variation, mark none

0 = No variation
1 = Worse in A.M.
2 = Worse in P.M.

B. When present, mark the severity of the variation. Mark "None" if NO variation

0 = None
1 = Mild
2 = Severe

19. Depersonalization and Derealization

0 = Absent	Such as:	Feelings of unreality
1 = Mild		Nihilistic ideas
2 = Moderate		
3 = Severe		
4 = Incapacitating		

20. Paranoid Symptoms

0 = None
1 = Suspicious
2 = Ideas of reference
3 = Delusions of reference and persecution

21. Obsessional and Compulsive Symptoms

0 = Absent
1 = Mild
2 = Severe

LEGAL ISSUES

PREMENSTRUAL SYNDROME, MENTAL ABNORMALITY, AND LEGAL RESPONSIBILITY

Laurence D. Houlgate, Ph.D.

Philosophy Department
California Polytechnic State University
San Luis Obispo, California

INTRODUCTION

I will leave questions of the specific definition and etiology of premenstrual syndrome (PMS) to the many others in this volume directly addressing these concerns. Instead, in this chapter I will examine the philosophical questions that arise when it is suggested that PMS be introduced into legal proceedings. I will begin with a hypothetical case, contrived to illustrate the issues, and then proceed to explicate these in terms of actual legal precedents.

LAWSON, CIRCUIT JUDGE (HYPOTHETICAL EXAMPLE)

After a morning and afternoon of wine drinking, Helen Barker and her husband, John, went to a party at the house of three acquaintances. During the evening, several fights broke out. In one of them, Mrs. Barker's jaw was injured when she was either struck or pushed to the ground. The time of the fight was approximately 10:30 p.m. After the fight, Mrs. Barker left the party. She told her husband that some men had molested her. He testified that she "looked like she was out of her mind." Other witnesses who saw her after the incident testified that her blouse was torn and her speech was unclear (but one of these witnesses added, "I heard every word she said"); that she was staggering and angry; and that she pounded on the mailbox with her fist. One witness testified that Mrs. Barker said, "I'm going to get my gun and come back" and that "someone is going to die tonight."

Half an hour later, at about 11 p.m., Mrs. Barker was on her way back to the party with a gun. One witness testified that she said she was going up there to kill her attackers or be killed. Upon her arrival at the address, Mrs. Barker fired a shot into the ground and entered the building. She proceeded to the apartment where the party was in progress, and fired five shots through the closed hallway door. Two of the shots struck Billy Ford, killing him. Helen Barker was arrested a few minutes later, several blocks away. The arresting officers testified that she appeared normal and did not appear to be drunk, that she spoke clearly, and that she had no odor of alcohol about her.

After the Government had presented the evidence of its non-expert witnesses, the trial judge ruled that there was insufficient evidence relevant to the issue of "pre-meditation" to go to the jury. Since this mental element is an essential component of the crime of murder, a verdict of acquittal was directed on this particular charge. The question remaining for the jury to decide was whether she should be convicted of second-degree murder and the offense of carrying a dangerous weapon.

In response to these charges, Mrs. Barker asserted the defense of insanity. The expert witnesses called in her defense testified that Helen Barker was suffering from a mental abnormality. The medical label given was "premenstrual syndrome" (PMS). The experts agreed that PMS is an abnormal condition of the mind (some argued that it was biochemical in origin) which can substantially impair a woman's ability to control her behavior. It was also testified that PMS is a condition that can be exacerbated by alcohol, leading to episodes of greater intensity, and would also be exacerbated by a blow to the head. In his instructions to the jury, the trial judge said: "The law provides that a jury shall bring in a verdict of not guilty by reason of insanity if, at the time of the criminal conduct, the defendant, as a result of mental disease or defect, either lacked substantial capacity to conform her conduct to the requirements of the law, or lacked substantial capacity to appreciate the wrongfulness of her conduct." The judge further stipulated that mental disease includes "any abnormal condition of the mind, *regardless of its medical label*, which substantially affects mental or emotional processes and substantially impairs behavior controls" (the processes and capacity of a person to regulate and control her conduct and her actions).

Some of the experts called by the Government said that Mrs. Barker's behavior on the night of the party was not consistent with PMS. In the words of one Dr. Johnson, "She was just plain mad." Others argued that even if her behavior was consistent with PMS, she certainly could have controlled her conduct. In spite of this testimony, the jury returned a verdict of "Not guilty, by reason of insanity."

Although the preceding case is hypothetical, those who are familiar with insanity defense cases in United States law will recognize it as quite similar to the facts and finding in *U.S. v. Brawner* (471 F. 2d, 1972). The most salient difference between the two is that the defendant in *Brawner* suffered from epilepsy, whereas in my imaginary case, Helen Barker suffers from PMS. Moreover, in *Brawner*, "the experts agreed that epilepsy *per se* is not a mental disease or defect," but a neurological disease which is often associated with a mental disease or defect. They further agreed that Brawner had a mental, as well as a neurological, disease (*U.S. v. Brawner*, p. 970). In my hypothetical case, the question of whether PMS is a mental disease or a neurological disease is not raised by the experts, although the jury sides with those experts who argued that Mrs. Barker has an "abnormal condition of the mind" that satisfies the judge's definition of mental disease.

The difference between the two are largely irrelevant, for in both the *Brawner* and in my hypothetical cases, serious conceptual and normative questions are raised about mental abnormality and the criminal law: What is mental abnormality? What value judgments are assumed or implied in the definition of mental disease? What is legal insanity? How should the definition of legal insanity incorporate reference to mental disease or defect? What is legal responsibility? Under what conditions should a person be excused from legal responsibility? Why, in general, do we think that persons who suffer certain kinds of mental abnormality ought to be excused from legal responsibility for their conduct? When should a legal excuse "completely" relieve a person from legal responsibility for his or her conduct and when should it merely "diminish" a person's responsibility so that he or she still stands to be convicted, but of some lesser offense?

Although I cannot answer all of these questions here, some answers must be attempted if we hope to resolve the question whether PMS ought to be allowed to excuse or at least partly relieve a woman from responsibility. PMS has not yet been tested as a defense in a criminal case in the United States, and it has rarely appeared in civil law [see, e.g., *In re Irvin,* 31 B.R. 251 (Bankruptcy, 1983)]. In the latter cases, it has not been recognized as a defense. Nonetheless, it is wise to be prepared in advance. Moreover, I find that the issues raised by the phenomenon of PMS alert us to the more general questions that arise in considering the connection between mental abnormality and responsibility, and are well worth exploring for this reason alone.

FORMS OF RESPONSIBILITY

The sentence, "D is responsible for x" has a number of different uses. First, we sometimes use it to say that something D did or failed to do was *the cause* of the occurrence of x. For example, John, while asleep in a narrow bed, rolls over, tumbles out of the bed, tipping the bedside table and breaking a vase that is set upon it. If we say that John was responsible for breaking the vase, we may mean only that he (and not someone else) caused the vase to fall and break. In saying this, we do not imply or suggest that John should be blamed, or that he should be made to pay for the vase, or that breaking the vase was in any way his fault. In such cases, if John wishes to defeat the suggestion that he was responsible for (caused) the breaking of the vase, he only needs to show that no actions he performed (consciously or unconsciously) led to the breaking of the vase (e.g., "Mary pushed me out of bed!"). He would not show that he broke the vase unintentionally, or that he took precautions to ensure that it would not get broken, for in both of these cases, he implies something that he now wishes to deny; namely, that an action or bodily movement of his caused the vase to break. Following H.L.A. Hart, I shall call this first form "causation-responsibility" (Hart, 1968, p. 214).

Second, in the context of a violation of the criminal law, the assertion "D is responsible for x" is typically used to express D's *liability* to punishment. If I assert that Jones is responsible for the death of Smith, I usually mean to say more than Jones caused or brought about Smith's death. I mean that a certain range of conditions is satisfied, conditions that are normally taken to be sufficient for Jones' liability to punishment. I call these cases "liability-responsibility," and I note here two of the most important of the implied conditions.

The first of these conditions are the mental or psychological criteria of responsibility. These are the conditions discussed in the law books under the heading *mens rea.* They include such items as the sanity and maturity of the defendant, and whether or not her conduct was intentional, reckless, or negligent. Thus, if Jones wishes to avoid legal liability-responsibility by proving that she lacked a necessary mental element at the time of her act, then we would expect to hear such defenses as "She was legally insane," or "She did it by accident," or "She did it by mistake."

Another element which is required for responsibility is summed up in the Latin phrase *actus reus*. These words signify the presence of a mental factor in human conduct that is different from the presence of intention, knowledge, or foresight. Persons who lack the requisite *actus reus* are typically those who are physically compelled by another, whose control is impaired by disease, who are in a drunken stupor, who are suddenly deprived of consciousness, or who are somnambulistic or in a state of automatism (Hart, 1968, p. 96). Unlike those cases in which the act is done by mistake or by accident, it is contended that in these cases there is no "act," or at least the bodily movements "are not subordinated to the agent's conscious plans of action: they do not occur as part of anything the agent takes himself to be doing" (Hart, 1968, p. 105). (For more on *mens rea* and *actus reus*, see chapter by Sadoff, this volume.]

In addition to causation and liability, the concept of responsibility is sometimes used to assert that a person does or does not have a certain range of capacities of understanding, reasoning, and control of conduct. For example, if I say of a person who is mentally defective that he is not responsible for his actions, then I mean either that he does not have the ability to understand what legal rules or morality require, or that he is unable to deliberate and reach decisions concerning these requirements, or that he cannot conform his conduct to such decisions when made. These capacities admit of degrees. As Hart has remarked, "responsible for his actions" in this sense refers not to a legal status, but to certain complex psychological characteristics of persons. "A person's responsibility for his actions may intelligibly be said to be 'diminished' or 'impaired' as well as altogether absent, and persons may be said to be 'suffering from diminished responsibility' much as a wounded man may be said to be suffering from a diminished capacity to control the movements of his limbs" (Hart, 1968, p. 220).

Although Hart's observation that someone can suffer diminished responsibility in the sense of a lessened degree of capacity is correct, this should not be confused with the attempt by someone to offer a *legal defense* of diminished responsibility. In the latter case, what is being said is that one is (or should be) liable to punishment for an offense that is less serious than the one with which he is charged. Hence, we must be careful to distinguish between the descriptive judgment that a person lacks sufficient capacity to conform his/her conduct to the law from the normative judgment that his/her legal liability should be less than (diminished from) that originally charged.

To summarize, there are three senses of the words "D is responsible for x" that are relevant to the law: causation-responsibility, legal liability-responsibility, and capacity-responsibility. Only the latter two are relevant to the defense of mental abnormality. When Helen Barker claims that she is not responsible for the death of Billy Ford, her claim is either that she should not be liable to punishment for his death, or that she lacks the capacity to conform her conduct to the requirements of the criminal law: "I was not, at the time of the shooting, responsible for my actions." However, the latter assertion would normally be put forth as proof that one of the psychological conditions of liability-responsibility has not been satisfied.

TYPES OF MENTAL ABNORMALITY

What are we to make of the assertion that Helen Barker suffered from mental abnormality at the time she killed Billy Ford? In the criminal law, there are four varieties of mental abnormality of a sort relevant to excusing or exempting someone from legal liability-responsibility (Gross, 1975, p. 476). First, there is *mental illness*, defined as "a disease of the mind, by virtue of a sufficiently definite pathology and sufficiently pronounced morbidity" (Gross, 1975, p. 476). A second type of mental abnormality is *intoxication,* whatever its source. Third, there is *mental defectiveness,* widely defined as a deficiency of mental capacity required to control behavior. These deficiencies are usually those of intelligence. The key word is "defect," and the contrast is to the notion of "illness." In thinking of mental defectiveness, the analogy is not to a person with a broken arm, but to a person with no arm at all. Fourth, there are types of wide separation of consciousness and action that exist during hypnosis, somnambulism, and epileptic seizure. As noted in the preceding section, these are the factors that are relevant to the *actus reus* condition of liability-responsibility. Following Gross' system of classification, I shall refer to the entire class under the heading *automatism.*

How are we to classify PMS? Is it one of the four types noted here, or is it so different from each of these that we require a fifth category? It does not appear to be mental illness, despite the finding in my hypothetical case. PMS lacks a definite pathology; that is, although women who report the relevant symptoms are reporting something that is statistically deviant, PMS does not have "disease" status at the present time. If we are to ascribe the concept of disease to the deviant behavior or functioning, then there must be "an explanatory scientific theory on the basis of which judgements of correct and incorrect functioning can be made" (Macklin, this volume). There is as yet no such generally accepted theory for premenstrual syndrome, and thus no basis for saying that there is a deviation from design or correct functioning in PMS cases.

PMS is not intoxication, although some women suffering from PMS may behave in ways that resemble the behavior of persons who are intoxicated. Moreover, some women report that their PMS symptoms are exacerbated by alcoholic intake.

Third, PMS is not mental defectiveness, for unlike cases in this category, the condition is cyclic: symptoms appear and disappear each month. Finally, although some cases of PMS bear resemblance to cases of automatism (in that women lose consciousness, or while conscious, lack muscular control), these cases are extremely rare.

Another distinction relevant to the proper classification of types of mental abnormality is that between extrapsychic and intrapsychic origins of the relevant impairment of mental capacity. Thus, it is sometimes important to know whether the origin of the impairment is external to the mind of the actor. External interventions include drugs, alcohol, hypnotic suggestions, blows on the head, emotional shock, and even such biological factors as an extra chromosome, a brain tumor, or a hormone deficiency. Of course, a person may do something to herself or allow another to do something to her that causes the mental impairment; e.g., voluntarily imbibing the alcohol which incurs the intoxication or willingly submitting to hypnosis. The origin of the resulting impairment remains extrapsychic. Although a person's liability will not extend to the actions taken while drunk or while in the hypnotized state, one can be made liable for the conduct that produced the loss of mental capacity.

It might be suggested that if PMS is to excuse a woman from liability for wrongful conduct, then the origin of PMS impairment must be shown to be extrapsychic; e.g., where a biological factor (estrogen excess) is held to be the cause. However, there are those who would argue that the origins of PMS symptoms are entirely within the mind of the actor. Even if this is true, however, it does not imply that the PMS sufferer is in some measure responsible for her illness. Her abnormality can be purely intrapsychic (having no identifiable biological source) and yet the etiology of the illness *may* make it quite clear that one who suffers PMS cannot reasonably be expected to do such things as would probably have prevented the onset of the symptoms. Suppose that a young woman has a long history of brief but severe mood disturbances in the premenstruum (e.g., she has delusions, hallucinations, shows paranoia, is suicidally depressed). There is a complete absence of such symptoms after menstruation. Suppose further that it is proved that her symptoms are intrapsychic. It does not follow from this finding alone that she is responsible either for these disturbances of mood, or for any anti-social act she may commit during these periods.

THE INSANITY DEFENSE

Even if PMS is eventually classified as a type of mental abnormality, it does not follow that we should excuse all women who commit crimes while suffering from PMS on the basis of mental abnormality. This excuse is applicable only when certain conditions of incapacitation are met. In the criminal law, these conditions have been formulated as rules which govern the defense of legal insanity. These rules look mainly to mental illness and defectiveness, but the conditions for excusing someone under them have a rationale which extends to *any* of the four kinds of mental abnormality listed in the previous section and may be found to extend to PMS.

There are four versions of the insanity defense that have developed in the criminal law. The first version dominates among American jurisdictions. It is known as the M'Naghten rules, introduced in England well over a century ago. In its original form, M'Naghten states that a person has a defense of insanity if he/she did not know the nature and quality of the act he/she was doing, or did not know that it was wrong, because he/she was "laboring under a defect of reason from disease of the mind (*M'Naghten*, 8 Eng. Rep. 718, 1843). The rationale of this rule is that a person who is unable to possess such knowledge (because of disease of the mind) cannot choose *not* to do what is legally prohibited. He or she has no effective choice to do otherwise than what was done.

Still, it is said that M'Naghten is too narrow. It does not cover the situation in which a person knows what he/she is doing, knows that he/she ought not be doing it, but cannot restrain himself/herself from doing it. Hence, we have a second version of the insanity defense, the so-called "irresistible impulse" rule, which is normally put forth as a supplement to the M'Naghten provisions. It is law in about one-third of United States jurisdictions, and it says that a person has a complete defense if she cannot restrain herself from doing what she knows to be wrong. The rationale for this rule is the same as that provided for the unsupplemented M'Naghten formula: We ought not to punish those who could not choose to do otherwise than they did.

The third version of the insanity defense is known as the Durham rule. It has been adopted in four United States jurisdictions. It says nothing about a person's capacity to discern the differences between right and wrong. It simply says that mental disease or defect is the basis for an excuse when it produces criminal conduct. If there is no mental disease or defect, or if the mental disease or defect did not produce the criminal act, then there is no defense (on the basis of insanity).

The rationale that underlies the Durham rule is essentially the same as the one that buttresses M'Naghten and the irresistible impulse rules: We ought not punish those who could not help what they did; the idea being that a person whose conduct is caused, determined, or produced by a mental disease or defect could not do otherwise. However, there is some reason to doubt the application of this rationale. Suppose that I have a mental disease and suppose that I commit an illegal act *because* I have the disease, in the sense that I probably would not have committed the act if I had been normal. Does it follow that I ought to be excused for my act? I think not, *unless* it is true that I could not have chosen to do otherwise. This is clarified by recognizing two separable elements in such situations. First, my act may be produced by my mental disease; and second, I may have been able to choose to do otherwise than I did. The concept of mental disease is such that to say that a person has a mental disease is not (by definition) to say that he or she cannot choose to do acts other than those chosen as a result of the mental disease. Mary may beat her child, seriously injuring him, because of a psychotic wish to kill her father, but it does not follow that she could not have chosen to do other than beat her child. Her psychosis may have "caused" her to do this, but it is at least possible that she could have made another choice, resisting the impulse to beat her child.

The fourth and final version of the defense of legal insanity is the one used in my hypothetical case. It is adapted from the American Law Institute rule used in *U.S. v. Brawner* (471 F. 2d 969, 1972). It says that a person need only be seriously mentally ill or mentally defective *at the time* of the criminal act in order to raise a defense of insanity. Unlike the Durham rule, there is no requirement in *Brawner* that there be a causal connection between the disease or defect and the conduct; they need only be contemporaneous. It is on this last point that the rule gets into difficulty. From the fact that a person is mentally ill at the time of his criminal conduct, it does not follow that he cannot have helped what he did. Simply because I have chicken pox at the time of the burglary, it does not follow that I could not have helped committing the burglary. Why, then, should we think that if I have a type of mental disease at the time of the burglary, I could not have helped but commit the burglary? There is no contradiction in saying that I was mentally ill at the time I committed the act *and* I could have chosen not to have done it.

On the basis of the preceding review, I am inclined to think that the M'Naghten rules, supplemented by the irresistible impulse provision, come closest to capturing the moral basis for recognizing a mental abnormality as an excuse. M'Naghten focuses not only on a person's lack of knowledge of the nature and moral quality of one's act, but also focuses on her *capacity* to know. "In a just legal system conduct ought to be treated as legally culpable unless reasonable opportunity exists to become aware of its legal interdiction" (Gross, 1975, p. 473). Where a person's mental abnormality deprives them of the ability to appreciate the harmfulness of their conduct, appreciation of the harm itself, or knowledge that the law prohibits what they are doing, then they cannot help what they do. If I do not know that what I am doing is morally or legally wrong, then I can still be held liable, for it might be said that I *should* have known this. But if, because of a lack of personal resources, I *could not* have known that what I was doing was morally or legally wrong (when the moral or legal prohibition is a reason for refraining), then there is no basis for saying that I should have known this. I ought to do only what I am capable of doing. The same considerations apply as well to the irresistible impulse supplement to M'Naghten.

CONCLUSIONS

I am hesitant to draw conclusions and make summary statements where few conclusions are to be drawn and there is so little agreement among the experts about the precise nature and cause of the phenomenon that is under investigation, "premenstrual syndrome." Hence, what I say below is hypothetical; that is, I proceed *as if* certain things are known to be true about PMS.

One concern in this paper has been to answer the question why a person is not responsible in the sense of being legally liable to punishment for his conduct: "What are, or should be, the conditions for legal liability?" I have stressed the point that before we raise the general medical question — "What states of mental abnormality leave a person in a condition in which she is not legally liable?" — and the more specific question — "Is PMS one of these states?" — we must have some general understanding of the nature of the conditions for legal liability-responsibility. In this regard, a person is liable to punishment or blame only when he or she possesses the requisite *mens rea* or *actus reus*.

The most promising cases of *mens rea*-related defenses is mental disease, and of the *actus reus* cases, automatism seems the most likely category. And yet PMS seems to resemble neither of these mental abnormalities. Of course, a woman suffering from PMS may also have a mental disease, but PMS is not itself a mental disease. Again, a woman suffering from PMS may have automatism as one of her symptoms. Moreover, the automatism may be such that she is unable to conform her conduct to the requirements of the law. If this occurs, then she has a defense; but in this case, it is the automatism that furnishes her with the excuse, not the PMS. There are other features of PMS (e.g., anxiety, depression, bloating), but none of these symptoms is in itself a defense; that is, we do not extend an excuse from liability to persons who did what they did out of anxiety or depression. In sum, although the expression "because I had PMS" might function as an *explanation* of someone's conduct, it cannot (yet) be classified as a mental abnormality of the sort that satisfies the conditions for legal liability-responsibility. That is, when we learn that a woman who committed a crime suffers from PMS, this information merely tells us that she experiences one or more of a range of symptoms commonly associated with the premenstrual syndrome. However, since there is as yet no evidence that women who experience such symptoms typically are unable to control their conduct, we ought not put PMS on the list of mental abnormalities that suffice to excuse a person from criminal responsibility (liability).

REFERENCES

Gross, H., 1975. Mental abnormality as a criminal excuse. In: J. Feinberg and H. Gross (Eds.), *Philosophy of Law*. Dickenson Publ. Co., Belmont, CA, pp. 466-476.

Hart, H.L.A., 1968. *Punishment and Responsibility: Essays in the Philosophy of Law*. Oxford University Press, New York, NY.

THE INSANITY DEFENSE IN CRIMINAL LAW

Robert L. Sadoff, M.D.

Department of Psychiatry
School of Medicine
University of Pennsylvania;
Center for Studies in Social Legal Psychiatry; and
Forensic Psychiatry Clinic
University of Pennsylvania
Philadelphia, Pennsylvania

INTRODUCTION

The insanity defense in criminal law is an important aspect of the discussion of premenstrual syndrome (PMS) because some criminal cases have utilized premenstrual syndrome as a defense to criminal responsibility. Does PMS lead to insanity? Can, or should, PMS be utilized as the basis for an insanity defense in criminal matters? Insanity cannot be equated with mental illness. Insanity is a legal concept exculpating (i.e., excusing) from criminal responsibility an individual whose mental illness at the time of the alleged criminal act led to a particular state of mind consistent with the test of criminal insanity in that particular jurisdiction. The definition of insanity has varied from one jurisdiction to another. Furthermore, since the Hinckley trial in 1982 (discussed below), changes in the insanity defense have occurred throughout the country, and the standard continues to evolve. Insanity negates the *mens rea* or guilty intent portion of criminal behavior which always consists of both the act *(actus reus)* and the intent *(mens rea).*

HISTORICAL DEVELOPMENT OF THE INSANITY CONCEPT

In its efforts toward a humane management of individuals charged with crime, since the 13th century, the criminal law has recognized a mental condition that would negate guilt. Bracton, a Roman cleric and judge, initiated "the wild brute test," wherein the determination would be made whether the individual had a mental state equivalent to that of a "wild brute" when the crime was committed (Whitlock, 1968). If that were the case, the defendant would be exculpated from guilt. Refinements in this very crude test occurred in the 16th century with Matthew Hale and William Coke, who elaborated on a condition called *non compos mentis,* which included mental retardation ("natural fool"), alcoholism (drunkenness), or acquired illness through injury or unexplained causes. Their concept included a totality of lack of understanding in order to exculpate (Whitlock, 1968).

It was not until 1800, and the case of Hadfield, that Erskine presented a modern view of insanity. He called for the delusion test, indicating a partial loss of mental ability rather than a total unawareness (*R. v. Hadfield*, 1800, 27 State Trials, 12/81). The argument indicated that Hadfield had a delusion that affected his behavior when he attempted to kill the king. Hadfield was acquitted by reason of insanity and sent to a hospital for treatment rather than to prison for punishment. Other cases in the early 19th century supported the delusion test, including the M'Naghten case in 1843 (*R. v. M'Naghten*, 1843, 10 Clark and Finney, 200).

The case of Daniel M'Naghten was most significant in the history of insanity pleadings. Although M'Naghten was found not guilty by reason of insanity on the basis of the delusion test, Queen Victoria prompted Parliament to consider a new law, which was more stringent, to keep people from being so readily found insane. From her request, the judges evolved what are now known as the M'Naghten Rules of Insanity. These rules state [10 Clark and Finney, 200, 8 English Reports 718 (H.L. 1843)]:

> "To establish a defense on the grounds of insanity, it must be clearly proved that, at the time of the committing of the act, the party accused was laboring under such a defect of reason, from disease of the mind, as not to know the nature and quality of the act he was doing; or, if he did know it, that he did not know he was doing what was wrong."

It should be noted that the authors of the M'Naghten Rules were influenced by the great 19th century American forensic psychiatrist, Isaac Ray, through his classic work, *A Treatise on the Medical Jurisprudence of Insanity*, originally published in Boston in 1838 and in London the following year.

Today, the M'Naghten test exists as the test of criminal responsibility in the majority of states in the United States. Some states have added an irresistible impulse test to the M'Naghten test, indicating that even if the person were able to know the nature and quality of his act, or to know that what he was doing was wrong but could not keep from doing the act because of an "irresistible" impulse, then he would be exculpated (*Davis v. U.S.*, 1897, 165 U.S. 373). The irresistible impulse addition never stands alone, but is always a complement to the M'Naghten test or a variant thereof.

The question now is, How does one differentiate an irresistible impulse from an unresisted impulse? A means for making this differentiation is "the policeman at the elbow" test. It poses the question of whether the person standing with a gun and ready to shoot would have shot if a policeman had approached or come "to his elbow." If he would have shot anyway with the policeman "at the elbow," then the impulse is seen as "irresistible;" if he would not have shot, the impulse is seen as "resisted." This is probably the difference of conscious motivation versus unconscious motivation and impulse control.

Another major change in the jurisprudence of insanity occurred in 1954, when Judge David Bazelon promulgated the Durham decision. This stated very simply, "An accused is not criminally responsible if his unlawful act was the product of mental disease or mental defect" (*U.S. v. Durham*, 1954, 214F, 2d, 862). That rule was modeled after the earlier New Hampshire tests of 1869 (*State v. Pike*, 1869, 49 N.H. 399, 6 Am. R. 533) and 1871 (*State v. Jones*, 1871, 50 N.H. 369, 398, 9

Am. R. 242-264), which were also influenced by Dr. Isaac Ray. Durham went through a number of changes through its 18-year history, until it was finally abolished by the 1972 Brawner decision *(U.S. v. Brawner*, 1972, 471 F, 2d, 969), which established the American Law Institute Model Penal Code in Washington, D.C. (American Law Institute, 1972). This two-part test was developed by a committee of the American Law Institute (ALI) established to study the problems of the insanity defense. They emerged with the following formula:

> "A person is not responsible for criminal conduct if, at the time of such conduct, as a result of mental disease or defect, he lacked substantial capacity either to appreciate the criminality (wrongfulness) of his conduct or to conform his conduct to the requirements of law. As used in this article, the terms, 'mental disease or defect' do not include an abnormality manifested only by repeated criminal or otherwise antisocial conduct."

The ALI Model Penal Code specifically excluded antisocial personality or psychopaths from those individuals who could be exculpated on the basis of insanity. The ALI test also included a more modern, three-part mental state rather than the one-part cognitive state of the 19th century M'Naghten test. The three parts of the personality included in the ALI test are the cognitive, the conative or emotional, and the volitional aspects.

John W. Hinckley, Jr., was tried in 1982 on the basis of the ALI Model Penal Code of Criminal Insanity. He was found not guilty by reason of insanity, because the jury believed that he met the requirements of that particular test at the time he shot the President of the United States and three other men. At the time of the Hinckley trial, the ALI Model Penal Code was in effect, not only in Washington, D.C., but also in every federal jurisdiction in the country. It was also utilized in a number of states, but not as many as have the M'Naghten test of insanity. There were other variants of M'Naghten and other attempts at modifying insanity or abolishing the test altogether during the past century. However, the Hinckley verdict stimulated more interest and excitement about the insanity defense than had been seen since the 1843 acquittal of Daniel M'Naghten. Survey polls regarding Hinckley indicated that the majority of Americans watching the trial, although not familiar with every detail, believed the verdict was unjust, inaccurate, or inappropriate. They worried that Mr. Hinckley would be set free and that his exculpation was inappropriate for the behavior he had shown.

A hue and cry arose either to abolish the insanity defense to prevent such further miscarriages of justice, or to modify it sufficiently to decrease its applicability or its successful utilization in the future. Congress held hearings in Washington following the Hinckley verdict, and many states acted to modify their legislation with respect to the insanity defense. Three states — Montana (*Montana v. Korell*, 690P, 2d, 992, Mon. Sup. Ct., 1984), Wyoming, and Idaho (Idaho Session Laws, 1982, CH368, SB1396) — abolished the insanity defense and returned to a former test of *mens rea*, which said that a person would be found criminally unresponsible only if he had such a severe mental illness or defect that it rendered him unable to form the proper intent to commit the crime charged. This was also the intent of the American Medical Association (AMA) in its break from the American Psychiatric Association (APA) and the American Bar Association's (ABA) proposal to modify the insanity defense. In this instance, the AMA supported the abolition of the insanity defense, whereas the ABA and APA supported the preservation of insanity in a modified form.

In separate deliberations, the APA and the ABA proposed similar changes for the insanity defense *(Mental Disability Law Reporter,* 1983, Vol. 7, No. 2, March-April, pp. 136-147). Both agreed to accept the concept of insanity as valid and viable in the criminal law. Both groups also chose to reject the "guilty but mentally ill" proposals that were later enacted in over a dozen states. Guilty but mentally ill, a concept initiated in Michigan in 1975 following the McQuillan case *(People v. McQuillan,* 1974, 392 Mich., 511, 221 N.W., 2d, 569), established a new verdict for the jury. They may find, in addition to "guilty as charged," "not guilty as charged," or "not guilty by reason of insanity," a fourth alternative, "guilty but mentally ill." This meant that the person had a particular type of mental illness, but it was not sufficient to meet the test of insanity in that jurisdiction.

Pennsylvania, for example, retained the M'Naghten test of insanity, which had been extant in Pennsylvania for a number of years. They chose to adopt the "guilty but mentally ill" doctrine by giving a new definition to "mentally ill" in this context. For these purposes, in Pennsylvania (General Assembly of Pennsylvania, 1981, Senate Bill 171, Act 286), a person found guilty but mentally ill must be mentally ill and meet the test of ALI or, having "lacked substantial capacity, either conform his conduct to the requirements of law or to appreciate the criminality of his behavior." Having been found "guilty but mentally ill," the defendant is then mandated for treatment in one of the state hospitals before being returned to the criminal justice system or to prison.

In addition to rejecting the guilty but mentally ill doctrine, both the ABA and the APA proposed a new test of insanity, following the recommendations of Law Professor Richard Bonnie *(Mental Disability Law Reporter,* 1983, Vol. 7, No. 2, March-April, p. 15):

> "A person charged with a criminal offense should be found not guilty by reason of insanity if it is shown that, as a result of mental disease or mental retardation, he was unable to appreciate the wrongfulness of his conduct at the time of the offense.
>
> "As used in this standard, the terms mental disease or mental retardation include only those severely abnormal mental conditions that grossly and demonstrably impair a person's perception or understanding of reality and that are not attributable primarily to the voluntary ingestion of alcohol or other psycho-active substances."

Primarily, the concern of the ABA and the APA was to remove the volitional component of the ALI test. The arguments against including volitional aspects of one's personality in the insanity test primarily reflect the inability of psychiatrists to accurately predict or assess the volitional component. Some argue that by removing the volitional component of the insanity defense, we have removed those individuals with addictive illnesses or compulsive disorders over which they have little or no control (Rachlin, Halpern, & Portnow, 1984). Specifically, pathological gambling, drug abuse, and alcohol abuse, as indicated, would be removed from the illnesses or conditions necessary for insanity. We must also consider the "dyscontrol syndrome," as proposed by Elliott (1978) in discussing conditions involving loss of volitional control. Elliott indicates the diagnosis is made primarily by history and involves neurological dysfunction of the brain, allowing violent behavior to occur without conscious control.

Recently, the federal government has enacted a new insanity law [The Insanity Defense Reform Act of 1984, Section 20 (a) and (b)], replacing the ALI test in the federal jurisdictions. This test is similar to the proposals of the ABA and APA, but it adds the concept of "nature and quality of the act" to the lack of appreciation of the wrongfulness of conduct. In essence, the new federal test states that a person would not be criminally responsible if, at the time of the commission of the acts, the defendant, as a result of severe mental disease or defect, was unable to appreciate the nature and quality or the wrongfulness of his acts. In addition, the new federal legislation places the burden of proof on the defendant to a clear and convincing degree, rather than the former burden on the prosecutor beyond a reasonable doubt. In addition, the new federal legislation prohibits the expert witness psychiatrist or psychologist from testifying to the ultimate question of insanity, but allows expert psychiatric testimony to develop the mental illness and the personality dynamics of the defendant.

Experienced attorneys and observers of the insanity defense have often stated that the wording of the test does not particularly matter when the jury ponders the guilt or innocence of the defendant. What seems to be important is whether the jury can identify with or sympathize with the defendant. A number of cases have been successfully pled as insanity where the defendant showed little or no mental illness *per se*, but did have sufficient social and emotional redeeming factors (i.e., justifiable homicide, self defense, or euthanasia) to satisfy the jury. For example, a woman in Detroit set her husband afire while he was sleeping. This occurred following years of his physically and emotionally abusing her. The jury sympathized with her for her plight and for her abuse, and found her temporarily insane. In another case, a young man killed his brother, who had been paralyzed from the neck down following a motorcycle accident in New Jersey. The young man, who acceded to his brother's pleadings, was found to be temporarily insane, as the jury did not have euthanasia as a viable defense. Two young boys in Philadelphia, who killed their abusive alcoholic father after several years of torture to them and to their mother, were also found temporarily insane by a jury. And finally, a young woman in Kentucky who aborted herself was found to be insane by the jury.

Perhaps the most recent such case in which the jury sympathized or identified with the defendant was the case of a resident of South Philadelphia, who had picked up a bag of money that dropped in front of his car from the doors of a Purolator armored truck that had hit a pothole in Philadelphia. He picked up the money and spent some of it on friends, but most was recovered. At trial, he was acquitted on the basis of insanity. When the jury was polled, they indicated that they would have done the same thing as the defendant, thus identifying with him.

INSANITY IN RELATION TO PREMENSTRUAL SYNDROME

What has all this to do with PMS? The changes in the insanity defense have limited the use of insanity for such conditions as premenstrual syndrome. There have been cases in England [*R. v. Craddock*, 1981, 1CL49; *R. v. Smith*, 1982, Crim. L. R. 531 (CA)] in which this condition was utilized successfully in acquitting a woman of criminal responsibility. The issue has been raised in the United States as well (*People v. Santos*, 1982, 1K046229 Criminal Court New York). Should PMS form the basis for an insanity acquittal? I do not believe we know enough about PMS at this juncture to state categorically that it is of sufficient magnitude to be the basis for acquittal in criminal behavior. It may form a part of the total mental picture that may be argued, either for insanity or for diminished capacity or diminished responsibility (Arenella, 1977) within the criminal law. The concept of diminished capacity provides for a lesser charge than the one initially imposed, or may provide for a lesser degree of homicide if specific intent is vitiated by the PMS and its attendant emotional impairment.

Another means of approaching PMS in criminal trials is through the defense of automatism in which the defendant claims no memory of the event in question. Automatism implies the individual acted as an "automaton" with no conscious control of behavior. There is no evidence for coma or lack of consciousness, but the individual has no memory of the behavior and acted without conscious will. This is a rare event and may be proven by use of combined polygraph and hypnosis or sodium amytal interviews. The polygraph is used to prove the presence of amnesia; and the hypnosis or sodium amytal, to help the individual recapture lost memory of the event. All interviews are recorded on unerasable videotape for possible viewing subsequently at trial. The problem, however, may lie in the lack of admissibility of the procedure in court due to the limitation of admissibility of such evidence. The Frye test (*Frye v. U.S.*, 1923, 293F 1013), promulgated in 1923, limited the admissibility into evidence to those procedures which are scientifically valid and accepted by the majority of professionals utilizing the procedures or those who are familiar with them.

SUMMARY AND CONCLUSIONS

In summary, PMS is still sufficiently unclear with respect to mental illness that it would not serve, in my opinion, as a basis for insanity in the criminal law. PMS may be a factor, along with other mental states, to be argued as the basis of a diminished capacity in particular cases. However, changes in the insanity defense have restricted the volitional aspect in favor of the cognitive factor, which remains the basis of impairment in the insanity defense. It is the volitional aspect, however, which may be the more viable factor in PMS. The volitional aspect, currently removed from most tests of insanity, remains as the critical factor in diminished capacity and automatism cases, both of which appear infrequently at the trial stage. These factors are mostly argued at the pretrial stage in order to obtain the most favorable negotiated plea. They are very complex issues, not completely understood by the jury, and are better argued at the pretrial stages of the criminal proceedings.

PMS may present an analogous parallel to the dyscontrol syndrome, noted above, in that both have organic substrates that may lead to uncontrolled violent behavior under certain conditions.

The attorney for the defendant has the obligation to obtain the best legal outcome for his client in criminal cases. This usually means the lightest possible sentence or an outright acquittal. The mental health professional has the obligation to properly diagnose and treat the defendant with mental illness or with other emotional difficulties. PMS is a diagnosis that is currently unclear with respect to impulse control, behavior, and treatment. This may present a conflict of management of the PMS defendant between the attorney and the consulting mental health professional. Treatment is most important to the psychiatrist or psychologist, even if it must be accomplished in a correctional setting or in a hospital.

Beyond the ethical requirement that a lawyer use all legal means available to defend a client, should PMS be used as a legal defense? PMS should be used as a legal defense whenever the condition is so extreme or severe that there is a reasonable conclusion by recognized experts that this particular individual, experiencing symptoms from her premenstrual syndrome, could not form the specific intent to commit the act charged, or her behavior was so affected that she lacked substantial capacity to control her behavior as a direct result of the PMS. The implication here is that the PMS was the controlling influence over the criminal behavior and not an incidental finding. One must search carefully for other motivating factors that could account for the criminal behavior or more likely account for the behavior noted. The mere existence of the PMS does not make the defense. There has to be a sequence of the following findings:

1. The presence of premenstrual syndrome.

2. A severe form of PMS that has been shown in this individual to affect her behavior, her judgment, and her cognitive awareness of her immediate environment.

3. That it was this impairment in judgment or control caused by the severity of her PMS that led to the criminal behavior.

4. Absent PMS, this particular individual would not have committed the crime or the behavior she did at the particular time.

If the PMS defendant is found guilty of the crime charged, she may be treated in a prison, in a hospital, or on probation as an outpatient. If she is acquitted as "not guilty by reason of insanity," she may be committed to a hospital for treatment if the judge believes she meets the criteria for commitment in that jurisdiction. In most states, the criteria include the presence of mental illness and "dangerousness" to self or others. Is the PMS individual mentally ill? She may or may not be, depending on the definition of mental illness and whether she has other conditions that meet the criteria for mental illness. Is PMS *per se* a mental illness? Most people think it is not, but there is no bar to a woman having PMS also having a serious mental illness, such as psychosis or depression or schizophrenia.

The question of dangerousness is most perplexing to mental health professionals since most psychiatrists believe they cannot accurately predict dangerousness except in limited circumstances. They may have an ability to predict imminent violence or to predict behavior that is consistent with a pattern of previously established behavior in that individual (Monahan, 1982).

Further research will clarify the true nature of PMS and its relation to behavior. In the meantime, the law is best advised to remain conservative in its application of scientific principles in criminal trials. The individual with PMS should be evaluated as carefully as any other individual without PMS to determine whether her condition can be applied to the tests of insanity, diminished responsibility, or automatism as stated in the criminal law. At this juncture, each case must be evaluated individually with respect to criminal responsibility.

REFERENCES

American Law Institute, 1972. *Model Penal Code,* Section 4.01, p. 66. Official Draft, May 4, Philadelphia, PA.

Arenella, P., 1977. The diminished capacity and diminished responsibility defenses: Two children of a doomed marriage. *Columbia Law Review 77:* 6.

Elliott, F. A., 1978. Neurological factors in violent behavior (the Dyscontrol Syndrome). In: R. L. Sadoff (Ed.), *Violence and Responsibility.* Spectrum Publications, New York, NY, pp. 59-86.

Monahan, J., 1982. *The Clinical Prediction of Violent Behavior.* NIMH, Washington, D.C.

Rachlin, S., A. L. Halpern, and S. L. Portnow, 1984. The Volitional Rule, personality disorders and the insanity defense. *Psychiatric Annals 14:* 139-147.

Ray, I., 1838. *A Treatise on the Medical Jurisprudence of Insanity.* Little, Brown, and Company, Boston, MA.

Whitlock, F. A., 1968. *Criminal Responsibility and Mental Illness.* Butterworths, London, p. 13.

PREMENSTRUAL SYNDROME AND CRIMINAL RESPONSIBILITY

Christopher Boorse, Ph.D.

Department of Philosophy
University of Delaware
Newark, Delaware

INTRODUCTION

In 1980-81, two British women escaped murder convictions by arguing that their legal responsibility was diminished by premenstrual syndrome (PMS). In a fit of rage Sandie Craddock, an East London barmaid with 45 prior convictions, stabbed a fellow barmaid three times through the heart (*Regina v. Craddock*, 1981, 1 C.L. 49; see also Apodaca & Fink, 1984; Carney & Williams, 1983). Christine English, after a quarrel with her lover, crushed him to death against a utility pole with her car (*Regina v. English*, an unreported decision of the Norwich Crown Court on November 10, 1981; see also Apodaca & Fink, 1984, p. 54; Carney & Williams, 1983, p. 261). With the aid of testimony by Dr. Katharina Dalton, the world's most prominent advocate for PMS victims, each woman was convicted only of manslaughter due to PMS-diminished responsibility. Most remarkably, neither woman was punished for her killing: Craddock received probation; English, a 12-month conditional discharge with a driving ban. About a year after her conviction, Craddock (now Smith) was re-arrested for an equivocal attempt to murder a policeman; convicted on three new charges, Smith again argued PMS to mitigate her sentence and again received probation. These judgments were approved on appeal. According to magazine stories and Dalton (see her chapter, this volume), Craddock and English are only two of the many British and Canadian defendants to reduce their criminal responsibility by pleading PMS.

Inspired by such precedents, the lawyer for Shirley Santos, a New York woman charged with assault in 1981 for badly beating her 4-year-old daughter, used PMS to argue that Santos was unconscious of her actions. This argument apparently influenced the prosecutor and judge to accept a guilty plea to harassment, a nonfelony (*People v. Santos*, No. 1K046229, November 3, 1982, Crim. Ct. N.Y.). [For discussion of the Santos case, see Apodaca & Fink (1984, p. 64); Carney & Williams (1983, p. 253); Holtzman (1984)]. *Santos*, the first American case involving a successful "PMS defense," brewed a storm of controversy in the popular press.[1] Many physicians and women with severe premenstrual symptoms hailed a new era in which a crippling disorder would receive long overdue respect. Law review articles defended the new use of PMS to support a denial or diminution of criminal responsibility.[2] Many feminists, however, were appalled at the return of the concept of "raging hormones" as a device to deny women the status of responsible adults. Critics saw the criminal application of PMS as a backward step that could negate sex equality and consign women to second-class status in the eyes of employers, the law, and the public [see the remarks by Elizabeth Holtzman in Switzer (1983, p. 126); e.g., "Allowing women to plead some special kind of insanity because of physical reactions to their menstrual cycle is not only medically unjustified, but dangerous to the legal rights of all women"]. Elizabeth Holtzman, the Brooklyn D.A. in charge of the Santos case, stated that PMS exists only as symptoms, not a syndrome, and that these symptoms have no significance for criminal law (Holtzman, 1984, p. 3). Much of the public, including many menstruating women, views the PMS defense with skepticism or derision, and some see it as one more abuse of insanity pleas to excuse patently guilty defendants.[3]

The present chapter surveys legal and philosophical issues concerning the use of PMS (and similar conditions) as an excuse in criminal law. Other legal contexts to which PMS, like any mental abnormality, may be relevant — such as employment discrimination, child custody, civil commitment, or competency in contracts and wills — are ignored. However, PMS may in the end prove more relevant to such contexts, since it will be argued that PMS is, at present, of little significance to criminal law.

---

[1] Popular press articles on PMS include Allen (1982), Angier & Witzleben (1982), Chambers (1982), Clark & Shapiro (1981), Cohen (1981), Cumming (1984), Eagan (1983), Gray (1981), Heneson (1984), Henig (1982), Herbert (1982), Hopson & Rosenfeld (1984), Lauersen & Stukane (1982), O'Roark (1981), Press (1982), Sommer (1984), Switzer (1983), and Vinocur (1983).

[2] An article by Wallach and Rubin (1971) is both the most favorable and the most comprehensive, and predates all the above cases. The authors accept the most extreme claims about premenstrual psychiatric symptoms, including PMS psychosis; consequently, they find PMS relevant to all the mental abnormality excuses of the criminal law, even M'Naghten insanity. Wallach and Rubin are ideological feminists. They are also unreliable on psychiatric matters, as is shown, for example, by their statement that "psychosis, schizophrenia, and paranoia. . . are frequently the very mental disorders which accompany" PMS (Wallach & Rubin, 1971, p. 241). Schizophrenia is a type of psychosis; further, it is a primary diagnosis and cannot be viewed as secondary to PMS. What is possible, if controversial, is that PMS occasionally — not "frequently" — has mental effects similar to schizophrenia. Favorable conclusions are also reached by Apodaca and Fink (1984), Carney and Williams (1983), Pahl-Smith (1985), and Taylor and Dalton (1983). To date, law review skepticism about PMS is limited to Holtzman (1984) and Press (1983). Press rejects the claim of PMS psychosis and therefore of PMS insanity. However, he considers that PMS may support a claim of diminished capacity even under the *Frye* rule.

[3] For example, 71-81% of responding readers in a *Glamour* article entitled "This is what you thought about pre-menstrual syndrome as a legal defense" (January, 1983, p. 15) apparently rejected PMS as any form of criminal excuse; 3% felt its use in the criminal courts is a hoax; and 65% of the same group claimed to have PMS.

PREMENSTRUAL SYNDROME: RECENT COURT DECISIONS

Information in the following section is primarily taken from Apodaca and Fink (1984), Brahams (1983), Carney and Williams (1983), Mulligan (1983), and Taylor and Dalton (1983).

Regina v. Craddock (1981, 1 C.L. 49)

Sandie Craddock, a 30-year-old barmaid, had a record of 45 previous convictions, many for inexplicable outbursts of violence (Apodaca & Fink, 1984, p. 62), when she was tried in 1980 for suddenly stabbing another barmaid to death. Craddock had also attempted suicide 25 times and been frequently committed to mental hospitals. While in prison awaiting trial, she made two further assaults and two more suicide attempts.

Examining Craddock and her history before trial, Dr. Katharina Dalton, the leading British crusader for recognizing PMS as a disabling disorder, used official records and Craddock's diaries to show a periodicity in her acts of violence. Dalton found that Craddock's crimes occurred at intervals of 29.04 $\pm$ 1.47 days and her suicide attempts at 29.55 $\pm$ 1.45 days (Carney & Williams, 1983, p. 259; chapter by Dalton, this volume). From this information, Dalton diagnosed Craddock as having severe PMS and treated her with massive doses of progesterone; Craddock's personality and behavior became calm and stable (Carney & Williams, 1983, p. 259; chapter by Dalton, this volume).

The prosecution accepted Dr. Dalton's diagnosis as a basis for diminished responsibility, reducing the charge to manslaughter. After jury conviction on this charge, the court further cited PMS as a factor mitigating sentence and put Craddock on probation for continued progesterone treatment. Thus, Craddock's homicide trial illustrates a double use of PMS: once to reduce murder to manslaughter, and once to avoid punishment for manslaughter. As a result, the defendant received no confinement for an unexcused killing and was released on probation for drug therapy.

Regina v. Smith [No. 1/A/82 (Crim. App., April 27, 1982)]

Craddock, who had changed her name to Smith, was free of further crimes or acts of violence for about a year, with one exception. In October of 1980, having missed four progesterone injections through administrative error, Smith threw a rock through a window and then reported herself to the police. The authorities granted her a conditional release on resumption of progesterone treatment.

Over the next eight months, Dalton progressively reduced Smith's dosage. In June of 1981, allegedly during her paramenstruum (Carney & Williams, 1983, p. 260), Smith again slashed her wrists, then took some bizarre and ambivalent steps toward killing a police officer whom she claimed to have insulted and slapped her in 1978. ["Paramenstruum" is Dalton's term (1984, p. 4) for the four days preceding plus the four days following the onset of menstrual flow.] Smith sent an anonymous threatening letter, assembled from newspaper fragments, to the officer; she called the police station to repeat her threat and inquire about the officer's schedule; and the next morning she appeared outside the police station carrying a knife. She was convicted by a jury of two counts of threatening a police officer and one count of carrying a weapon. The court again placed Smith under probation and Dalton's supervision, citing PMS.

On appeal, Smith's counsel asked the court to recognize a defense of irresistible impulse due to a specific, innocent, and remediable medical condition (Carney & Williams, 1983). The English Court of Appeal, continuing the traditional English ban on irresistible-impulse defenses (Walker, 1968, pp. 104-111), refused to admit PMS as a substantive defense. The court stated that it was contrary to the purpose of criminal law to acquit and discharge a defendant who was still a threat to society. It did not, however, criticize the use of PMS in *Craddock* for diminished responsibility (Mulligan, 1983, p. 224), and it approved the trial court's use of PMS to mitigate the sentence to probation with medical supervision.

Regina v. English (An Unreported Decision of the Norwich Crown Court on November 10, 1981)

In sharp contrast to Sandie Smith/Craddock, Christine English, a 37-year-old divorced mother of two, had no record of criminality or violent acts when she killed her lover, Barry Kitson, in December 1980. However, English had suffered severe post partum depression after the birth of her second son, had been sterilized, and had attempted suicide. Kitson, whom she met in 1976, was a married, unemployed alcoholic six years younger than herself. Their relationship was marked by frequent quarrels, including a familiar pattern of physical violence by Kitson during drinking bouts followed by promises of reform. In the United States, a lawyer for English might have argued battered-woman syndrome (BWS) instead of or in addition to PMS.[4]

On the day of the killing, Kitson refused English's offer of dinner and admitted he had a date with another woman. After a violent morning row, English located Kitson in a pub where they quarreled again. English followed him out of the bar and drove him around Colchester in an attempt to find the other woman. After heavy drinking in another pub and further violence, Kitson asked English to take him home with her. English refused, and yet another fight ensued. Kitson left the car saying, "I hate you and I never want to see you again!" English drove away, but returned in an effort to make peace. When she found him again, he made a V sign at her (the British version of the American finger). English then smashed him against a lamp post with her car. His lower body crushed, Kitson died in the hospital two weeks later. Immediately after the incident, English, hysterical but clear-headed and remorseful, was taken to a police station; on leaving at 5 a.m., she began to menstruate.

English, like Craddock/Smith, offered a diminished responsibility plea to manslaughter, using a diagnosis of PMS supported by Dalton and a Broadmoor psychiatrist, Dr. John Hamilton. Their testimony portrayed English as emotionally stressed and provoked by Kitson's aggressive behavior. Both physicians also agreed that English's failure to eat for nine hours before the crime helped to cause her action, since it might have induced hypoglycemia and, according to Dalton, a reactive surge of adrenalin. Another psychiatrist, Dr. Paul D'Orban, testified for the prosecution. As in *Craddock* and *Smith*, the judge, acting under the diminished responsibility provision of the Homicide Act 1957, accepted

---

[4] Besides being novel psychological syndromes of dubious admissibility in criminal defense, PMS and BWS are similar in their possible relevance to provocation/self-defense situations. They are also similar in the courtroom dominance of a single expert — Dalton for PMS, Lenore Walker for BWS.

English's plea, finding that she acted under "wholly exceptional circumstances" (Carney & Williams, 1983, p. 261).[5] English received no sentence, only a one-year conditional discharge with a ban on driving.

People v. Santos [November 3, 1982, No. 1K046229 (Crim. Ct. N.Y.)]

In 1981, Shirley Santos, a Brooklyn mother, called an ambulance for her 4-year-old daughter, after beating her badly enough for two weeks' hospitalization. Santos was charged with second-degree assault and endangering the welfare of a child, both felonies. Her explanation of the incident was: "I don't remember what happened. . . I would never hurt my baby. . . I just got my period." Legal-Aid attorney Stephanie Benson argued in a pretrial hearing that PMS, together with fasting, made Santos so hypoglycemic that she was unconscious of her actions in beating the child. In other words, Benson's legal theory was PMS-induced automatism.

The presiding judge of the criminal court stated that the defense was credible, explaining that if mental disturbances are admissible evidence, physical disturbances should also be allowed. In the end, felony charges were dropped by the prosecution in return for a guilty plea to harassment, a misdemeanor. Both attorneys claimed that this result vindicated their disparate views of the merits of the PMS defense, but no authoritative statement was made by the court. Santos received no sentence, fine, or probation, although she did lose custody of her daughter in a separate family court proceeding.

An interesting sidelight on the *Santos* case is that Dalton, who had never examined Santos, stated to one interviewer that Santos did not have PMS (Apodaca & Fink, 1984, p. 64, note 128). In the *Smith* trial, however, Dalton expressly compared a PMS sufferer to a baby batterer and endorsed the idea that such women can act automatically, without intent, and without later memory of their actions (Carney & Williams, 1983, p. 262, note 77). Another sidelight is that Santos disavowed Benson's PMS defense (Norris & Sullivan, 1983, p. 278).

In re Irvin [31 B.R. 251 (Bkrtcy. 1983)]

The following summary is based entirely on the court's opinion.

The only reported American case in which a judge wrote an opinion on a PMS defense is, ironically, a bankruptcy proceeding. In spite of its being a non-criminal case, it is unique and concerns a debt arising from a crime, and therefore will be discussed here. Jamie Lynn Irvin filed for bankruptcy to discharge, among other debts, a $5,200 judgment obtained by Betty Ann Lovato in a civil damage suit. The damages

---

[5] Apart from PMS itself, it is hard to see how English's circumstances were "exceptional." Verbal and physical fights were typical of the English-Kitson relationship, as they are of many couples'. In any case, English, like any woman, is responsible for choosing a violent alcoholic married man as her lover and remaining with him. Nor are obscene gestures "exceptional." Surely, the court did not mean to hold that murder is a natural reaction to obscenity. Except for PMS, English no more seems a "victim of circumstances" (W. S. Gilbert, *Ruddigore*, Act II, duet of Despard and Margaret) than any other criminal defendant. Her excuse is limited to premenstrual "spleen and vapours."

were for Lovato's injuries in a 1979 incident when Irvin stabbed Lovato in the back, chest, and hands with a steak knife. In the 1983 action, Lovato argued that Irvin's debt to her was non-dischargeable, under a provision of the bankruptcy code barring discharge of debts resulting from "wilful and malicious" actions. Irvin claimed PMS as a defense to wilfulness and malice in stabbing Lovato.

Irvin and Lovato, who lived together off and on for about two years between 1977 and 1979, had a stormy relationship with many jealous quarrels. Irvin threatened Lovato three times at knifepoint. During a separation, she broke into Lovato's home and hid under her bed, armed with a knife and tomahawk, with which she attacked Lovato as she slept. Irvin's prior roommates described many previous threats of suicide and murder by knife, drugs, or automobile, occurring several times weekly. One roommate claimed to have been threatened by Irvin at knifepoint a hundred times, to have suffered broken bones from her beatings, and to have had a shotgun held to her head for two hours in an effort to force her to reveal infidelity or plans to abandon Irvin. Irvin once traveled to Germany and attacked this woman with a knife, nearly severing her arm. In the 1979 incident, after a joint counseling session with a clinical psychologist who was exploring the connection between Irvin's violence and PMS, Irvin forced her way into Lovato's car, pursued her on foot, and stabbed her with a knife she had concealed during the counseling session. Irvin then imprisoned Lovato for five hours to discuss their relationship and construct a cover story for the hospital. She later pled guilty to attempted assault, an offense involving an intent to do bodily harm.

Irvin testified that on the day of the assault she began menstruating, was confused and frightened, and experienced her behavior during the assault as by another person. Psychiatrist David Muller testified to the (obvious) facts that Irvin was highly sensitive to rejection, had difficulty dealing with anger constructively, and had episodes of extreme rage and depression. Dr. Muller diagnosed Irvin as having Borderline Personality Disorder aggravated by PMS, and he rated her logical decision-making ability on the day of the crime at 25-30% of normal. A gynecologist agreed that Irvin had PMS, but stated that this was true of almost all menstruating women.

Judge Gueck presumed malice from the wrongfulness of Irvin's actions. Interpreting the term "wilful" to mean deliberate or intentional, he then rejected Irvin's claim that PMS negated her intention and will. The court did not believe that Irvin's violence and loss of control were caused by PMS, since she had a past history of continual violence with no clear correlation to her menstrual cycles. Finally, the judge applied the general acceptance test to reject PMS as a substantive defense [*In re Irvin* (31 B.R. 251, Bkrtcy. 1983), p. 261]: "There is insufficient evidence presented in the within action to establish that premenstrual syndrome is sufficiently defined and accepted in the medical community to be an acceptable defense." (PMS evidence had already been admitted over vigorous objection by Lovato's counsel.) Quoting various sources, the court found that PMS is a poorly defined disorder with uncertain cause, one that is difficult to diagnose, and one that has never been accepted as a substantive defense in British or American courts.[6]

---

[6] The court's recent scientific sources were a selection of articles by Dalton and her book, *Once A Month* (1979), as well as articles by Gonzalez (1981), and Reid and Yen (1981). The court also cited Wallach and Rubin (1971). Some of the court's reasons for PMS's failure to meet the general acceptance test are arguably irrelevant. Obscurity of pathogenesis of a disorder *[In re Irvin*

Other Cases

Besides the above cases, Gray (1981) mentions two Canadian women accused of shoplifting who avoided penalties via PMS. In one case, the charges were dropped following psychiatric consultation; and in the other, the woman received a discharge for treatment with diuretics. Dalton (see her chapter, this volume) cites additional cases of defendants accused of arson; forging a prescription; infanticide; shoplifting; and false emergency calls. Additional offenses are mentioned in her list of 38 premenstrual offenders in 1982. Dalton implies that the disposition of these cases was influenced by her diagnosis of PMS and subsequent progesterone therapy, but gives few details of the proceedings. Norris and Sullivan (1983, Chapters 11 and 12, and pp. 27-28), in a historical survey of menstrual disorders, identified (among other famous women) Lizzie Borden as a PMS sufferer. Norris and Sullivan also mention three mid-19th century criminal acquittals for obstructed or disordered menstruation (p. 270).[7]

PREMENSTRUAL SYNDROME: CURRENT SCIENTIFIC VIEWS

Even on the most sympathetic reading, PMS is a clinical syndrome of which the definition, symptoms, pathophysiology, causes, treatment, and prevalence are all highly controversial.

Definition

Although changes in the bodies and minds of menstruating women have been noted for many centuries, recent concern with PMS as a medical syndrome began in a 1931 article by R.T. Frank. Frank described "premenstrual tension" as a feeling of "indescribable tension and a desire to find relief by foolish actions difficult to restrain" (Frank, 1931, p. 1053). In the ensuing 50 years, many more physical and psychological symptoms have been added to Frank's "tension" and the name broadened to "syndrome."

By definition, phenomena labeled as PMS share the periodicity of the female menstrual cycle. Leading researchers require that the monthly symptoms begin in the luteal phase (the two weeks between ovulation and bleeding) and remit during or shortly after the cycle's

---

(31 B.R. 251, Bkrtcy. 1983), p. 261] is no bar to its acceptance in medicine and should not be in law, else many common medical disorders (peptic ulcer, hypertension, most cancers) would be inadmissible. Nor should courts exclude disorders about which "many scientific questions remain" (Court's quote from Dalton, p. 261), since this is the universal condition of science. What should count heavily is the definition and psychological effects of a disorder. On this basis, it is argued below that Judge Gueck was correct to hold PMS inadmissible under the *Frye* rule.

[7] Since *Irvin,* PMS has been referred to in *State v. Lashwood* [384 N.W.2d 319 (S.D. 1986)]. The Supreme Court of South Dakota found PMS evidence insufficient to overturn pleas in a forgery case because the defendant knew right from wrong and could help in her own defense. Premenstrual depression is mentioned in passing in *Phelan v. Hanft* [471 So.2d 648 (Fla. App. 3 Dist. 1985)], a medical malpractice case. Neither of these opinions contains substantive discussion of PMS.

end, which in normal women is the menstrual flow. Thus, Sutherland and Stewart (1965, p. 1180) defined the syndrome as "any combination of emotional or physical features which occur cyclically in a female before menstruation, and which regress and disappear during menstruation." Dalton (1982) has defined PMS as "the presence of monthly recurrent symptoms in the premenstruum or early menstruation with a complete absence of symptoms after menstruation."[8] The clause on postmenstrual remission differentiates PMS from dysmenorrhea (menstrual discomfort, cramps), which is considered a distinct entity.

A newer definitional trend adds a severity condition to distinguish PMS, a medical disorder, from normal premenstrual changes. Thus, Rubinow and Roy-Byrne (1984, p. 163) define PMS as "the cyclic occurrence of symptoms that are of sufficient severity to interfere with some aspects of life and which appear with a consistent and predictable relationship to menses." In another authoritative literature review, Reid (1985, p. 5) defines PMS as:

> ". . . the cyclic recurrence, in the luteal phase of the menstrual cycle, of a combination of distressing physical, psychological, and/or behavioral changes of sufficient severity to result in deterioration of interpersonal relationships and/or interference with normal activities."

Definitions for research purposes, in aiming at a population of women with "severe" PMS, may frame even stricter criteria. An example of this approach is the definition of Steiner and Haskett (see their chapter, this volume) that is shown in Figure 1. The application of such criteria narrows the PMS population to the clearest and severest cases. This approach minimizes false positives, focusing on a smaller and more homogeneous population, but naturally maximizes false negatives, women with some form of PMS who fail the criteria.

For a discussion of PMS as a criminal excuse, these differences in definition are of crucial importance. A condition typical of women can scarcely constitute a defense to crime. A rare condition in a minority of severely impaired women can. Confusion between broad and narrow concepts of PMS is partly due to the term "syndrome," which in medicine usually refers to a cluster of abnormal phenomena, but can also refer to a cluster of normal ones.

Wherever necessary for clarity below, normal PMS, the type and intensity of symptoms experienced by typical premenstrual women, will be designated as "n-PMS." Pathological PMS — the severe impairment of a minority of premenstrual women — will be designated as "p-PMS."

Symptoms

The list of symptoms associated with PMS — that is, showing cyclicity in some women — runs to over 150. Commonly reported physical symptoms include (Reid & Yen, 1981, p. 86):

---

[8] A curious inconsistency in some of Dalton's discussions is her simultaneous insistence that PMS symptoms be confined to the "premenstruum" and attribution of "paramenstrual" symptoms to PMS. The "paramenstruum" includes four days of menstrual flow, which is the whole flow in most women. At any rate, it should be recognized that premenstruum plus paramenstruum is about 14 + 4 = 18 days, or two-thirds of a woman's life.

RESEARCH DIAGNOSTIC CRITERIA FOR PMS

A through D are required.

A. At least 5 of the following are required for definite diagnosis and 4 for probable diagnosis as part of a current episode.

   1. Irritable, hostile, angry, short-fused.
   2. Tense, restless, jittery, upset, high-strung, unable to relax.
   3. Decreased efficiency, fatigue.
   4. Dysphoric, marked spontaneous emotional lability, crying.
   5. Lowered motor coordination, clumsy, prone to accidents (cut finger, break dish, etc.)
   6. Distractable, confused, forgetful, difficulty in concentration, lowered judgement.
   7. Change in eating habits (cravings, overeating, etc.)
   8. Marked change in libido.

B. Overall disturbance is so severe that at least one of the following is present:

   1. Serious impairment socially, with family, at home, at school or work.
   2. Sought or was referred for help from someone or took medication (especially tranquilizers and/or diuretics) at least once during a premenstrual period.

C. Premenstrual dysphoric symptoms for at least six of the nine preceding menstrual cycles.

D. Symptoms only during the premenstrual period with relief soon after onset of menses.

Fig. 1. Definition of PMS used by Steiner and Haskett (see their chapter, this volume).

headache	increased thirst or appetite
breast swelling and tenderness	sweet or salt craving
abdominal bloating	acneiform skin eruptions
edema of extremities	constipation
fatigue	

Less common are (Rubinow & Roy-Byrne, 1984, p. 170):

oliguria	vertigo
joint and muscle pain	paresthesias and tremors
insomnia or hypersomnia	lack of coordination
nausea	seizures

It is noteworthy that most of the above are symptoms rather than signs; that is, they are established by patient report rather than by objective physical examination. Common psychological symptoms include (Rubinow & Roy-Byrne, 1984, p. 170):

irritability	impulses to violence
anger	paranoia
depression	confusion
anxiety	difficulty in concentration
emotional lability	psychotic ideas

Prevalence

The prevalence of PMS is uncertain. Clearly, though, it varies greatly with the definition of PMS, especially the number of symptoms required and their severity. On the broadest definition, as many as 90% of menstruating women have PMS; that is, their luteal phase regularly includes one of the above symptoms (Reid & Yen, 1981, p. 86). Reid and Yen (1981, p. 85) describe PMS as "a major clinical entity affecting a large segment of the female population." They estimate that 20-40% report some temporary mental or physical incapacitation, while 5-10% are impaired to a degree that Reid counts "severe." Thus, Reid's (1985, his Fig. 1) recent survey of literature divides menstruating women as follows:

no premenstrual symptoms	10-15%	
mild symptoms	50%	
moderate symptoms	30%	PMS
severe symptoms	5-10%	PMS

Reid defines the latter two groups (35-40%) as PMS. Rubinow and Roy-Byrne's (1984, pp. 164-165) critique of PMS research indicates that these prevalence data should be regarded as methodologically "soft." In any case, the division of symptom severity into "mild," "moderate," and "severe" is vague and may depend as much on patients' self-report habits as on their experience of the symptoms themselves.

Causes

As to the pathophysiology and etiology of PMS, a multitude of theories has been proposed, none of which can be regarded as established. Reid (1985) classifies the theories into estrogen excess or progesterone deficiency (the position of Dalton, 1984); generalized fluid retention due to the action of aldosterone, vasopressin, prolactin, or dietary factors; vitamin B6 deficiency; hypoglycemia; endogenous hormone allergy; and psychogenesis. Reid states that existing theories fail to connect PMS symptoms to known variations in the ovarian hormones (estrogen and progesterone) that direct the menstrual cycle. In addition, basic facts assumed by theorists are often disconfirmed by later studies, as with the claim that PMS patients show generalized fluid retention. Reid and Yen (1981, pp. 95-96) favor an ingenious hypothesis that interprets PMS symptoms as a withdrawal syndrome from cycling endogenous opiates (endorphins).

At present, however, there is no consistently demonstrable hormone abnormality in PMS patients, nor any other objectively measurable physiological abnormality.

Treatment

Various current treatments for PMS are based on the above theories, including diuretics, vitamin B6, and progesterone, as well as purely symptomatic drugs such as aspirin or bromocriptine. In general, these treatments either have not been given serious therapeutic trials (double-blind and placebo-controlled), or such trials have shown slight or no superiority of drug to placebo (Rubinow & Roy-Byrne, 1984, pp. 166-168). It is widely agreed that placebo treatment is unusually effective in PMS, and sympathetic discussion alone can make PMS symptoms more bearable. It is possible that the dramatic therapeutic success claimed by clinicians such as Dalton is an effect of the physician-patient relationship itself — the warmth and concern of a committed therapist. Alternatively, progesterone may have generalized tranquilizing action (see chapter by O'Brien, this volume), or it and other drugs may work by suppressing the ovarian cycle altogether (Muse, Cetel, Futterman, & Yen, 1984; and chapters by O'Brien and by Sampson, this volume).[9]

SOME PHILOSOPHICAL ISSUES

Numerous conceptual and ethical issues surround the question of PMS as a criminal excuse. Although none can be pursued here in adequate depth, it is helpful to mention them before undertaking legal analysis.

Is Premenstrual Syndrome a Medical Disorder?

Insanity tests and some forms of diminished capacity apply to defendants with "mental disease," which would require PMS to be at least a medical disorder. A number of objections to viewing PMS as a medical disorder may be imagined, but most have no force. For example, PMS is clinically defined and lacks known pathology or pathophysiology, but this situation is common in medicine. Examples of such presently "functional" disorders include migraine, narcolepsy, and irritable colon. There is no doubt that almost all the symptoms listed above are standard manifestations of medical diseases. Only two important objections to describing PMS as a medical disorder require discussion.

One objection is the apparently high prevalence of PMS symptoms in menstruating women. It is unusual in medicine for a disease to affect the majority of the species, sex, or age group. One might cite atherosclerosis, dental caries, and functional decline in old age, but the paucity of such cases raises the question of whether these processes are rightly called diseases at all. Insofar as n-PMS affects a majority (or 90%) of menstruating women, it seems more analogous to normal effects of one physiologic function on another; e.g., pain in teething, fatigue after exercise, the disabilities of pregnancy, or transient menstrual anemia. Such normal physiologic deficits may be viewed as design defects in the human species — one might say the same of menstruation itself — but not as medical disorders. However, narrower definitions of p-PMS that cover only a fraction of menstruating women (especially on the order of 5-10%) readily allow p-PMS to be classified as medically abnormal. Even if such women differ only in degree from other women, medicine offers many examples of disorders that are quantitative abnormalities (hypothyroidism, Cushing's syndrome, dwarfism, anemia, macrocytosis).

The other objection is that PMS may be not one disorder, but many disorders. Attempts have been made to divide PMS into subtypes based

---

9 The issue of progesterone's tranquilizing action is important in that English courts have probably taken the effects of progesterone therapy to confirm Dalton's hormone-deficiency theory. But any criminal behavior, however caused, can be suppressed by drug treatment. Major antipsychotic drugs (used in the U.S.S.R. on dissidents) will do the trick, and conventional addictive drugs like heroin or cocaine might also work. Drug suppression of crime does not show the crime was caused by drug deficiency. Sampson (her chapter, this volume) provides data on progesterone doses that suppress the menstrual cycle. Dalton's patients from the judicial system are maintained on progesterone doses high enough to produce this effect (Dalton, 1984).

on primary symptoms (Abraham, 1980; Moos, 1969) or temporal pattern, although such schemes may leave more than half of all women as mixed cases (Reid, 1985, his Fig. 2).[10] Again, however, medicine often divides diseases into subtypes — diabetes mellitus, pneumonia, and cancer are examples. Since the disease, however subclassified, remains pathological, for purposes of legal analysis it makes no difference whether PMS is one disease or many. At the same time, the caveat must be entered that conceptions of disease for medical and legal purposes are not necessarily equivalent. One of the best recent discussions of this vexed question is that of Moore (1984, chapter 5).

Is Premenstrual Syndrome a Mental Disease?

Legal tests for insanity or diminished responsibility are usually framed in terms of "mental disease." In medicine, the question "Physical or mental?" is both obscure and oversimplified. It is obscure in that a disease can be classified as mental or physical in the sense of clinical features, primary pathology, or etiology. These classifications do not coincide. Clinical features determine the inclusion of a disorder in a psychiatric classification such as the *Diagnostic and Statistical Manual of Mental Disorders* (Edition 3, 1980; DSM-III), but such disorders may have physical etiology and/or primary pathology. Examples of organic diseases with psychiatric effects include brain tumors, stroke, Alzheimer's disease, neurosyphilis, liver cancer, renal failure, hypothyroidism, lead poisoning, and alcohol or LSD intoxication. In general, all major types of organic disease (infection, tumor, trauma, metabolic disturbance, toxins, etc.) can affect central nervous system (CNS) tissue and produce psychiatric symptoms. [See Rose (1970) for a brief survey of organic conditions with legally significant psychiatric effects.] Conversely, psychogenic psychopathology can have organic clinical effects. Examples of wholly or partly psychogenic disorders with organic effects include peptic ulcer, ulcerative colitis, bronchial asthma, eczema, hypertension, and anorexia nervosa. Of the eight possibilities generated by physical/mental and etiology/pathology/clinical features, medical examples of each type exist, and many diseases are of mixed type.

For theoretical purposes, the most fundamental classification is by causes; i.e., by etiology or pathology. On this interpretation, the alternative "Physical or mental?" is oversimplified. The causation (etiology and pathogenesis) of a disease may be multifactorial, reflecting the interaction of genetic, environmental, psychological, and social factors.

At a minimum, for example, the pathway to p-PMS symptoms may include effects of the factors shown in Figure 2. The cause of the *disorder* p-PMS — what differentiates women who report *severe* life disruption by cyclic premenstrual symptoms — may be any one of these factors or a mixture of several. Women with p-PMS may have a primary hormonal abnormality. Equally, they may have atypical individual psychology that makes them react to a universal cyclic physiologic stressor with a mental crisis; or they may suffer from a mixture of these and other factors. At present, it is unknown what factors explain

---

[10] Reid's most common types A and B are onset of symptoms at the middle (A) or the beginning (B) of the luteal phase, with a sharp decline at menstruation. Group C is like A plus an isolated peak at ovulation, while Group D is symptom-free only from the end of menses to ovulation, thus having "only one good week" in the month.

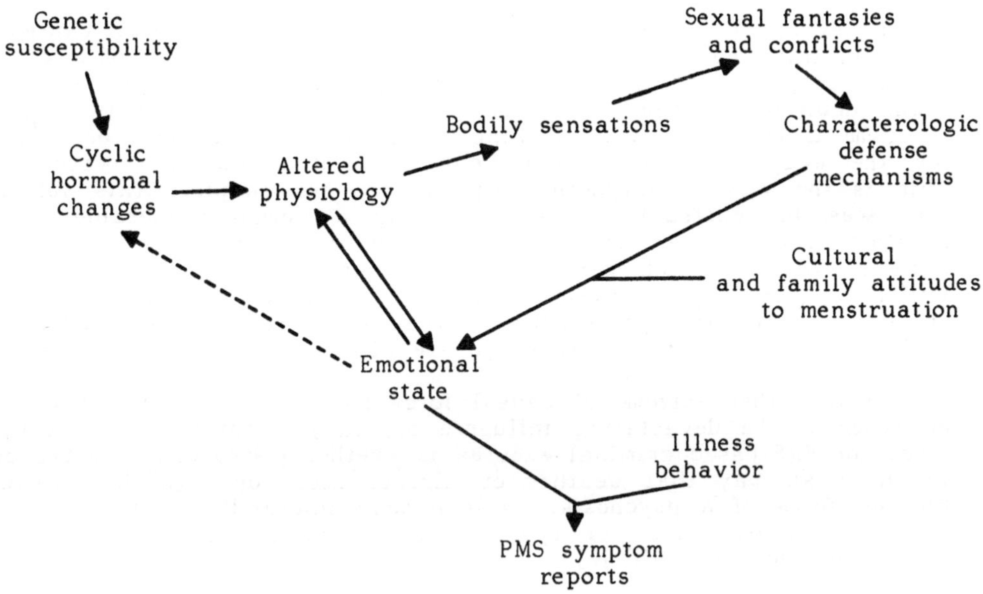

Fig. 2. Interrelations among vulnerability factors predisposing to p-PMS.

the variance in the feelings and emotions of premenstrual women.[11] Fortunately, the legal category "mental disease" does not exclude organic diseases in any case, and therefore the question "Physical or mental?" is unnecessary to the resolution of issues about PMS and criminal responsibility.

Does Premenstrual Syndrome Cause Crime?

Whether PMS causes crime depends partly on the analysis of causation. In the weakest sense — cause as a necessary condition — it seems clear that p-PMS is a cause of some crimes. Dalton and Taylor (1983, pp. 274-276) cite various studies showing that roughly 50% of crimes and psychiatric admissions by women fall into the 8-day paramenstruum. Given a 28-day cycle, such data, if correct, show that paramenstrual status doubles the risk of crime or psychiatric breakdown in certain women.

---

[11] For psychological approaches to PMS, see chapters in this volume by Blechman & Clay, Ericksen, Ruble & Brooks-Gunn, and Sampson. Even Reid and Yen (1981, p. 97), who are mainly oriented to physiology, concede, "There is little doubt that core psychological characteristics may modulate an individual's interpretation or expression of premenstrual symptoms. . ." From a psychoanalytic standpoint, menstruation is ideally suited to activate unconscious fantasies of castration and impregnation which are at the core of a woman's psychosexual identity. Psychoanalysis is perhaps the only major discipline not represented at the NSF-EVIST Conference. Recent discovery of "baboon PMS" reported in a *New York Times* article (June 4, 1985) may strengthen a physiological explanation of human n-PMS, but does not necessarily bear on human p-PMS.

However, other internal and external factors are also causes of crime in this weak sense: fatigue, hunger, weather, time of day, etc. Normal people can handle these stresses; impaired people sometimes break down under them. To view p-PMS as a necessary-condition cause of crime is consistent with viewing it as only an occasion, or trigger, for the eruption of permanent weaknesses of a woman's personality. This is the view of Gwyneth Sampson (see her chapter, this volume), who sees premenstrual status as making a woman vulnerable to the Achilles' heel of her personality. Such weaknesses may be psychopathological, in which case they may count toward reducing criminal guilt; or they may be morally culpable, in which case they will not. In either case, the possibility is that PMS does not so much cause violence as trigger it in women who are already predisposed to violence.

At the other extreme of causal force from that of a mere necessary condition is the devastating influence of, say, a psychosis. A central issue for PMS-based criminal excuses is whether p-PMS causes crime only in the weak way that weather or alcohol does, or with the more full-blooded force of a psychosis, or with some intermediate force. [For a sophisticated discussion of types of causation in medicine, see Meehl (1977) and Murphy (1976)].]

Should Disorders That Cause Crime Excuse It?

This is the main moral issue underlying the insanity defense and other psychiatric legal excuses, and it can be given only a few introductory remarks.

First, some moral philosophers believe both that any cause of action for which the agent is not responsible excuses the action and that all action is ultimately caused by events for which the agent is not responsible. Such philosophers conclude that no one is morally responsible for any action — a position known as "hard determinism." [12] Hard determinism destroys the moral basis of criminal law; although many psychiatrists are hard determinists, court testimony based on this viewpoint subverts the law. Philosophers opposing hard determinism fall into two groups. One group denies causal determinism and embraces uncaused free will. Although jurists often assume that this position is the only basis for criminal law, in contemporary philosophy a much more popular position is "soft determinism." Soft determinists hold that moral responsibility for action requires only causal determination of the action by the agent's own character and will.

In this chapter, it is assumed that the framework of criminal law and punishment is ethically justified, via soft determinism or otherwise. Naturally, if no one deserves punishment, then PMS victims do not; the issue for discussion is whether p-PMS should be an excuse within criminal law. Within the law, psychiatric excuses rest on the idea that diseases — by contrast with normal mental causes — excuse conduct. Why some diseases excuse conduct and what kinds of disease should do so is controversial. Several recent writers argue that the moral basis of the insanity defense is disease-caused irrationality, which requires a certain kind and level of disease (Fingarette, 1972; Moore, 1984). The position assumed below is that causation by disease *per se* is

---

[12] For a brief survey of the issues of determinism and moral responsibility, see Taylor (1967). Still useful are Hook (1958) and Morgenbesser and Walsh (1962). For current references on this and other philosophical topics, see *The Philosopher's Index*.

morally important only in that diseases are innocent causes; i.e., in that people are not blameworthy for their diseases. It does not follow that actions caused by such diseases as necessary conditions are blameless, as Houlgate correctly observes (see his chapter, this volume). Rather, moral exculpation by disease requires a fairly severe disruption of basic cognition and volition, as in traditional psychiatric legal defenses.

A third fundamental issue is whether organic mental abnormality is a stronger excuse than psychogenic. This issue affects the merits of the *Durham* insanity test and diminished responsibility, and the merits of p-PMS under either. If a psychogenic mental disorder excuses as well as an organic one, then the *Durham* rule and the concept of diminished responsibility threaten the collapse of law. On the other hand, if organic disorders have moral preference, whether p-PMS qualifies for these defenses depends on whether it is a hormonal or psychogenic disorder. No resolution of this crucial issue about psychiatric excuses is undertaken here.

PREMENSTRUAL SYNDROME AS A CRIMINAL EXCUSE

In spite of the controversy, p-PMS presents few novel issues as a mental abnormality affecting criminal responsibility. Certainly, there is, or should be, no question of a *sui generis* "PMS defense." Perhaps the closest analogues to p-PMS are other female reproductive phenomena such as *post partum* depression (see Kane, 1980, pp. 1343-1348) and menopausal psychiatric symptoms.[13] In any case, established forms of psychiatric excuse in law apply uncontroversially to other endocrine hormonal disorders (e.g., myxedema madness, diabetes mellitus, hyperthyroidism; see Reiser & Whisnant, 1980, pp. 1917-1929), other quantitative abnormalities (e.g., psychotic depression), and other disorders with mixed physical-mental causation (e.g., schizophrenia on the diathesis-stress or genetic-environmental model). [For a survey of theories on the etiology of schizophrenia, see Weiner (1980).] For legal purposes, the only novel psychiatric features of PMS are its cyclicity and supposed wide prevalence. The firestorm of debate over the PMS trials discussed above is best explained as due to three factors: (i) skepticism about the facts of p-PMS symptomatology claimed by researchers such as Dalton; (ii) rampant confusion between broad and narrow conceptions of PMS (i.e., between n-PMS as a near-universal syndrome of normal changes and p-PMS as an uncommon medical disorder); and (iii) the flaws in the famous cases themselves. It is argued below that the outcomes of these cases make no sense on any legal or psychiatric theory.

As for (i), the only thing one can presently say about the severe psychiatric symptoms claimed by Dalton and others to beset otherwise normal women is that their verification awaits further research. In many cases, such research may show ordinary primary psychopathology

---

[13] In England, by acts of 1922 and 1938, infanticide of a baby by its mother in its first year is a separate crime equivalent to manslaughter. This special rule for infanticide is intended to recognize *post partum* mental disturbance (formerly called "lactational insanity") and is akin to diminished responsibility (see O'Donovan, 1984; Walker, 1968, pp. 125-137). Some of the same mental symptoms are reported for menopause as for PMS, such as depression and emotional lability. It is disputed whether menopause really raises the incidence of such symptoms (see Reiser & Whisnant, 1980, pp. 1924-1925).

in women with p-PMS, in which case PMS recedes to a secondary diagnosis or cyclic aggravating factor, losing much of its mystery. This result seems especially likely in apparent cyclic psychoses; indeed, some of the references cited below concern premenstrual exacerbations of underlying psychosis.

As for (ii), legal excuses based on mental abnormality probably cannot apply to a disorder that affects a huge segment of the public, such as 85% of menstruating women 25-50% of the time. Psychiatric defenses are intended for exceptional defendants, not typical ones. If *(per impossibile)* it were shown that most premenstrual women act unconsciously or without knowing what they are doing, they would qualify for the defenses of automatism or M'Naghten insanity, respectively. No such fantastic claim is made even by the most enthusiastic PMS advocates. Other psychiatric tests of responsibility have vague degree-of-impairment language (discussed below) that seems sure to be interpreted to reject PMS defenses by typical premenstrual women. The specter of PMS as a generic female excuse, branding all women criminally insane half the time, is a bogey created by the press. No PMS researcher holds this absurd position.

In reviewing forms of legal excuse for which p-PMS might qualify, one must recall some features of criminal law. The most basic requirement for a crime is a voluntary act (or omission where there is a legal duty to act) — an act directed by the agent's will (see LaFave & Scott, 1972, pp. 177-191).[14] A crime is classically seen as consisting of a physical movement (the *actus reus*) and one or more accompanying mental states (the *mens rea*), together perhaps with certain effects and/or circumstances. Statutory or common law defines types of crime by specifying these "elements" precisely — physical act, mental state, effects, and circumstances. For example, robbery consists of a (1) trespassory (2) taking and (3) carrying away of the (4) personal property (5) of another, from (6) his presence or person, with (7) intent to steal, (8) by force or intimidation (LaFave & Scott, 1971, p. 692). In most jurisdictions, first-degree murder (except felony murder) consists in causing the death of another living human being *(actus reus)*, with a specific type of malice — a premeditated and deliberated intent to kill *(mens rea)* (LaFave & Scott, 1972, pp. 528-568).

A defendant cannot be convicted of a crime unless all of its elements are proved beyond reasonable doubt. This traditional rule of criminal procedure was made a constitutional requirement of due process in *In re Winship* (1970, 397 U.S. 358), and further interpreted with respect to what is an element in *Mullaney v. Wilbur* (1975, 421 U.S. 684) and *Patterson v. New York* (1977, 432 U.S. 197). The *Patterson* decision upheld the possibility of placing the burden of proving a form of diminished responsibility on the defendant. However (despite widespread confusion on this point), defendants may be acquitted on insanity in spite of all the elements being proved. It has been convincingly shown [e.g., by Fingarette (1972) and by Moore (1984)] that typical insane defendants do have the *mens rea* elements of

---

14 In the terminology of the Model Penal Code 1.13(2) and some other authors, the criminal "act" is a bodily movement and voluntariness is a mental element [2.01(1)]. An alternative view is that without voluntariness, there is not even an act, so that voluntariness is incorporated into *actus reus* and *mens rea* elements are additional. The choice between these approaches will not affect the analysis in this text. For some discussion of the alternatives, see LaFave and Scott (1972, pp. 177-181).

their crimes as those elements are ordinarily defined in common sense and law. Thus, the best view is that the insanity defense is *sui generis*, marking out a class of offenders who, despite their acts, lack moral guilt and therefore deserve a medical-custodial rather than a penal disposition.[15]

Complete Defenses to Criminal Guilt

A complete defense exonerates the defendant from all guilt and punishment. In the unique case of insanity, insane defendants are normally committed to mental hospitals after acquittal.

Automatism or Unconsciousness. In the rare, independent defense of automatism, a defendant argues that her behavior occurred unconsciously or with significantly clouded consciousness. Medical conditions that have supported automatism defenses include epileptic seizures, concussion, brain tumor, sleepwalking, and diabetic hypoglycemia (see LaFave & Scott, 1972, pp. 337-341). The defense argument in *Santos* was a claim of automatism due to hypoglycemia induced by PMS and fasting. In addition, a "blackout" during menstruation was accepted by a 1943 Georgia court to negate civil liability of an automobile driver (*Edwards v. Ford,* 1943, 69 Ga. App. 578, 26 S.E. 2d 306).[16]

The relation between automatism and the insanity defense is unclear in several ways. Automatism negates the voluntariness of an act; i.e., it negates an element of the crime, whereas insanity at least need not so function. On this analysis, a reasonable doubt about automatism must suffice to acquit, whereas the burden of proving insanity may be placed on the defendant (*Leland v. Oregon,* 1952, 343 U.S. 790). Unlike post-insanity commitments, no procedure exists for committing automatistic defendants; hence, such defendants are set free, a prospect that led one recent British court to refuse an automatism defense [*Regina v. Sullivan* (British Court of Appeal, 1982), discussed in Brahams (1983)]. On the other hand, some courts have ruled that "mental disease" must be a chronic disorder (Goldstein, 1967, p. 117), so that transient mental disturbances are left to automatism or excluded altogether.

Insanity. Insanity is a complete defense to any criminal charge, but is unique in being normally followed by court commitment. Although the roots of the insanity defense reach back to the origins of Western law (Herrmann, 1983; Walker, 1968, 1973), the four alternative current tests have arisen since 1843. All require the act of the accused to be

---

15 Confusion between the *mens rea* and *sui generis* views of insanity is partly caused by an ambiguity of *mens rea:* The prescriptive Latin meaning is simply "evil mind" (which the insanity defense declares the insane to lack), but the phrase is also used by lawyers as a descriptive shorthand for the defined mental elements in crimes (which the insane possess). The insanity defense is a moral judgment that in insane offenders, a *mens rea* element is not *rea;* that is, a mental element that would be evil in a normal person is not evil in the insane.

16 Other older cases involving premenstrual symptoms concern denial of disability benefits to a PMS victim, revocation of a real estate license for shoplifting, child custody, and acquittal for rape of a premenstrual woman (see Apodaca & Fink, 1984).

caused by mental disease. All except the product rule add further severity requirements for mental disease to constitute insanity.

Several legal obstacles exist to qualifying p-PMS as a mental disease for insanity. First, courts, lawyers, and psychiatrists often operate under a tacit agreement that "mental disease" requires psychosis [see Goldstein (1967, p. 48); Wallach & Rubin (1971); and the Model Penal Code (Section 4.01, Appendix B, Tentative Draft No. 4, 1955)]. Nothing in the language of standard insanity tests justifies this assumption, since the concepts of "disease" and "mental" do not imply it. Diseases in medicine range from lethal (bronchogenic carcinoma) to trivial (eczema, ringworm, hay fever); there is no severity requirement in the idea of disease. Lesser psychiatric disorders are "mental" in every sense that psychoses are; i.e., clinical features, etiology, and pathology. Indeed, it is widely believed that psychoses are more physically caused than neuroses or personality disorders, and such was the uniform assumption of alienists in the latter half of the 19th century. The Victorian term "mental disease" simply served to characterize a medical specialty in diseases with major clinical effects on the mind.

Secondly, in insanity trials many courts require "mental disease" to be a chronic condition, not a temporary one (see Goldstein, 1967, p. 117). This rule is a practical convenience, supporting a presumption that the disorder causing the criminal act continues at trial and justifies post-trial commitment. It also helps to weed out spurious pleas of "temporary insanity" due to minor transient disturbances. But the chronicity rule makes no theoretical sense: A defendant whose mind was temporarily deranged, through no fault of her own, is as morally innocent as a chronic mental patient. In legal theory, only mental state concurrent with the act matters to guilt; the accused's mental health before and after the crime is irrelevant. The chronicity rule is therefore wrong on principle. Even if accepted, it should be interpreted to include regularly recurring episodic mental impairments such as manic-depressive psychosis, epilepsy, or (if severity requirements are met) p-PMS.

On the other hand, an obstacle cited by several writers does not exist. The idea that "mental disease" as traditionally interpreted excludes hormonal disorders is implied by Taylor and Dalton (1983, pp. 280-281). Apodaca and Fink (1984, p. 67) flatly state that a hormonal disorder cannot be a mental disease or defect; Carney and Williams (1983, p. 264) state that PMS cannot be a mental disease or defect because it is a physiological disorder; and Pahl-Smith (1985, p. 260) says, "PMS is a physiological problem, not a disease of the mind," although she foresees that PMS might be "correlated" to mental disease. No leading authority on the insanity defense excludes organic mental disorders, including endocrine disorders, from any traditional insanity test. The defense requires mental manifestations of a disease (clinical features or psychopathology), but the disease can be organically caused (etiology or primary pathology). A rule excluding organic psychopathology would be historically and ethically perverse. The idea of the insanity defense is that a certain degree of innocent mental derangement negates guilt. Organic diseases can cause exactly the same mental symptoms as "functional" ones, and such patients are no more responsible for their underlying disease. Any differences would surely favor the organic defendant.

It will be assumed below that p-PMS, although possibly a hormonal disease, is a "mental disease" within the meaning of insanity and diminished responsibility tests as ideally read. The serious obstacle to p-PMS as a criminal excuse is whether p-PMS psychiatric symptoms rise to the proper levels of severity.

(1) The M'Naghten Rule. The oldest and most famous contemporary test of insanity is the M'Naghten rule. It was formulated in 1843 by British judges in answers to five questions posed by the House of Lords during the furor over the acquittal of Daniel M'Naghten, a paranoid Scot who killed Prime Minister Robert Peel's secretary in an attempt to kill Peel. The M'Naghten answers are internally inconsistent, were not and could not have been the basis of M'Naghten's acquittal, and appear to concern only "partial insanity."[17] Nonetheless, in a striking irony of legal history, the main M'Naghten rule became the authoritative law of insanity in England and in most American states. The test excuses a defendant who has (*M'Naghten's Case*, 8 Eng. Rep. 718):

> ". . . such a defect of reason, from disease of the mind, as not to know the nature and quality of the act he was doing, or if he did know it that he did not know he was doing what was wrong."

[For a survey of the right-wrong test before *M'Naghten*, see Platt and Diamond (1966).]

The M'Naghten rule is often called the knowledge test, or right-wrong test, because of its focus on the accused's knowledge of the wrongness of his act. Both its cognitive emphasis and its use of moral concepts have evoked bitter criticism by psychiatrists since the rule's formulation.[18] Under the usual interpretations of "wrong" and of "knowledge," a literal reading of the rule seems to excuse only a tiny minority of psychotics — those, for example, with delusions so severe that they do not know that they are killing a human being. ["Wrong" is typically read to mean either "considered wrong by society" or "legally wrong," with the latter the English interpretation; see Goldstein (1967, pp. 51-53); LaFave & Scott (1972, pp. 278-279).] However, courts often do not apply the rule literally and may allow psychiatrists to testify that a defendant did not "appreciate" the significance of his act as a normal person would; i.e., have "emotional" or "affective" knowledge of its nature, quality, or wrongfulness.

In the United States, as its framers intended, the M'Naghten rule often leads to conviction, even death, for psychotic criminals. Hence, it is unlikely that M'Naghten can excuse p-PMS defendants. Even when

---

17 The judges' answers are inconsistent on whether the knowledge called for in the test is of wrongfulness or illegality. The trial testimony was relevant to an irresistible impulse or a delusion test as much as to the right-wrong test; in any case, the judges' answer to question 4 states that the accused is guilty if he would be guilty were his delusion true, and M'Naghten's paranoid delusions do not meet the test for valid self-defense. The truth-of-delusion rule is also inconsistent with the main rule, since one could have a delusion which would not, if true, legally excuse the act, but which one falsely believes does excuse it legally and morally. Finally, the judges' answers twice explicitly restrict themselves to "persons who labor under such partial delusions only, and are not in other respects insane" (*M'Naghten's Case*, 8 Eng. Rep. 718).

18 One of the first and most vociferous critics was Isaac Ray, in later editions of his *Treatise on the Medical Jurisprudence of Insanity*. For later criticisms by psychiatrists and lawyers, see references in LaFave and Scott (1972, pp. 280-283).

"knowledge" is broadened to emotional appreciation, a psychotic delusion or at least affective blunting is usually necessary for M'Naghten acquittal. The issue of PMS psychosis is presently controversial, with a few investigators reporting cyclical psychotic episodes in women without underlying conventional psychosis [on PMS psychosis, see Altschule & Brem (1963); Berlin, Bergey, & Money (1983); Dennerstein, Judd, & Davies (1983); Endo, Daiguji, Asano, Yamashita, & Takahashi (1978); Glick & Stewart (1980); Kane, Daly, Wallach, & Keeler (1966); Ota, Makai, & Gotoda (1954); Teja (1976); Williams & Weekes (1952)]. Dalton (see her chapter, this volume) reports treating 22 women with "premenstrual psychosis" in 1982 alone. However, even Dalton does not believe PMS will support a M'Naghten insanity defense (Taylor & Dalton, 1983, p. 279).

(2) Control ("Irresistible Impulse") Tests. A minority of American states supplement the M'Naghten rule with one of a family of control tests (LaFave & Scott, 1972, pp. 283-286). Control tests excuse defendants who, from mental abnormality, are wholly or largely unable to control their actions. Where M'Naghten deals with cognition, control tests deal with volition. Thus, the M'Naghten and control tests are sometimes viewed as assimilating insanity to two standard kinds of legal excuse, deriving from Aristotelian ethics (Aristotle, translated by Ostwald, 1962, pp. 52-57): ignorance and compulsion. Other commentators insist that all insanity tests are *sui generis*. [For a discussion of the analogy between insanity and either ignorance or compulsion, see Fingarette (1972) and Moore (1984).]

Although control tests are often called "irresistible impulse," the name is misleading. Most courts do not require the behavior in question to be impulsive, nor (outside of military courts) must it be wholly irresistible (LaFave & Scott, 1972, p. 285). A typical formulation is one from the New Mexico Supreme Court (*State v. White*, 1954, 270 P.2d 727,731):

> "Assuming defendant's knowledge of the nature and quality of his act and his knowledge that the act is wrong, if, by reason of disease of the mind, defendant has been deprived of or has lost the power of his will which would enable him to prevent himself from doing the act, he cannot be found guilty."

Affective psychoses are the clearest example of conditions that pass a control but not a knowledge test — for example, *post partum* psychotic depression in which a mother kills her children. As with M'Naghten, nothing in the language of the test requires psychosis. In principle, lesser disorders — neuroses, perversions, or various personality disorders — may make the defendant unable to "control" her actions. Little information is available on how often non-psychotic diagnoses allow successful control-insanity pleas, although many discussions mention kleptomania.

The major criticism of control tests is of their assumption that some defendants cannot control their actions, while others can but merely fail to do so. Psychiatrists and jurists agree that to distinguish an irresistible from an unresisted impulse is difficult in practice; many critics also claim that it makes no theoretical sense. Since typical control tests do not require that the act be fully irresistible, an additional element of theoretical vagueness enters the test. The degree of loss of self-control which shall exculpate remains unexplained.

(3) The American Law Institute (ALI; Model Penal Code) Test. The American drafters of the Model Penal Code formulated a test that fuses a broadened M'Naghten with a control test. Until recently, this ALI rule was applied in almost all Federal jurisdictions and roughly one-third of the states; its popularity fell precipitously after its use to acquit John W. Hinckley, Jr. The ALI rule reads (Model Penal Code, 1962, Sec. 401, Proposed Official Draft):

> "A person is not responsible for criminal conduct if at the time of such conduct as a result of mental disease or defect he lacks substantial capacity either to appreciate the criminality [wrongfulness] of his conduct or to conform his conduct to the requirements of law."

A second clause was intended to exclude psychopathy. This test amounts to M'Naghten with the "nature and quality" wing suppressed and "appreciate" for "know"; with an alternative control test; and with both wings explicitly weakened to lack of "substantial capacity." The major criticism of the ALI rule, besides the problems of any control test, is the vagueness of "substantial capacity."

What are the prospects for p-PMS defendants passing a control test like the one in the ALI rule? Several emotional symptoms of p-PMS — anxiety, rage, emotional lability, and especially the feeling of being "out of control" — strongly suggest a reduction in the premenstrual woman's (actual or perceived) self-control. On the other hand, "substantial incapacity" is a vague standard. Whether such a defense should succeed depends on the intentions of the framers of control tests regarding the degree of dyscontrol. It also depends on whether one agrees with the recent decisions by both the American Bar Association (ABA) and the American Psychiatric Association (APA) to oppose volitional tests of insanity. Practically speaking, the assumption of many judges and psychiatrists that insanity requires psychosis, together with jury reluctance to find premenstrual dyscontrol sufficiently severe for acquittal, make it unlikely that any p-PMS control defense will succeed.

Taylor and Dalton (1983, pp. 274-276) argue for the existence of p-PMS dyscontrol insanity. However, one important part of their evidence is correlational studies linking female crime to the menstrual cycle. As explained earlier, such correlations may show a weak causal influence; i.e., that premenstrual changes contribute to antisocial behavior in some women. But mere contributory causation cannot be sufficient for legal compulsion or loss of control. Many mental, physical, and environmental factors favor criminal behavior. Similar or stronger correlations exist between crime and: weather (temperature, humidity); time of day; level of fatigue; hunger or satiety; sexual tension, etc. Each of these factors also has demonstrable endocrine effects, altering blood levels of such hormones as cortisol, epinephrine, and insulin in dramatic and predictable ways — which is more than can presently be said for p-PMS. As examples of the correlations, rape or attempted rape occurs twice as often per hour between 6 P.M. and midnight (34% of total incidents) as between 6 A.M. and 6 P.M. (33%). The same is true of aggravated assault (40% vs. 41%; McGarrell & Flanagan, 1985). This time effect equals the PMS effect in the studies quoted by Taylor and Dalton (1983). Age is also a potent factor. Robbery is about three times as likely to be committed by persons aged 25-29 as by those aged 45-49, and 50% more likely still in the group aged 20-24 (McGarrell & Flanagan, 1985, pp. 468-469, 473). As for season, rape is about 40% more likely in August than in February (*FBI Uniform Crime Reports 1984*, pp. 14, 7). A *reductio* of this statistical approach is that it would make the criminal law treat men more leniently than women. Men are over six times as likely as women to be arrested for non-negligent homicide, and about five times as likely to be arrested for violent crimes or crime in general (McGarrell & Flanagan, 1985, pp. 474 and 476). If a 5:1 ratio does not create a "testosterone defense," it is hard to see why a 2:1 ratio should create a "progesterone defense."

Despite associated endocrine and psychological "syndromes," it seems absurd to exonerate criminal defendants for the effects of weather, hunger, or lust. No court would or should excuse defendants for the following crimes and (newly christened) syndromes:

CSS	Circadian stress syndrome	Evening assault
MDS	Meteorologic decompensation syndrome	Hot weather murder
NDS	Nutrition deprivation syndrome (fames uxorialis)	Wife beating
PNTS	Post-naval tension syndrome	Rape by a sailor
VHS	Vernal hyperkinetic syndrome (spring fever)	Student rioting
CED	Catastrophic economic dysthymia (unemployment)	Robbery
ODS	Object desertion syndrome	Murder of ex-wife

The point is simple: Causal influence of a factor, even when mediated by an endocrine process, does not negate and may not even limit criminal responsibility. On the contrary, criminal law expects everyone to meet stress with increased self-control, and it must take more, not less, care to punish anti-social acts where typical temptation to them is strong.

(4) The Durham (Product) Rule. The simplest and broadest insanity rule is the product test. It was first accepted by Judge Doe of New Hampshire following a correspondence with Isaac Ray (Moore, 1984, pp. 224-228), the American physician whose text on legal insanity also inspired M'Naghten's acquittal (Diamond, 1956). Judge Bazelon of the Washington, D.C. Court of Appeals adopted the New Hampshire test between 1954 and 1962. As applied in the Washington court, the test excused any criminal defendant whose act was "the product of mental disease or defect;" i.e., was caused by psychopathology (*Durham v. U.S.*, 1954, 214 F. 2d 862, pp. 874-875). The idea of causation in the *Durham* rule was explained in a 1957 case (*Carter v. U.S.*, 252 F. 2d 608, p. 617) as the standard one in law — a necessary condition "but for" which the act would not have occurred.[19]

The intent of the court in adopting the *Durham* rule was to give more scope to contemporary psychiatry than traditional tests allowed. Nonetheless, by 1962 Judge Bazelon was sufficiently dissatisfied with

---

[19] In civil and criminal law, a necessary condition of a result R is called a "cause in fact" of R. A further condition is required for a person to be legally responsible for R: Not only must his conduct be a cause in fact of R, but R must not differ too much from what he intended or risked by that conduct. If the extra condition is satisfied, his conduct is called the "legal" or "proximate" cause of R (LaFave & Scott, 1972, pp. 256-267 and references on p. 248, Note 7).

psychiatric testimony to rule that psychiatric and legal concepts of "mental disease" were not necessarily equivalent. He held that for legal purposes, a "mental disease or defect" must be one that "substantially affects mental or emotional processes and substantially impairs behavior controls" (*McDonald v. U.S.*, 1962, 312 F. 2d 847, p. 851). With this "substantiality" requirement, the product test became similar to the ALI substantial capacity rule, which replaced it in Bazelon's court in 1972 (*U.S. v. Brawner*, 1972, 471 F. 2d 969).

It seems clear that under the pure (1954-62) product test, p-PMS can excuse criminal behavior. There is no good reason (other than its absence from the official DSM-III classification) for denying p-PMS (if it exists) the title of mental disease, and no reason to deny that premenstrual status is in some women a necessary-condition cause of crime. Whether the effects of PMS are substantial in the 1962-72 sense depends, as with the ALI rule, on what "substantial" means.

It also seems clear — although this point is often missed — that the pure product test rests on a moral error and is legally disastrous. Literally interpreted, it excuses virtually all criminal behavior. Almost every criminal could be given a DSM-I or DSM-II diagnosis, although DSM-III tightened the diagnostic criteria considerably. Further, almost every criminal's mental disorder is a necessary condition for his crime, in the sense that it is almost always true that the act would not have occurred if the criminal were a normal person. In the eyes of most psychiatrists, completely normal people do not commit serious crimes.

Ethically speaking, an act is surely not excusable merely because a disease is one of its necessary conditions. A blow, a broken promise, a theft are not blameless because, but for the agent's mild cold or acne-ridden face, he would not have acted as he did. The moral significance of mere causal influence by disease is that a person is (usually) blameless for having the disease. One cannot conclude that he is blameless for whatever the disease "causes" as a necessary condition; i.e., whatever he would not have done without it. The same argument would excuse all acts occasioned by similarly blameless conditions such as unemployment, marital strife, or disappointment in love. Ordinary ethics, like law, require us to act properly in many difficult circumstances for which we are blameless, of which disease is only one. The fact that a disease has mental as well as physical effects seems, in principle, to make little difference here. For disease to negate moral responsibility, it must not only be a necessary condition of the act, but also severely disrupt the agent's mental abilities in the manner of traditional insanity tests.

Except for the possibility of primary PMS psychosis, the upshot of this section is that p-PMS cannot support an insanity plea — nor has such a plea been made in a real case. Even p-PMS does not seem to involve the cognitive defect of the M'Naghten rule or the level of dyscontrol in the control or ALI rules. The pure product test excuses p-PMS defendants, but only because it excuses essentially all defendants and so is an unacceptable insanity test.

Partial Defenses to Criminal Guilt

In many jurisdictions, by either statute or judicial decision, mental abnormality less than insanity is a criminal defense. Almost always such "diminished capacity" or "diminished responsibility" results in conviction on a lesser charge — manslaughter instead of murder, or second-degree instead of first-degree murder. For crimes without degrees or without a lesser included offense (where logic would excuse the defendant altogether), courts usually refuse to admit diminished capacity.

Diminished responsibility or capacity is like the insanity defense in allowing mental abnormality, supported by expert psychiatric testimony, to reduce criminal guilt. These pleas are unlike the insanity defense in three ways. First, a plea of partial responsibility usually ends in conviction of some crime. Second, unlike the insanity defense, a successful partial responsibility plea does not result in routine hospitalization or court supervision of treatment. The defendant's disorder, and that part of the gravity of the offense which it excuses, escape judicial control. Third, under the more common "elements" (*mens rea*) version, logic requires that the burden of disproving diminished capacity be upon the prosecution.

Even by comparison with insanity, confusion plagues judicial opinions and scholarly discussions about diminished capacity or responsibility. Two of the clearest discussions are Fingarette and Hasse (1979) and Arenella (1977). The best analysis separates these partial defenses into two rationales: the *elements (mens rea)* approach and the *degree of moral guilt* approach.[20] Some sources call these, respectively, "diminished capacity" and "diminished responsibility," which is a helpful but not universal terminology. The former term is misleading in that, as will be seen, the issue is not the defendant's capacity to be in a particular mental state, but whether she was or was not in it.

Elements (Mens Rea, Diminished Capacity) Approach. In this original and most common variant, mental abnormality negates a mental state essential to a crime. All crimes (except strict liability offenses and perhaps negligence offenses) are defined as including specific mental elements. A defendant's mental disorder, although not enough for legal insanity, may make her unlikely or unable to entertain mental states such as intention, knowledge, premeditation, or malice. If the state is an element of the crime charged, the defendant by definition has not committed the crime and cannot be convicted of it — although she may be guilty of a lesser crime that does not require the element in question. Consequently, if psychiatrists can testify to the absence of the mental state, it would seem that such testimony must be admitted.

This rationale for considering mental abnormality less than insanity is, at bottom, a matter of basic law. As LaFave and Scott (1972, p. 331) state:

> "The logic of the partial responsibility doctrine would appear to be unassailable. The reception of evidence of the

---

20 Arenella omits the strict incapacity approach that Fingarette and Hasse document and expose; he shows that the diminished capacity approach metamorphosed, in California, into diminished responsibility, but he does not explain why this metamorphosis must occur. From the two discussions together, one can therefore see *three* versions of the *mens rea* elements approach: (1) incapacity (defendant *could* not have had the state, hence did not); (2) absence (defendant *did* not have the state); and (3) diminished capacity (defendant was *less able* to have the state than a normal person). As explained below, diminished responsibility is a logically unrelated fourth approach — a mini-insanity defense.

> defendant's abnormal mental condition, totally apart from the defense of insanity, is certainly appropriate whenever that evidence is relevant to the issue of whether he had the mental state which is a necessary element of the crime charged. Were it otherwise, major crimes specifically requiring a certain bad state of mind would, in effect, be strict liability offenses as applied to abnormal defendants."

This reasoning is what remains of psychiatric excuses in law if, as currently is advocated by some, the insanity defense is abolished.

A second common, although less overwhelming, argument for diminished capacity is that it merely extends to mental disorder the usual rules for voluntary alcohol intoxication (Fingarette & Hasse, 1979, chapter 8; LaFave & Scott, 1971, pp. 327-328). The argument is stated in *State v. Noel* (1926, 133 A. 274, 285) and *U.S. v. Brawner* (1972, 471 F. 2d 969,999).

Although estimates vary as to how many American jurisdictions accept the elements approach to partial responsibility, Robinson (1984, p. 474) states that most do. Besides frequent confusion of diminished capacity with insanity, some courts reject this approach for practical reasons. Such courts fear that juries will be unable to grasp psychiatric testimony regarding subtle differences between states of mind, or that diminished capacity will cause compromise verdicts or inadequate protection of the public from abnormal defendants (see Lindman & McIntyre, 1961, pp. 356-357). Nonetheless, it seems obvious that the "principle of legality" — that defendants cannot be guilty of crimes unless their acts have been defined as criminal, or *nullum crimen sine lege* (LaFave & Scott, 1972, p. 7) — entails that lack of essential mental elements of a crime, from psychiatric disorder or any other source, negates guilt. The only debatable aspect of the approach is the admissibility of psychiatric evidence. Unless psychiatric testimony is somehow irrelevant or unreliable on the issue of mental elements, the *mens rea* approach to partial responsibility is arguably a constitutional necessity, and furthermore, the burden of disproof must rest with the prosecution (Krausz, 1983). The "principle of legality" (*nullum crimen sine lege*) would seem to be the most basic due-process right of all.

Before illustrating this approach with cases, one must mention that many courts have encrusted two illogical restrictions on the elements rationale. First, the doctrine of "specific intent," originally developed for similar purposes in the law of intoxication, is commonly applied: Mental abnormality may negate specific intents but not general intent, sometimes described as "the intent necessarily entering every crime" (*Crosby v. People*, 1891, 27 N.E. 49, Illinois S. C., pp. 52-53). The purpose of the limitation is to avoid total acquittal of the intoxicated or abnormal offender in crimes without lesser degrees. One problem with the doctrine is that the specific-general distinction is so obscure that leading textbook writers recommend its demise (see Hall, 1960; LaFave & Scott, 1972, p. 358; Williams, 1961, p. 49; and Model Penal Code, 2.02, Comment, Tent. Draft No. 4, 1955). There is one fairly clear definition (LaFave & Scott, 1972, p. 202) — that "specific intent" is an intent to do some further act; e.g., breaking and entering with intent "to commit a felony therein" in the definition of burglary, or assault with intent "to rape." But this definition does not give the desired result. In cases of robbery, burglary, or tax evasion, to name a few, no "floor crime" may exist once mental abnormality negates the specific intent (LaFave & Scott, 1972, p. 331). The more serious problem is that the logic of the elements approach cannot be restricted to "specific" intents. Any mental state essential to a crime might be negated by mental abnormality, in which case acquittal is required by basic law.

A second limitation some courts apply is to require psychiatric testimony to show that the defendant was incapable of having the required mental state (Fingarette & Hasse, 1979, chapters 6-8, especially pp. 97-99). This rule may have arisen by inadvertence. In any case, there is a large difference between arguing that a defendant was incapable of having, say, an intent to kill and merely arguing that she did not do so. Obviously, incapacity proves absence, but not conversely. In particular circumstances, a defendant's motivation may raise reasonable doubt of his intent, e.g., to rape without proving the massive psychological injury that would be necessary for incapacity to so intend. As several courts have clearly stated, there is no justification on the elements rationale for focusing on capacity, since the legal issue is the presence or absence in fact of the elements of the crime.[21]

Since California is the American state that has most fully explored diminished capacity, it is convenient to illustrate the *mens rea* approach by discussing a few celebrated California cases. Recently, California voters abolished the diminished capacity defense by referendum on June 8, 1982, under the title "The Victims' Bill of Rights" (Proposition 8, 1982 Cal. Legis. Sess. 1164, West). As careful analyses (Arenella, 1977; Fingarette & Hasse, 1979) have shown, however, most of the California cases, although described in terms of the elements approach, really rest on a diminished responsibility rationale. One that truly fits the elements approach is *Wells* (1949, 202 P.2d 53, *cert. denied,* 338 U.S. 836), involving a prisoner accused of assaulting a guard, a capital offense that by statute required malice. Wells sought to negate malice by psychiatric evidence that he was in a state of high tension with abnormal fears for his personal safety, and therefore had an honest but unreasonable belief that he acted in self defense. This argument is a rare instance where a psychiatrically described state of mind is directly relevant to a legal mental element.

Later cases, however, were primarily homicide cases[22] with psychotic defendants in which the California Supreme Court used psychiatry, in effect, to redefine the traditional elements of murder: premeditation and deliberation, malice, and the intent to kill (Arenella, 1977, pp. 839-849; Fingarette & Hasse, 1979, pp. 119-133). Apart from felony murders, American law typically defines first-degree murder as involving these three elements. Second-degree murder is the same without premeditation or deliberation, or with an intent only to do serious bodily harm, or with extreme recklessness. Voluntary manslaughter, in turn, subtracts malice, which means that the killing was done in a "heat of passion" on reasonable provocation, or else with an "imperfect" defense such

---

21 For example, in *People v. Crittle* [1973, 212 N.W. 2d 196 (Mich. S. Ct.)], the court said that proposed jury instructions on drunkenness "all have one thing in common. They refer to a *capacity* standard. Their test is not Justice Cooley's — 'The crime cannot have been committed when the intent did not exist.' It is obviously a different standard and not to be followed." (See also Arenella, 1977, p. 839, Note 67.)

22 The diminished capacity defense has been applied to non-homicide crimes. In California, cases included battery on a police officer, burglary, robbery, rape, arson, and check bouncing (see Arenella, 1977, p. 843, Note 88; Fingarette & Hasse, 1972, p. 129, Note 37).

as unreasonable self defense or public duty (LaFave & Scott, 1972, pp. 571-586).[23]

Gorshen (1959, 336 P.2d 492) was, on the surface, a classic first-degree murder: The defendant, ordered home by his foreman for drunkenness, announced he would go home, get his gun, and shoot the foreman, which he then proceeded to do in the presence of a police officer. Gorshen's psychiatrist diagnosed him as a chronic paranoid schizophrenic with sexual hallucinations, whose work to him symbolized virility. This testimony, and the psychiatrist's judgment that Gorshen's action was caused by pathologic unconscious processes, convinced the Supreme Court to reduce the conviction from first- to second-degree murder, thus taking psychiatric testimony about motive to negate premeditation and deliberation. The Court went one step further in *Conley* (1966, 411 P.2d 911), in which the defendant, again intoxicated, killed his lover and her husband three days after the end of the affair. As in *Gorshen*, Conley stated his intentions and bought and practiced with a rifle on the day of the crime. The California Supreme Court held that Conley did not act with malice if he did not understand his "social obligation to act within the law." Finally, in *Mosher* (1969, 461 P.2d 659), the Court held that psychiatric testimony could also prove absence of the intent to kill.

The above cases, as Arenella shows, involve psychiatric testimony that "explain[s] why the accused entertained the requisite [mental state] rather than proving its absence" (Arenella, 1977, p. 831). On ordinary definitions of premeditation, malice, and intent to kill, the psychotic killers had these elements. The California Supreme Court's decision to redefine them to reduce the defendant's convictions was motivated, as the court conceded, by dissatisfaction with California's M'Naghten insanity test (see *People v. Berry*, 1955, 282 P.2d 861; and *People v. Daugherty*, 1953, 256 P.2d 911). The court was not really applying evidence of mental abnormality to disprove mental elements of crimes according to their ordinary definitions. Instead, it was making an ethical judgment as to how mental disorder should mitigate criminal responsibility — the second approach examined below. The upshot of analysis of the first (elements) approach is that — although mandated by basic law and constitutional principle — it has rare literal application (Arenella, 1977, pp. 831, 844-847; Fingarette & Hasse, 1979, pp. 66-70). Abnormal defendants, like intoxicated defendants, almost always intend to do what they do, often plan their acts beforehand, and often act with "malice" as the law defines that term. Cases where mental abnormality genuinely negates a mental element of crime are rare.

What are the prospects for using p-PMS to negate a mental element of a crime? The answer depends partly on the facts of PMS psychopathology, which are in dispute. Even if premenstrual psychosis exists, a literal view of the elements approach is no more helpful to psychotic PMS defendants than it would be to non-PMS psychotics like Wolff,

---

23 "Malice," the "element" that differentiates murder from manslaughter, is a notoriously confusing concept that many authorities suggest abandoning. Malice cannot easily be explained as a mental state. In a typical jurisdiction, malice is the mental element of murder — either intent to kill, intent to do serious bodily injury, extreme recklessness, or participation in a felony from which death results — *in the absence of justification or excuse* (LaFave & Scott, 1972, pp. 528-530). Thus, murder is not really manslaughter plus malice; rather, manslaughter is murder with excuse. Malice is the phlogiston of homicide: Its absence is the presence of the oxygen of excuse.

Goedecke, or Gorshen. If psychosis is almost always consistent with premeditation, malice, and intent to kill, diminished capacity will rarely aid a premenstrual killer. A more promising PMS-based mental disturbance is unconsciousness or a "dissociative reaction," claimed by Dalton (this volume) and some others to be common in p-PMS and related to hypoglycemia. Such a state might produce the kind of detached, automatistic behavior necessary for an automatism defense, while in milder form it might be used to argue lack of intent in crimes requiring clear-cut goals; e.g., theft crimes.

The clearest way that p-PMS (perhaps even n-PMS) could negate *mens rea* elements is simply by corroborating emotional turmoil. For example, the difference between first- and second-degree murder is premeditation and deliberation, which are usually held to require "a cool mind capable of reflection" (LaFave & Scott, 1972, p. 563). PMS might support a premenstrual defendant's claim to have killed impulsively and passionately, thus reducing her guilt to second-degree murder and preventing a death penalty. Such evidence might especially help to rebut circumstantial evidence of motive (e.g., life insurance) or block adverse inferences from behavior such as concealment.[24] Or, somewhat as in *Wells*, PMS-based emotional turmoil might support an honest though unreasonable belief in self-defense. In homicide, many jurisdictions allow such an "imperfect" defense to reduce guilt to manslaughter. Further, emotional turmoil may help a woman show that she acted inadvertently, in distraction and confusion, rather than with a certain intent. Shoplifting is an offense where such a claim could be true, as well as other theft crimes, which require an intent to permanently deprive the owner of the property (LaFave & Scott, 1971, pp. 637-642). Many crimes may offer a similar choice between two interpretations: distracted or impulsive behavior vs. action for a sinister purpose.

Although these examples seem to give PMS wide legal scope, in fact they go little beyond the common-sense idea that premenstrual women are tense and easily upset. Recognizing p-PMS as an extreme of this normal pattern may strenghten the inference, but it is an inference familiar to the ordinary juror.

One caveat to this generous view of PMS testimony is that the *mens rea* approach ought to require only a reasonable doubt about a mental element for acquittal. Considering their mantle of authority, psychiatrists who testify about severe emotional turmoil should be controlled by the strict admissibility criteria discussed below, lest every premenstrual woman be guaranteed emotional frenzy by sympathetic experts. Another troublesome issue with PMS-diminished capacity, as with voluntary intoxication (Fingarette & Hasse, 1979, pp. 101-104), is how to penalize women for negligently entering situations where an emotional storm causes foreseeable damage. On the above reasoning, one might acquit a premenstrual woman of tax fraud for filing a false return. However, common sense suggests some countervailing negligence liability for picking the worst time of her cycle to file. Less frivolous cases can be imagined without difficulty.

---

[24] For example, in a recent Texas case, one housewife hacked another to death with an ax, striking her 41 times, then returned to church pretending nothing had occurred. The jury believed her plea of self defense in spite of the number of blows and the concealment, but pre-existing emotional upset and confusion might have strengthened her claim of panic. A popular account of this case is found in Bloom and Atkinson (1983).

Degree of Moral Guilt (Diminished Responsibility) Approach. This second — and conceptually distinct — approach rests on a *de novo* moral judgment that mental abnormality ought to reduce criminal responsibility. On this approach, diminished responsibility is a junior insanity defense. Like insanity, it partially excuses an abnormal defendant, not because she has not committed the crime as defined (the elements approach), but in spite of her doing so. A major difference is that no procedures exist for routine commitment of the diminished-responsibility defendant for medical treatment.

For a time, an explicit diminished-responsibility rationale emerged in California, as illustrated by cases like *Wolff* (1964, 394 P.2d. 959). Wolff was a teenager found schizophrenic (indeed, legally insane) by all the experts at trial. After days or weeks of planning, Wolff killed his mother by beating her with an ax handle and strangling her, in order to be able to bring girls home to rape or photograph them nude. He was tried and convicted under the M'Naghten test; the court then reduced his conviction from first- to second-degree murder, reasoning as follows. The difference between first- and second-degree murder marks a "difference in the quantum of personal turpitude." However, the quality (the extent and depth) of Wolff's premeditation was reduced by his youth and mental disorder. In understanding and reflecting on his action, his realization of the "enormity of the evil" was "materially vague and detached," and so he could not "maturely and meaningfully reflect" on its gravity. Similar reasoning in two later cases reduced equally classic first-degree murders to second degree. Goedecke, who carefully and systematically executed his family and faked their discovery the next day, was diagnosed as a schizoid personality and held to have acted in a "disassociative state" (*People v. Goedecke*, 1967, 423 P.2d 777). Nicolaus, a delusional killer of his children, believed himself to be Frankenstein (*People v. Nicolaus*, 1967, 423 P.2d 787).

Wolff and its progeny show the California court creating by decision what a few jurisdictions have established by statute: a rule for reducing homicides caused by serious mental abnormality. The sole American statutory step in this direction is the Model Penal Code provision that a killing is manslaughter, not murder, if committed "under the influence of extreme mental or emotional disturbance for which there is reasonable explanation or excuse" [Model Penal Code, Sec. 210.3(1)(b)]. This provision, adopted in states such as New York [N.Y. Penal Law, Sec. 125.25(1)(a); McKinney, 1975], liberalizes the traditional "objective" test for provocation in manslaughter.[25] By the objective test (see LaFave & Scott, 1972, pp. 573-582), heat of passion makes a killing manslaughter only if the provocation could have caused a reasonable man to lose control, and only if the reasonable man would not have "cooled off" in the time between provocation and killing. The Model Penal Code shifts from reasonable persons to defendants whose passions have "reasonable explanation or excuse." While it is unclear exactly when mental disorder counts as such an explanation or excuse in states like New York, the rationale for a subjective test of passion, if fully pursued, surely implies that passions caused by psychopathology for which the accused is not culpable qualify. Indeed, the New York Appellate Court stated in *People v. Patterson* (1976, 347 N.E. 2d 898, pp. 907-908):

---

[25] This was the provision at issue in *Patterson v. N.Y.* (1977, 432 U.S. 197). For a discussion of a recent trial in which extreme emotional disturbance was an issue, see Gaylin (1982).

"An action influenced by an extreme emotional disturbance is not one that is necessarily so spontaneously undertaken [as in traditional "heat of passion"]. Rather, it may be that a significant mental trauma has affected a defendant's mind for a substantial period of time, simmering in the unknowing subconscious and then inexplicably coming to the fore. The difference between the present New York statute and its predecessor and its ancient Maine analogue can be explained by the tremendous advances made in psychology. . . and a willingness of the courts, legislators, and public to reduce the level of responsibility imposed on those whose capacity has been diminished by mental trauma."

The British Homicide Act of 1957 [5 & 6 Eliz II, Ch. 11, Sec. 2(1)], applied in the trials of Sandie Smith and Christine English, includes a pure diminished-responsibility defense. It states that a person is guilty of manslaughter rather than murder if:

"he was suffering from such abnormality of mind (whether arising from a condition of arrested or retarded development of mind or any inherent causes or induced by disease or injury) as substantially impaired his mental responsibility for his acts and omissions in doing or being a party to the killing."

Whatever its drafters' intent, the phrase "mental responsibility" expresses a moral concept, not a psychiatric one. Responsibility is not a psychiatric status; it is susceptibility to moral blame or legal guilt. The British statute seems to state that any mental disorder (or other "abnormality") that makes a killer much less blameworthy than a normal killer reduces the charge. Both the English and the Model Penal Code provision apply only to homicide; general statutory rules reducing charges for abnormal defendants do not exist in Anglo-American law. There is, however, a general diminished-responsibility provision in the German Criminal Code (Sec. 21; see Kadish & Paulsen, 1975, p. 612).

Should PMS qualify as a "reasonable explanation or excuse" for "extreme emotional disturbance," or as "substantially impairing mental responsibility"? For n-PMS, the answer seems to be no on both counts. There is no evidence that the Model Penal Code drafters or the legislatures of states like New York intended to immunize ordinary premenstrual women against murder convictions. In the British Homicide Act, the phrase "abnormality of mind" is plausibly taken to exclude such women as well. *Regina v. Byrne* (1960, 2 Q.B. 396,403) defined "abnormality of mind" to include any "state of mind so different from that of ordinary human beings that the reasonable man would term it abnormal." p-PMS, as described by its advocates, seems to fit this definition, but not n-PMS. Given the current extraordinary sensitivity to women's status, a conferral of special criminal immunities on all or most women should be made explicitly by legislatures. On the ethical merits, n-PMS has little exonerative appeal for obvious reasons about to be mentioned.

p-PMS — if it exists — can sensibly be called a mental abnormality, and can be viewed as an aspect of the offender's subjective situation creating a "reasonable explanation or excuse" if other mental abnormalities are similarly viewed. To admit PMS under either formula while excluding ordinary psychopathology seems unjust to the ordinary abnormal defendant, unless, as queried above, p-PMS is organic and organic disorders are stronger excuses. But if English courts include sexual psychopathy as a mental abnormality reducing sex murder to manslaughter, the mental tension of a severe PMS sufferer may be similarly irresistible.[26]

The two primary questions of ethics and legal policy appear to be these. First, does p-PMS rise to a "substantial" enough level of irrationality or emotional dyscontrol for an immunity to guilt for murder? As earlier suggested, the chief moral significance of psychopathology short of insanity is that it is innocent mental disturbance. But other sources of equivalent mental disturbance may be equally innocent — unemployment, marital discord, separation, physical illness, poverty — and the basis of criminal law is threatened if these innocent stressors substantially excuse persons from controlling their behavior in spite of them. Second, diminished-responsibility provisions pose the issue of whether virtually all killers can be given a psychiatric diagnosis. Categories such as explosive personality or psychopathy (intermittent explosive disorder and antisocial personality disorder, DSM-III) — not to mention DSM-I's (1952) "dyssocial" personality, a category tailor-made for members of organized crime — make one wonder whether the Homicide Act of 1957 allows the crime of murder to occur at all. In the language of *Wolff*, surely no professional killer can "maturely and meaningfully reflect on the gravity" of murder for hire, realize the "enormity of [its] evil," or commit the crime in other than a "materially vague and detached" frame of mind. A person who could so reflect would not be a hit man; few psychiatrists would diagnose hit men as having a normal personality.

Thus, while p-PMS may fit diminished responsibility, it may do so at the cost of destroying such fundamental legal concepts as the existence of murder. Diminished responsibility threatens the collapse of homicide in the same way as the *Durham* rule threatens the collapse of all criminal law. While some moralists welcome this result, others wish to accommodate the moral significance of mental disorder by less drastic means. A crucial question in this debate is whether physical disorders are stronger excuses than mental disorders. If defendants with pheochromocytoma, pellagra, or hypothyroidism are less culpable than defendants with psychopathy, sexual sadism, or explosive personality — are less responsible for their disorders or less responsible for controlling their effects — then the relevance of p-PMS to criminal guilt importantly depends on whether it is a "hormonal disease." On the other hand, if physical versus mental causation of emotional turmoil or character defect is morally irrelevant, then even p-PMS as a basis for immunity to murder may owe more to medical mythagogy than to rational legal policy.

Mitigation of Sentence

Generally speaking, courts have wide discretion in punishing crimes. Although statutes specify minimum and maximum sentences for an offense, judges use aggravating or mitigating circumstances to place an individual defendant's sentence within that range, and may also suspend sentence. A defendant's penalty may be mitigated by youth, lack of prior criminal record, position in the community, laudable motives, or — for present purposes — physical or mental abnormality.

---

26 In *Regina v. Byrne*, the court held that its definition covers a sexual psychopath's inability "to exercise will-power to control his physical acts" in killing and mutilating his victim. This is an example of diminished responsibility based on a concept of irresistible impulse.

Reducing punishment because of medical disorder is a kind of diminished responsibility approach, but an informal one that occurs after trial.[27]

Presumably, *ceteris paribus,* a crime partly caused by a blameless medical disorder is less culpable than a crime not influenced by a comparable innocent cause. (It is not obvious that medical disorders short of insanity have greater excusing power than other innocent necessary conditions of crime.) To the extent that criminal punishment rests on moral guilt — the modern *retributive* theory of punishment — abnormal defendants should be punished less severely for a crime than normal ones without comparable innocent excuses. This does not mean that they should not be punished at all. On the retributive view, criminal conviction reflects a moral judgment that the defendant is partly at fault for not resisting her disorder and behaving lawfully in spite of it. If the disorder is so severe that no one could reasonably be expected to resist it, the defendant should be acquitted of any crime, as in the insanity defense. In a penal system based on moral guilt, then, abnormal offenders normally deserve punishment, although less than normal offenders lacking similar excuses. What is senseless is to "double-count" the abnormality by first reducing the charge and then reducing the sentence as well. That procedure implicitly rejects substantive criminal law's grading of the crimes themselves.

The other major theories of punishment are *consequentialist* (or, broadly, *utilitarian*), justifying punishment by its beneficial social effects. These effects include crime prevention via *incapacitation* of the offender; *special deterrence* of the offender himself after punishment; *general deterrence* of other potential criminals; and perhaps moral *reform* of the offender and moral *education* of the public (LaFave & Scott, 1972, pp. 271-273). [The philosophical literature on punishment is vast; for a brief introduction, see Benn (1967, Vol. 7, pp. 29-36).] Utilitarians since Bentham (1970, p. 161) have argued that punishing mentally abnormal persons fails to serve most of these purposes and is therefore useless suffering. A clear exception is incapacitation (in prison), which protects the public against normals and abnormals alike. For PMS defendants, Taylor and Dalton (1983, p. 286) suggest confinement in a medical facility for the 8-day paramenstruum, with freedom the remainder of the month.

Special deterrence is classically argued to fail for the insane offender because he is too cognitively or too emotionally impaired to calculate rationally the costs of further crime. However, this argument does not apply to defendants with lesser impairments. Except for the possibility of PMS psychosis, a woman with even p-PMS seems psychologically intact enough for past punishment to aid her self-control.

General deterrence is classically said to fail for insane defendants because normal persons, not viewing themselves as insane, do not identify with them. To exempt the insane from punishment is therefore, from a utilitarian standpoint, cost-free. Whether or not this is a good argument for grossly psychotic offenders, it is wholly unconvincing for offenders with lesser pathology. It is incredible that potential normal criminals not only distinguish themselves from abnormal ones, but do so so easily and with such confidence in courts' agreement that they suffer no extra fear at abnormals' punishment. The argument is even worse

---

[27] An extreme example of using mental disorder to mitigate punishment is Clarence Darrow's "insanity defense" for Leopold and Loeb, which was conducted entirely at a post-trial penalty hearing (August 22, 23, and 25, 1923).

for a condition such as PMS, where much of the public believes (however wrongly) both that PMS is a criminal excuse and that almost all women have it. Commentators favorable to PMS excuses ignore both this problem and general deterrence itself. A broader general deterrence issue is the weakening of all criminal sanctions by celebrated cases where the law is seen as irrationally or unjustly merciful. Rightly or wrongly, cases like those of John Hinckley, Dan White, and Christine English generate contempt for law itself and thereby limit whatever deterrent effect comes from the endorsement of law by conscience.

In sum, a moral desert view of punishment justifies leniency for non-psychotic abnormal offenders, including women with p-PMS, but not when such leniency is already built into substantive law via diminished responsibility. Utilitarian views of punishment have much more trouble justifying a general rule of mitigation, and their apparent sacrifice of general deterrence to mitigation is especially dangerous for defendants with PMS and similar disorders whom the public perceives as just like themselves. On neither approach can one agree with Carney and Williams that "Under no circumstances should courts punish a defendant for PMS-induced conduct" (Carney & Williams, 1983, p. 267).[28] On the contrary, both retributive and consequentialist views suggest that typical p-PMS defendants deserve punishment, while n-PMS defendants do not even deserve mitigation.

THE ADMISSIBILITY OF PREMENSTRUAL SYNDROME EVIDENCE

The above analysis of PMS as a criminal defense ignores the issue of the scientific status of PMS research — an issue that may render the results of the analysis moot. Under standard rules for novel scientific evidence, including expert psychiatric testimony, PMS is of dubious admissibility.

The first standard requirement for any evidence is relevance to a legal issue in the trial. Evidence is relevant if it tends to make a legally significant fact more probable or less probable (McCormick, 1972, p. 437; see also Federal Rules of Evidence 401). As described above, some mental symptoms reported by PMS patients and their physicians are themselves legally relevant facts, with respect to *mens rea* elements of some crimes or to insanity or diminished responsibility. Testimony about PMS and its effects on a given woman, therefore, is certainly sometimes relevant if true.

---

[28] Apodaca and Fink (1984, p. 65) also conclude, "Imprisoning a defendant who is suffering from PMS when the crime was committed fails to accomplish any one of these purposes [of punishment in American law]." In a footnote, they concede that imprisonment does serve the purpose of prevention by incapacitation; their real objection is the injustice of punishing crimes caused by hormonal disorder. Their position agrees with Taylor and Dalton (1983, pp. 284-286). These writers' discussions of punishing PMS women have two flaws. First, they minimize the importance of degrees of causal influence and the possibility that punishing PMS women is partly deserved (retribution) and can strengthen their self control (special deterrence). Second, they wholly ignore general deterrence, arguably the strongest utilitarian reason for punishment. Brahams' argument (1983) that PMS defendants should not be imprisoned because of prison overcrowding is a general argument against punishing any new defendant and needs no serious rebuttal.

Three traditional requirements for expert testimony, jointly called the *Dyas* test, concern lay competence, witness qualifications, and the state of the science [McCormick, 1972, pp. 29-31; *Dyas v. U.S.*, 1977, 376 A.2d 827,832 (D.C.), *cert. denied*, 434 U.S. 973]:

(1) The subject matter "must be so distinctively related to some science, profession, business, or occupation as to be beyond the ken of the average layman."

(2) The expert witness "must have sufficient skill, knowledge, or experience in that field or calling" that "his opinion or inference will probably aid the trier in his search for truth."

(3) "The state of the pertinent art or scientific knowledge" must not be such that it "does not permit a reasonable opinion to be asserted even by the expert."

Although some effects of the menstrual cycle are within the average layman's ken, no male has experienced the cycle and most women have not experienced p-PMS. Again assuming the truth of claims about p-PMS by researchers such as Dalton, expert testimony to this effect supplements lay knowledge and therefore satisifies condition (1). Condition (2) is no more problematic for PMS than for other medical or psychological disorders.

The difficulty with admitting PMS evidence is condition (3), the state of the science. Until recently, the standard test for novel science has been the *Frye* "general acceptance" test. The *Frye* rule was stated by a Federal appeals court in 1923 in excluding a lie detector test [*Frye v. U.S.*, 1923, 293 F. 1013 (D.C. Cir.)]. Since then, it has been used to exclude a variety of criminalistic techniques: voice spectrography [*U.S. v. Addison*, 1974, 498 F.2d 741,745 (D.C. Cir.)]; hair analysis [*U.S. v. Brady*, 1979, 595 F.2d 359, 362-3 (6th Cir.), *cert. denied*, 444 U.S. 862]; psycholinguistic text analysis [*U.S. v. Hearst*, 412 F.Supp. 893 (N.D. Cal. 1976) (Hearst II), *aff'd*, 563 F.2d 1331 (9th Cir. 1977)]; and some psychological diagnoses (battered woman syndrome) [*State v. Thomas*, 1981, 423 N.E. 2d 137; *Buhrle v. State*, 1981, 627 P.2d 1374, 1376-1378 (Wyo.)]. The *Frye* court wrote (293 F. 1014):

> "Just when a scientific principle or discovery crosses the line between the experimental and demonstrable stages is difficult to define. Somewhere in this twilight zone the evidential force of the principle must be recognized, and while the courts will go a long way in admitting expert testimony deduced from a well-recognized scientific principle or discovery, the thing from which the deduction is made must be sufficiently established to have gained general acceptance in the particular field to which it belongs."

The *Frye* rule that a piece of novel science pass beyond the "experimental" stage to general acceptance by the relevant scientific community was intended to be conservative, and it is attacked or defended for its conservatism by commentators. [More examples of the *Frye* rule in action and discussion of arguments for and against it can be found in Giannelli (1980); see also Dixon (1979); Moennsen (1984); Minton (1980).] How strict or loose it is in practice depends on how "general acceptance" and "scientific community" are defined. The proportion of experts in a given field who must accept the technique or theory has never been clearly stated. Most courts do not require unanimity [*Reed v. State*, 1978, 391 A.2d 364; *U.S. v. Addison*, 1974,

498 F.2d 741,745 (D.C. Cir.)], an impossible standard in scientific work, but seem instead to require a substantial majority. Still more uncertain is what "field" to classify a novel technique or theory into. At one extreme, if one tests general acceptance among practitioners of the new theory or technique themselves — polygraphy among polygraphers — acceptance is immediate. At the other extreme, if one requires acceptance by most workers in a broad discipline to which a theory belongs, such as medicine or psychology, then general acceptance is delayed by members who have no information about it. General acceptance by this standard is especially difficult if one includes all the fields the technique could be said to touch, such as physiology, psychology, linguistics, and electronics for a lie detector [*People v. King*, 1968, 266 Cal. App. 2d 437 (voiceprints)].

For novel mental disorders — e.g., post-traumatic stress disorder (see Erlinder, 1984; Ford, 1983; Packer, 1983),[29] rape trauma syndrome (see Buchele & Buchele, 1985; Massaro, 1985),[30] battered woman syndrome (see Blackman & Brickman, 1984; Cross, 1982; Thar, 1982; Walter, 1982),[31] and PMS — the relevant scientific community seems clear. Presumably, it consists of specialists in mental disorders; i.e., psychiatrists and clinical psychologists. The biomedical fields of endocrinology and gynecology are heavily involved in PMS research, since the cyclicity of the disorder lies in female endocrine glands. But since only the mental effects of PMS are legally relevant, it seems important to the goals of *Frye* to insist on general acceptance by specialists in mental disorder. Gynecologists, endocrinologists, internists, etc., have by training no more than an average physician's knowledge of mental processes, which should not be enough for expert testimony about legally crucial states of mind. As with any novelty, taking the relevant scientific group to be PMS researchers tends to nullify the test, since most researchers on any phenomenon are intellectually and professionally committed at least to its existence and importance.

---

[29] See also Note entitled, "Post-traumatic stress disorder as an insanity defense in Vermont," *Vermont Law Review 9:* 69-100, 1984.

[30] See also Note entitled, "The admissibility of expert testimony on rape trauma syndrome," *Journal of Criminal Law and Criminology 75:* 1366-1416, 1984; and "Expert testimony on rape trauma syndrome: admissibility and effective use in criminal rape prosecution," *American University Law Review 33:* 417-462, 1984.

[31] See also Notes entitled, "Criminal law — evidence — expert testimony relating to subject matter of battered women admissible on issue of self-defense," *Seton Hall Law Review 11:* 255-264, 1980; "Use of expert testimony in the defense of battered women," *University of Colorado Law Review 52:* 587-599, 1981; "Evidence: admitting expert testimony on the battered woman syndrome," *Washburn Law Journal 21:* 689-697, 1982; "Admissibility of expert testimony on the battered woman syndrome in support of a claim of self-defense," *Connecticut Law Review 15:* 121-139, 1982; "Expert testimony on the battered woman syndrome: a question of admissibility in the prosecution of the battered wife for the killing of her husband," *St. Louis University Law Journal 27:* 407-435, 1983; "A woman, a horse, and a hickory tree: the development of expert testimony on the battered woman syndrome in a homicide case," *University of Missouri at Kansas City Law Review 53:* 386-410, 1985; and "Battered women, straw men, and expert testimony: a comment on *State v. Kelly*," *Criminal Law Bulletin 21:* 125-155, 1985.

If the *Frye* rule is interpreted as suggested, no consensus exists on legally relevant mental symptoms of PMS. Within the NSF-EVIST Conference, much skepticism was voiced about the claims of advocates such as Katharina Dalton. Much of her data has been questioned on the basis of her lack of double-blind controlled trials. Among PMS researchers, there is wide disbelief in primary premenstrual psychosis, dissociative or automatistic states, hypoglycemia, and even in the actual versus reported severity of emotional distress. It is doubtful that most of the Conference participants supported any important role for PMS as a criminal excuse. At best, most researchers believe that p-PMS causes extreme emotional tension in a small minority of women. The larger mental health community of psychiatrists and psychologists is even less convinced of PMS-based mental disturbances that rise to the level of legal excuse. Thus, applying *Frye* to PMS means that PMS evidence is admissible only to show extreme emotional stress for the common-sense negation of *mens rea* elements and inadmissible otherwise.

The *Frye* test has been much criticized for excessive conservatism. An alternative "relevancy" approach has been followed by many courts and is argued by some to be incorporated in the Federal Rules of Evidence (see Giannelli, 1980, pp. 1228–1229). This approach, associated with McCormick, calls for balancing the probative value of the evidence against the dangers of admitting it, such as unfair prejudice, confusion of the issues, deception of the jury, or waste of time. It is hard to see, however, how probative value ("relevancy") of the evidence can be separated from its scientific reliability (Giannelli, 1980, p. 1235: "The probative value of scientific evidence. . . is connected inextricably to its reliability"); and the scientific reliability of novel psychiatric diagnoses can only be judged by scientists; i.e., by degree of acceptance. The issue between the two approaches should therefore be how much acceptance by the scientific community is required for admitting new medical science.

The most radical view is to admit any novel theory endorsed by a qualified physician or psychologist, and in practice some courts follow this rule. In its favor is the basic intellectual principle that truth emerges from the clash of all points of view, which provides a strong bias toward considering any possibly reliable evidence. Clearly, a general acceptance standard sometimes deprives a defendant of true evidence merely because its truth is not yet known by the witness's peers, and thus results in a false conviction. [This is the problem for novel psychiatric diagnoses, which are usually introduced by the defense. *Frye* causes the opposite problem — undeserved acquittals — for novel criminalistic science, which is usually introduced by the prosecution.] Conversely, defendants who benefit from false novel testimony are falsely acquitted. For the following two reasons, it seems likely that the proposed radical policy will lead to far more false acquittals than *Frye* does false convictions.

First, the volume of partly or wholly unsubstantiated medical theories is enormous even among serious investigators. The record of research on any mental disorder, such as schizophrenia, homosexuality, alcoholism, or PMS, shows countless unverified causal hypotheses, not to mention major changes in the description and classification of the disorder itself. The inevitable confusion, missteps, and false starts of empirical science are compounded in medicine and psychology by the major problem of unscrupulous researchers. Medicine is rife with diet doctors and renegade M.D.'s hawking megavitamins, herbal medicine, foot reflexology, iridology, Eastern religion, and other forms of "holistic" and cultist medicine (Stalker & Glymour, 1985).[32] The mental health disciplines are scarcely any more successful in silencing frivolous practitioners.

At the same time, where medical testimony bears on a *mens rea* element of the crime, the burden of disproving it beyond reasonable doubt must fall on the prosecution (*In re Winship*, 1970, 297 U.S. 358). But this is a logically impossible burden when an expert testifies to a crucial fact about a defendant's state of mind. A juror confronting a qualified expert's testimony has only three alternatives: (i) the evidence is reasonable; (ii) the expert is unreasonable; or (iii) the expert does not believe or understand his own testimony. But a juror cannot be justified in believing an expert unreasonable in his field of expertise, since the juror's ignorance of that field is the reason for expert testimony in the first place. Cases were a juror could be justified in conclusion (iii) are hard to imagine. Thus, as a matter of logic, given the *Winship* rule on burden of proof, testimony by an expert which, if true, disproves a mental element of crime should force acquittal.

Combining the two points, it is likely that for almost any mental element, some M.D. somewhere exists who will testify to its absence; but then the proposed liberal admissibility rule forces acquittal for any crime. Hypoglycemia and unconsciousness alone will do the trick. These considerations suggest some version of a *Frye* general acceptance test as essential to admissibility. In that case, for the moment, PMS evidence should be excluded except on the issue of emotional tension. On the other hand, if general acceptance is relaxed for any controversial diagnosis such as PMS, reliability mandates vigorous attacks on defense experts via cross examination and contrary experts. On no view of the search for truth ought an uncontradicted PMS defense be allowed to carry the day without prosecutorial opposition.

RECENT PREMENSTRUAL SYNDROME CASES REVISITED

In light of this analysis, the four cases cited above (*Craddock*, *Smith*, *English*, and *Santos*) in which PMS aided the defendant are multiply flawed. First, by the traditional American rules of admissibility of novel science, in none of the four cases ought PMS evidence to have been admitted. Neither Craddock-Smith, English, nor Santos contended merely that she had an emotional storm that negated a *mens rea* element. Santos' attorney planned a plea of automatism related to hypoglycemia, an effect of PMS as to which scientific consensus does not exist. Smith and English used PMS as an abnormality showing "substantial impairment" of responsibility, which presumably requires a clear distinction between their p-PMS and the premenstrual symptoms of ordinary women, as well as a clear description of how these mental symptoms made a major contribution to the crime. On neither issue are PMS researchers agreed, much less the mental health

---

32 An example of questionable medical theories influencing a criminal case is the murder trial of Dan White of April 24-May 22, 1979. White, who had killed a popular San Francisco mayor and city supervisor, successfully pled diminished capacity, in part on the basis of a "Twinkie defense" (gorging on junk food). A brief discussion of the trial and its medical testimony can be found in Hardyman (1978-79). The "Twinkie defense" was a major factor in California voters' rejection of diminished capacity by Proposition 8 [1982 Cal. Legis. Sess. 1164 (West)].

community. The *Frye* rule leads naturally to the result reached by Judge Gueck in *Irvin*. PMS evidence for Smith and English, as for other British defendants, was extraordinarily dependent on one practitioner, Katharina Dalton, whose claims about mental and criminogenic effects of PMS are widely regarded as extreme.

Second, in the three British cases, there is little evidence of a vigorous prosecution attempt to impeach defense experts. If PMS testimony is admitted, the uncertain state of research demands aggressive cross examination and contrary testimony by skeptical experts. Accounts of these trials mention a prosecution expert only in *English*, a psychiatrist who subsequently wrote to *The Lancet* defending the result (d'Orban, 1981; see also d'Orban, 1983; d'Orban & J. Dalton, 1980). Rebuttal evidence from different PMS researchers might have considerably reduced the force of Dalton's testimony in the *Craddock/Smith* and *English* cases.

Third, as contrary experts might have testified, the possibility of primary conventional psychopathology in defendants Craddock/Smith and English was real. Craddock/Smith would have been diagnosed by other psychiatrists as a psychopath, and her paranoid ideas about the policeman might even suggest an underlying psychosis. English's life was filled with violence long before she killed her lover, not only in her choice of a violent alcoholic lover, but also in a suicide attempt. No dynamically oriented psychiatrist would ignore the masochism in her personality. Emphasis on her suppressed violence, with or without a criminal sentence, might have aided English in achieving a degree of self-insight denied by attributing her sudden killing to raging hormones.

Fourth, in *Craddock* and *English*, PMS was apparently used not only to reduce murder to manslaughter, but also to avoid all punishment. This double-counting in effect nullifies the conviction; indeed, it leaves the defendant better off than after a successful plea of insanity, a doctrinally inexplicable result. Similarly, the appeals court in *Smith* rejected PMS as a substantive defense, yet approved probation under medical supervision for a woman with countless prior criminal convictions, including a homicide. Again, this result is a *de facto* insanity acquittal, but releases into society a defendant of proven dangerousness on the basis of a scientifically naive faith in progesterone therapy.

The British cases rest on a simplistic model of PMS and crime containing the following assumptions: (i) PMS is a hormone deficiency disease; (ii) this hormone deficiency alone causes severe temporary psychopathology; (iii) such psychopathology alone causes crime; (iv) PMS hormone deficiency is cured by progesterone therapy; and (v) it is unjust to punish crime caused by a treatable hormone disorder. Each of these assumptions is questioned above and elsewhere in this volume. Although PMS symptoms may have a hormonal cause, present evidence indicates it is not a progesterone deficiency, and progesterone treatment is either ineffective or may work by suppressing the menstrual cycle and tranquilizing the patient. PMS defendants may have other primary psychopathology; or their crimes may result from culpable character defects triggered by premenstrual stress, in which case punishment is appropriate on any penal theory.

Finally, for several reasons, the *Santos* case, despite its wide publicity, deserves no respect as a precedent. The use of PMS in a plea bargain meant that the defense was not presented at trial, where prosecution rebuttal and judicial analysis could occur. No written opinion was issued by the judge; his recorded comment that physical disorders as well as mental disorders should be relevant to criminal guilt merely restates settled law. Most troubling is the potential of defense attorney Benson's automatism argument to acquit virtually all defendants. If suitable medical testimony proves reasonable doubt about consciousness, any well represented defendant can, in principle, find an irresponsible physician to certify his "blackout" — the classic plea of the guilty offender.

It therefore seems appropriate for future courts to treat all PMS issues as matters of first impression, giving as little weight as possible to *Craddock, Smith, English,* and *Santos*. A thorough analysis of PMS in a criminal trial has yet to occur in either Great Britain or America. On the contrary, the heavy media exposure of these cases, together with their grave inherent defects, is a classic portrait of how not to establish a new criminal defense.

CONCLUSIONS

(1) The existence of PMS as a syndrome is controversial, as well as its prevalence, clinical features, etiology, and therapy. Despite broad consensus that most premenstrual women experience at least one of a group of physical and mental complaints, a unitary entity PMS may or may not exist. If it exists, it may need subclassification in unknown ways.

(2) Two conceptions of PMS require sharp distinction — normal PMS (n-PMS), which affects up to 90% of menstruating women, and severe or pathologic PMS (p-PMS), which affects a small minority. This distinction may calm the debate over PMS criminal defenses. PMS as a defense for all premenstrual women — universal monthly female insanity — is absurd and advocated by no PMS researcher.

(3) The distinction between n-PMS and p-PMS is currently arbitrary and rests on women's self-reports. Until biological markers or clear psychiatric deficits separate these two groups, it is uncertain whether they differ merely in self-perception or self-description. *A fortiori,* it is unclear whether women with p-PMS differ from normal women physiologically, psychologically, or both.

(4) Except for such uncertainties, there is no conceptual problem in calling p-PMS a medical disorder. Under the usual view of medical excuses in law, the exculpatory force of PMS depends simply on its mental symptoms, not on whether their pathogenesis is physiological or psychological.

(5) Data on increased premenstrual crime show, at most, a weak causal influence of menstrual events on crime. The strength of such influence and of currently known hormonal changes is no greater for PMS than for many other factors favoring crime; e.g., weather, fatigue, hunger, unemployment, separation, etc.

(6) At present, the only clear relevance of PMS to criminal defense is to corroborate emotional turmoil negating *mens rea* elements, especially premeditation or intent. Enough consensus exists on premenstrual emotionality for such expert testimony to be admissible under the *Frye* rule. Such a use of PMS is a slight, but only a slight, extension of common sense about menstruating women.

(7) If genuine, the most extreme reported premenstrual mental symptoms — psychosis and dissociative states — justify traditional insanity and automatism defenses. Insufficient consensus exists on PMS psychosis or dissociation for such testimony to pass the *Frye* test.

(8) In relevant jurisdictions, p-PMS reasonably qualifies for diminished responsibility (e.g., for the Model Penal Code "extreme emotional disturbance" or Britain's Homicide Act) if the same treatment is given to other non-psychotic mental and physical disorders. But the proviso threatens the foundations of criminal law. Again, there is insufficient consensus under *Frye*.

(9) Convicted PMS defendants should normally be punished. One reason is that available therapies are unproven. Another is that standard moral theories suggest that conviction, even of abnormal offenders, should normally entail punishment. The moral assumption of the *Durham* rule — that "but-for" causation of crime by disease negates moral guilt — is untenable.

(10) As is often observed, procedures are needed for judicial-medical control of defendants who use abnormalities to reduce guilt under diminished responsibility. Via civil commitment or otherwise, medical disorders serious enough to excuse crime are serious enough for court supervision.

(11) Admissibility of novel psychiatric diagnoses — e.g., rape trauma syndrome, battered woman syndrome, compulsive gambling, and PMS — might be much clarified by a committee of the American Psychiatric Association (or a joint APA-ABA committee) charged with assessing new syndromes. Courts are poorly equipped to judge scientific consensus and even less competent to judge novel science. As essays on PMS demonstrate, the problem is compounded by medical credulity and anti-prosecution bias on the part of legal commentators.

(12) If PMS is admitted in a criminal trial, psychiatrists must investigate conventional primary psychopathology. Defendants Smith and English might have been diagnosed with primary mental disorders, with PMS as an aggravating factor. Demoting PMS to a secondary diagnosis or cyclic stressor eases legal uncertainties about its status, reduces its mystery, and thereby can improve public confidence in law.

(13) In sum, PMS merits further medical and legal debate, but public controversy over PMS defenses is overblown. Few new legal issues are involved, only the application of familiar rules of responsibility to a poorly understood cyclic phenomenon in a small minority of women. Public controversy rests partly on confusing n-PMS with p-PMS, and partly on a handful of indefensible court cases. At this point, in criminal law, PMS has no monumental implications for feminism or the status of women.

REFERENCES

Abraham, G. E., 1980. Premenstrual tension. *Current Problems in Obstetrics and Gynecology 3:* 5-39.

Allen, J., 1982. Premenstrual frenzy. *New York,* November 1, pp. 36-42.

Altschule, M. D. and J. Brem, 1963. Periodic psychosis of puberty. *American Journal of Psychiatry 119:* 1176-1178.

Angier, N. and J. Witzleben, 1982. Dr. Jekyll and Ms. Hyde. *Discover,* November, pp. 28-34.

Apodaca, L. and L. Fink, 1984. Criminal law: Premenstrual syndrome in the courts. *Washburn Law Journal 24:* 54-77.

Arenella, P., 1977. The diminished capacity and diminished responsibility defenses: Two children of a doomed marriage. *Columbia Law Review 77:* 827-865.

Aristotle (translated by M. Ostwald), 1962. *Nicomachean Ethics, Book III, Chapter 1.* Bobbs-Merrill Co., Indianapolis, IN.
Benn, S. I., 1967. Punishment. In: P. Edwards (Ed.), *Encyclopedia of Philosophy, Vol. 7.* Macmillan, New York, NY, pp. 29-36.
Bentham, J. (J. H. Burns and H.L.A. Hart, eds.), 1970. *An Introduction to the Principles of Morals and Legislation [1789].* Athlone Press, London.
Berlin, F. S., G. K. Bergey, and J. Money, 1983. Periodic psychosis of puberty: A case report. *American Journal of Psychiatry 139:* 119-120.
Blackman, J. and E. Brickman, 1984. The impact of expert testimony on trials of battered women who kill their husbands. *Behavioral Science and Law 2:* 413-422.
Bloom, J. and J. Atkinson, 1983. *Evidence of Love.* Bantam Books, New York, NY.
Brahams, D., 1983. Epilepsy and legal insanity: *R. v. Sullivan. The Practitioner 227:* 421-423.
Brahams, D., 1983. Premenstrual tension and criminal responsibility. *The Practitioner 227:* 807-813.
Buchele, B. J. and J. P. Buchele, 1985. Legal and psychological issues in the use of expert testimony on rape trauma syndrome. *Washburn Law Journal 25:* 26-42.
Carney, R. M. and B. D. Williams, 1983. Recent decisions: Criminal law — premenstrual syndrome: a criminal defense. *Notre Dame Law Review 59:* 253-269.
Chambers, M., 1982. Menstrual stresses as a legal defense. *New York Times*, May 29, p. 46.
Clark, M. and D. Shapiro, 1981. The monthly syndrome. *Newsweek*, May 4, p. 74.
Cohen, S. S., 1981. The premenstrual syndrome. *Mademoiselle*, October, pp. 57-58.
Cross, M. B., 1982. The expert as educator: A proposed approach to the use of battered woman syndrome expert testimony. *Vanderbilt Law Review 35:* 741-768.
Cumming, C., 1984. Singing the PMS blues. *Women's Sports*, January, p. 54.
Dalton, K., 1979. *Once A Month.* Hunter House, Pomona, CA.
Dalton, K., 1982. Legal implications of PMS. *World Medicine*, April 17, pp. 93-94.
Dalton, K., 1984. *The Premenstrual Syndrome and Progesterone Therapy* (second edition). Year Book Medical Publishers, Chicago, IL.
Dennerstein, L., F. Judd, and B. Davies, 1983. Psychosis and the menstrual cycle. *Medical Journal of Australia 1:* 524-526.
Diamond, B. L., 1956. Isaac Ray and the trial of Daniel M'Naghten. *American Journal of Psychiatry 112:* 651-656.
Dixon, P. H., 1979. Evidence — admissibility of evidence — *Frye* standard of "general acceptance" for admissibility of scientific evidence rejected in favor of balancing test [*U.S. v. Williams*]. *Cornell Law Review 64:* 875-885.
d'Orban, P. T., 1981. Premenstrual syndrome: A disease of the mind? *The Lancet 2:* 1413.
d'Orban, P. T., 1983. Medicolegal aspects of premenstrual syndrome. *British Journal of Hospital Medicine 30:* 404-409.
d'Orban, P. T. and J. Dalton, 1980. Violent crime and the menstrual cycle. *Psychological Medicine 10:* 353-359.
Eagan, A. B., 1983. The selling of premenstrual syndrome. *Ms.*, October, p. 26.
Endo, M., M. Daiguji, Y. Asano, I. Yamashita, and S. Takahashi, 1978. Periodic psychosis recurring in association with menstrual cycle. *Journal of Clinical Psychiatry 39:* 456-466.

Erlinder, C. P., 1984. Paying the price for Vietnam: Post-traumatic stress disorder and criminal behavior. *British Columbia Law Review 25:* 305-347.
Fingarette, H., 1972. *The Meaning of Criminal Insanity.* University of California Press, Berkeley, CA.
Fingarette, H. and A. F. Hasse, 1979. *Mental Disabilities and Criminal Responsibility.* University of California Press, Berkeley, CA.
Ford, J. R., 1983. In defense of the defenders: The Vietnam vet syndrome. *Criminal Law Bulletin 19:* 434-441.
Frank, R. T., 1931. The hormonal causes of premenstrual tension. *Archives of Neurology and Psychiatry 26:* 1053-1054.
Gaylin, W., 1982. *The Killing of Bonnie Garland: A Question of Justice.* Simon and Schuster, New York, NY.
Giannelli, P. C., 1980. The admissibility of novel scientific evidence: *Frye v. U.S.*, a half-century later. *Columbia Law Review 80:* 1197-1250.
Glick, I. D. and D. Stewart, 1980. A new drug treatment for premenstrual exacerbation of schizophrenia. *Comprehensive Psychiatry 21:* 281-287.
Goldstein, A., 1967. *The Insanity Defense.* Yale University Press, New Haven, CT.
Gonzalez, E. R., 1981. Premenstrual syndrome: An ancient woe deserving of modern scrutiny. *Journal of the American Medical Association 245:* 1393.
Gray, C., 1981. Raging female hormones in the courts. *Maclean's* June 15, pp. 46-49.
Hall, J., 1960. *General Principles of Criminal Law* (second edition). Bobbs-Merrill Co., Indianapolis, IN.
Hardyman, D., 1978-79. The diminished capacity defense in California: An idea whose time has gone? *Glendale Law Review 3:* 311-321.
Heneson, N., 1984. The selling of PMS. *Science 84*, May, pp. 66-71.
Henig, R. M., 1982. Dispelling menstrual myths. *New York Times Magazine*, March 7, pp. 64-65.
Herbert, W., 1982. Premenstrual changes. *Science News*, December 11, pp. 380-381.
Herrmann, D.H.J., 1983. *The Insanity Defense: Philosophical, Historical, and Legal Perspectives.* Charles C. Thomas, Springfield, IL.
Holtzman, E., 1984. Premenstrual syndrome: The indefensible defense. *Harvard Women's Law Journal 7:* 1-3.
Hook, S. (Ed.), 1958. *Determinism and Freedom in the Age of Modern Science.* New York University Press, New York, NY.
Hopson, J. L. and A. Rosenfeld, 1984. PMS: Puzzling monthly symptoms. *Psychology Today*, August, pp. 30-35.
Kadish, S. and M. Paulsen, 1975. *Criminal Law and Its Processes* (third edition). Little, Brown and Co., Boston, MA.
Kane, Jr., F. J., 1980. Postpartum disorders. In: H. I. Kaplan, A. M. Freedman, and B. J. Sadock (Eds.), *Comprehensive Textbook of Psychiatry, Vol. 2.* Williams and Wilkins, Baltimore, MD, pp. 1343-1348.
Kane, Jr., F. J., R. J. Daly, M. H. Wallach, and M. H. Keeler, 1966. Amelioration of premenstrual mood disturbance with a progestational agent (Enovid). *Diseases of the Nervous System 27:* 339-342.
Krausz, F. R., 1983. The relevance of innocence: Proposition 8 and the diminished capacity defense. *California Law Review 71:* 1197-1215.
LaFave, W. R. and A. W. Scott, Jr., 1972. *Criminal Law.* West, St. Paul, MN.
Lauersen, N. and E. Stukane, 1982. Premenstrual syndrome: Can you win the hormone war? *Mademoiselle*, December, pp. 148-149.
Lindman, F. T. and D. M. McIntyre, 1961. *The Mentally Disabled and the Law.* The University of Chicago Press, Chicago, IL.

Massaro, T. M., 1985. Experts, psychology, credibility, and rape: The rape trauma syndrome issue and its implications for expert psychological testimony. *Minnesota Law Review 69:* 395-470.
McCormick, C., 1972. *Handbook of the Law of Evidence* (second edition by E. W. Cleary). West, St. Paul, MN.
McGarrell, E. F. and T. J. Flanagan (Eds.), 1985. *Sourcebook of Criminal Justice Statistics — 1984.* U.S. Department of Justice, Washington, D.C.
Meehl, P., 1977. Specific etiology and other forms of strong influence: Some quantitative meanings. *Journal of Medicine and Philosophy 2:* 33-53.
Minton, L. E., 1980. Expert testimony based on novel scientific techniques: Admissibility under the federal rules of evidence. *George Washington Law Review 48:* 774-790.
Moennsen, A. A., 1984. Admissibility of scientific evidence — an alternative to the *Frye* rule. *William and Mary Law Review 25:* 545-575.
Moore, M. S., 1984. *Law and Psychiatry: Rethinking the Relationship.* Cambridge University Press, Cambridge.
Moos, R. H., 1969. Typology of menstrual cycle symptoms. *American Journal of Obstetrics and Gynecology 103:* 390-402.
Morgenbesser, S. and J. Walsh (Eds.), 1962. *Free Will.* Prentice-Hall, Englewood Cliffs, NJ.
Mulligan, N., 1983. Recent developments: Premenstrual syndrome. *Harvard Women's Law Journal 6:* 219-227.
Murphy, E. A., 1976. *The Logic of Medicine.* Johns Hopkins University Press, Baltimore, MD.
Muse, K. N., N. S. Cetel, L. A. Futterman, and S.S.C. Yen, 1984. The premenstrual syndrome: Effects of 'medical ovariectomy.' *New England Journal of Medicine 311:* 1345-1349.
Norris, R. and C. Sullivan, 1983. *PMS: Premenstrual Syndrome.* Rawson Associates, New York, NY.
O'Donovan, K., 1984. The medicalisation of infanticide. *Criminal Law Review 1984:* 259-264.
O'Roark, M. A., 1981. Your once-a-month mood changes. *McCalls,* July, pp. 12-16.
Ota, Y., T. Mukai, and K. Gotoda, 1954. Studies on the relationship between psychotic symptoms and sexual cycle. *Folia Psychiatria et Neurologica Japonica 8:* 203-217.
Packer, I. K., 1983. Post-traumatic stress disorder and the insanity defense: A critical analysis. *Journal of Psychiatry and Law 11:* 125-136.
Pahl-Smith, C., 1985. Premenstrual syndrome as a criminal defense: The need for a medico-legal understanding. *North Carolina Central Law Journal 15:* 246-273.
Platt, A. and B. L. Diamond, 1966. The origins of the "right and wrong" test of criminal responsibility and its subsequent development: An historical survey. *California Law Review 54:* 1227,
Press, A., 1982. Not guilty because of PMS? *Newsweek,* November 8, p. 111.
Press, M. P., 1983. Premenstrual stress syndrome as a defense in crminal cases. *Duke Law Journal 1983:* 176-195.
Ray, I., 1838. *A Treatise on the Medical Jurisprudence of Insanity.* Little, Brown and Co., Boston, MA.
Reid, R. L., 1985. Premenstrual syndrome. *Current Problems in Obstetrics, Gynecology, and Fertility 8:* 1-57.
Reid, R. L. and S.S.C. Yen, 1981. Premenstrual syndrome. *American Journal of Obstetrics and Gynecology 139:* 85-104.
Reiser, M. and L. Whisnant, 1980. Endocrine disorders. In: H. I. Kaplan, A. M. Freedman, and B. J. Sadock (Eds.), *Comprehensive Textbook of Psychiatry III, Vol. 2.* Williams and Wilkins, Baltimore, MD, pp. 1917-1929.

Robinson, P., 1984. *Criminal Law Defenses.* West, St. Paul, MN.
Rose, E. F., 1970. Criminal responsibility and competency as influenced by organic disease. *Missouri Law Review 35:* 326-348.
Rubinow, D. R. and P. Roy-Byrne, 1984. Premenstrual syndromes: Overview from a methodologic perspective. *American Journal of Psychiatry 141:* 163-172.
Sommer, B., 1984. PMS in the courts: Are all women on trial? *Psychology Today,* August, pp. 36-38.
Stalker, D. and C. Glymour (Eds.), 1985. *Examining Holistic Medicine.* Prometheus, Buffalo, NY.
Steiner, M., R. F. Haskett, and B. J. Carroll, 1980. Premenstrual tension syndrome: The development of research diagnostic criteria and new rating scales. *Acta Psychiatrica Scandinavica 62:* 177-190.
Sutherland, H. and I. Stewart, 1965. A critical analysis of the premenstrual syndrome. *The Lancet 1:* 1180-1183.
Switzer, E., 1983. PMS: The return of raging hormones. *Working Woman,* October, pp. 123-127.
Taylor, L. and K. Dalton, 1983. Premenstrual syndrome: A new criminal defense? *California Western Law Review 19:* 269-287.
Taylor, R., 1967. Determinism. In: P. Edwards (Ed.), *The Encyclopedia of Philosophy, Vol. 2.* Macmillan, New York, NY, pp. 359-373.
Teja, J. S., 1976. Periodic psychosis of puberty. *Journal of Nervous and Mental Disease 162:* 52-57.
Thar, A. E., 1982. The admissibility of expert testimony on battered wife syndrome: An evidentiary analysis. *Northwestern University Law Review 77:* 348-373.
Vinocur, B. A., 1983. Help for premenstrual syndrome. *Saturday Evening Post,* April, pp. 34-37.
Walker, N., 1968. *Crime and Insanity in England, Vol. 1.* Edinburgh University Press, Edinburgh.
Walker, N., 1973. *Crime and Insanity in England, Vol. 2.* Edinburgh University Press, Edinburgh.
Wallach, A. and L. Rubin, 1971. The premenstrual syndrome and criminal responsibility. *UCLA Law Review 19:* 209-311.
Walter, P. D., 1982. Expert testimony and battered women: Conflict among the courts and a proposal. *Journal of Legal Medicine 3:* 267-294.
Weiner, H., 1980. Schizophrenia: Etiology. In: H. I. Kaplan, A. M. Freedman, and B. J. Sadock (Eds.), *Comprehensive Textbook of Psychiatry III, Vol. 2.* Williams and Wilkins, Baltimore, MD, pp. 1121-1152.
Williams, E. Y. and L. R. Weekes, 1952. Premenstrual tension associated with psychotic episodes. *Journal of Nervous and Mental Diseases 116:* 321-329.
Williams, G., 1961. *Criminal Law — The General Part* (second edition). Stevens, London.

CRIMINAL LAW, BIOLOGICAL PSYCHIATRY, AND PREMENSTRUAL SYNDROME: CONFLICTING PERSPECTIVES

C. R. Jeffery, Ph.D.

School of Criminology
Florida State University
Tallahassee, Florida

INTRODUCTION

This paper is primarily devoted to a discussion of premenstrual syndrome (PMS) and its relationship to criminal law and the insanity defense. However, it is not possible to discuss PMS and criminal law without first establishing the exact nature and extent of PMS.

At the Conference on PMS which generated the present volume, several major issues emerged relating to (1) moral, ethical, and legal issues; (2) definitional issues; and (3) research and treatment issues. A very brief discussion of these issues in relation to the major objective of this paper will be undertaken, with the observation that these issues are discussed in other papers in a more complete manner.

PMS involves such moral issues as the medicalization of PMS by labeling PMS a disease, and medical control of men over women by the application of the label "PMS" to some women (see chapters in this volume by Bell, Ericksen, Macklin, and Ruble & Brooks-Gunn). The issue raised is whether the label is a benefit or a burden. Is PMS a normal concomitant of the menstrual cycle, or is it a separate entity and a disease? If a disease, what sort of disease? Is PMS a mental disease, a psychological condition, or a physical disease involving hormones, neurons, and human physiology? Does the label imply paternalism and an assault on the feminist position? Are those suffering from PMS morally irresponsible for their behavior and thus excused for their behavior, or are they legally responsible and thus subject to punishment if they commit a crime? The heart of the legal argument encompasses such moral questions, since if we allow PMS as an excusing condition for those accused of crimes, we must first label, medicalize, and paternalize the women so labeled. Is it better to treat women with PMS or to condemn them? Are they sick people or criminals? Any label of sickness obviously places the labelee in an inferior position and subject to social control by others. If we do not treat the PMS patient, however, then we must resort to a legal/punitive response when she becomes assaultive and aggressive. Our response to behavior depends on whether we classify it as an illness or as criminal behavior.

Definitional issues concern the basic nature and existence of PMS. There is no agreement as to what PMS is or its prevalence in the female population. A consensus definition of PMS has not been agreed upon by endocrinologists, gynecologists, neurologists, or others dealing with it, and this would appear to mean that adequate diagnosis and evaluation of PMS is not possible at this time. The physicians present at the Conference (Halbreich, Norris, O'Brien, Reid, Rubinow, Sampson, Steiner, and Vergare) emphasized the lack of a scientific definition of PMS and the need for further research. In contrast, the psychologists and sociologists (Bell, Ericksen, and Ruble) emphasized the self-reporting approach to PMS, and noted that self reports, like all verbal behavior, are subject to social, cultural, and historical influences. Whether or not a woman reports that she has experienced PMS symptoms is a matter of psychological conditioning and socialization. It would seem that self reports and self-definitional processes cannot be used to indicate the presence or absence of PMS, or to identify PMS cases. We must separate what people say in a cultural context about PMS from what is or is not real about PMS as a biological condition. Such conflicts between psychological and biological approaches to PMS must be resolved before we can establish a scientific definition of PMS.

Research problems where PMS is concerned were emphasized by the medical members of the Conference. Because the concept of PMS has been so closely identified with the medical practice of one person, Dr. Katharina Dalton, PMS has not been adequately defined or researched. Dalton believes in the efficacy of progesterone treatment for PMS, as she defines the syndrome, but her view is not wholly shared by other medical researchers. The placebo effect is most prominent in the case of PMS. The need for placebo studies, double-blind studies, and prospective rather than retrospective studies was emphasized throughout the Conference.

Interdisciplinary research involving biology, psychology, sociology, law, and ethics was highly recommended. Reid discussed Vitamin B deficiencies and the endorphin hypothesis among possible alternative approaches to understanding PMS. Halbreich noted the relationship between PMS and depression, and Steiner emphasized the failure of lithium and prolactin as treatment alternatives to progesterone. Bird noted the need to study the brain in relation to its interactions with hormonal systems in order to build a neurological model of PMS.

We are left with no basic scientific understanding of PMS, nor do we have a proven research design or treatment regime for PMS. A neurological and endocrinological model of PMS is needed to replace the self-report studies and the clinical observations which have constituted one basis for our discussion of PMS so far. Without a basic understanding of the impact of the menstrual cycle on the brain and thus on behavior, we will be unable to discuss ethical and legal aspects of PMS. Much more interdisciplinary discussion and research must be undertaken before we can relate PMS to legal and ethical concerns.

The present chapter will discuss legal criminology versus scientific criminology, and then describe the several different schools of criminology and psychology. Criminal law in relation to biological diseases of the brain, as well as a medical model for the criminal justice system, will be reviewed. Finally, programs and policies for the future will be considered.

CRIMINAL LAW AND HUMAN NATURE

Legal Criminology

Mentalism

The legal position is based on historical precedent and the use of political power and force. The criminal law is based on a mind-body dualism and mentalism. The mental element of the crime is the *mens rea*, whereas the physical behavior is the *actus reus*. The act must be caused by a mental element defined variously as a guilty mind, free will, volition, willful behavior, malicious behavior, or felonious behavior (Low, Jeffries, & Bonnie, 1981). *Mens rea*, like other non-physical events, is not known directly but only indirectly through behavior. If a person behaves like a criminal, it is assumed he/she intended to behave as a criminal. We see criminal behavior and we assume a criminal mind. (For more on *mens rea* and *actus reus*, see chapter by Sadoff, this volume).

The law states that behavior must be voluntary in order to be criminal, and therefore to involve moral responsibility and to warrant punishment. Involuntary behavior is defined as reflexes, convulsions, movements during unconsciousness, coerced movements, muscular contractions, concussions, or somnambulism (Model Penal Code, Section 2.01). The law draws a distinction between voluntary behavior and involuntary behavior, or between behavior caused by the mind and behavior caused by the brain. A muscular contraction caused by the stimulation of a motor neuron is regarded as involuntary. Reflexes likewise are involuntary. We must ask at this point if we are able to maintain this distinction of voluntary and involuntary behavior in light of the Pavlovian experiments connecting a stimulus "bell" to a response "salivation." Such conditioned reflexes show that the relationship between stimulus and response can be changed. We do know that motor behavior is controlled by motor neurons, whereas associational or inter-neurons that mediate conditioned reflexes also connect or are involved in what we call "voluntary behavior." Furthermore, operant conditioning involving greater complexities of neural structures and behavior is often referred to as "voluntary control of behavior."

Retribution

Criminal law is justified in terms of two different and contradictory theories and goals. The oldest is retribution or justice, the "eye for an eye" model. This theory goes back to tribal law which existed before state law came into existence. Tribal law can be interpreted as a primitive vengeful response to an injury, or it can be regarded, as some historians do, as a means of limiting revenge by stating that restitution must be limited to the injury, and that restitution and not revenge is the purpose of the law. With the development of state law from the 12th century on, the use of punishment developed in the form of executions and exile. The concept of punishment in its more modern form came from the German philosophers Hegel and Kant, who argued that the purpose of the law is justice, and justice is served when the punishment fits the crime. The purpose of criminal law is to punish the criminal, not to deter or reform. The law cannot be used as a means to an end, but only as an end, and that end is just retribution (Feinberg & Gross, 1980; Michael & Adler, 1933). This view of law is found in a modern form in the work of the legal philosopher, H.L.A. Hart (1968).

Utilitarianism

The Kantian/Hegelian view of law was seriously challenged by the utilitarians Bentham and Beccaria who, following the tradition put forth in philosophy by Aristotle and Aquinas, put forth the doctrine of deterrence. The purpose of law is to serve a social good, and the social good is to prevent criminals from committing more crimes (specific deterrence). The deterrence argument maintains free will and volitional behavior, along with moral blameworthiness; that is, we cannot execute the insane, but first we make them well and then we execute them. The purpose of punishment is not to right a wrong committed in the past, but to reduce the crime rate and to insure social order and harmony in the future (Michael & Adler, 1933).

Scientific Criminology

Both the theory of retributive justice and the theory of deterrence were seriously challenged in the 19th century by the scientific positivists as represented in the works of Darwin, Freud, Marx, Spencer, and Comte. The development of the behavioral sciences contradicted the basic view of human nature as found in legalistic philosophy. The work of the Italian School of Criminology (Lombroso, Garofalo, Ferri) is critical in this respect (Mannheim, 1970). Ferri (1967) wrote that scientific criminology was based on the scientific study of offenders and not on legal concepts of crime. The focus must be on the study of the offender and not on the study of criminal law. Criminal behavior is not the product of *mens rea,* free will, and voluntaristic mentalism, but rather is the product of biological, psychological, and sociological conditions of offenders. Ferri described in detail the great scientific meetings held between 1879 and 1895 wherein epilepsy, brain disorders, and other neurological conditions were discussed in relation to crime and criminal law. Ferri advocated indeterminate sentences where the judge would sentence on the basis of the offender's personality and needs and not on the basis of the crime committed. Judges would use scientific methods to classify and assign prisoners to hospitals for treatment. Prisons would be replaced with hospitals.

From 1890 to 1960, criminology, or the scientific study of the offender, developed in Europe and the United States, based on positivistic principles of science, treatment, and research. Only a few of the major figures in the development of a treatment/prevention model of criminal justice will be mentioned here. In 1933, Michael and Adler advocated that the criminal law be used for deterrence and rehabilitative ends, without the requirement of *mens rea* and moral guilt. Wootton (1963) advocated a similar position in which the criminal law would abandon *mens rea* and punishment in favor of a behavioral treatment approach to crime. Menninger (1968), in *The Crime of Punishment,* severely chastised the criminal law for its punitive approach to human behavior and its lack of scientific knowledge about human behavior. He stated that more crimes are committed against the criminal than by the criminal, and he advocated a scientific behavioral approach to justice. Kittrie (1971), in *The Right To Be Different,* rejected the punitive approach to crime, and he put forth a "therapeutic bill of rights," within which a treatment program could be developed to replace the "just retribution model" of justice.

Failure of Rehabilitation

Many treatment programs were established, first using psychoanalytic and psychological concepts, and later using sociological concepts concerning poverty, discrimination, and social justice. All of these programs were based on faulty psychiatric and sociological concepts, and all failed miserably (Jeffery, 1977, 1985). The failure of these rehabilitative programs was well summarized in the Martinson Report (Lipton, Martinson, & Wilks, 1975), which evaluated the impact of rehabilitation on the criminal justice system and concluded that "nothing works."

Just Retribution Reemerges

Starting with the Goldwater presidential campaign against Johnson in 1964, the conservatives put forth a "law and order" platform, or a get-tough-with-the-criminal approach to the crime problem. By 1969, Nixon was in the White House, and the punitive response to crime was renewed with unusual vigor. The instrument for this was the Safe Streets Act and the Law Enforcement Assistance Administration (LEAA), which was a federal program to fight crime by making use of the police-courts-prison system. Criminology and research into the behavioral basis for crime and criminality were ignored in favor of the retributive model. The prevailing view was that "bad men" (or women) must be put in prison for life or executed.

Lawyers, political scientists, economists, and philosophers joined in this return to the just retribution model, as illustrated in the writings of Ehrlich (1975), Fogel (1975), Morris (1974), van den Haag (1975), von Hirsch (1976, 1983), and Wilson (1975). The just retribution model is based on free will and moral choice, as well as punishment for the wicked. Coercive treatment is not allowed, behavioral science research is discouraged as dangerous, discretion by judges and parole boards is eliminated or limited, and long fixed sentences are used in place of indeterminate sentences based on the psychology of the offender.

As a result of LEAA projects and the retributive justice policies of the 1970's, we now have overcrowded prisons and prison violence in the form of murder, rape, and assaults, and more people are in prison than ever before. Many state prison systems are under court order for violating basic constitutional rights of inmates (*Corrections Digest, 1985;* Reid, 1985: 516 ff.). We now have returned to executions as a substitute for solving human behavioral problems. Behavioral research has been ignored and neglected, and recent advances in genetics and the brain sciences have not been utilized by the criminal law. Violence by the state leads to violence by its citizens. Retribution is not a very noble goal for our criminal law.

In the 1960's, the liberal position was one of rehabilitation and social intervention in order to reduce crime, whereas by 1984 the liberal position became indistinguishable from the conservative one taken by Presidents Nixon and Reagan. This is illustrated by the statement by Geraldine Ferraro, the nominee for Vice President by the Democratic party in 1984, a woman regarded by many as being very liberal. She stated, in her nomination-acceptance speech in San Francisco, that she was a former prosecutor who knew how to be tough on criminals and how to put criminals in prison.

SCHOOLS OF PSYCHOLOGY

Cognitive Psychology

Historically, psychology has been divided between the rationalists and the empiricists. The rationalists, from Plato to Kant, hold that man has an innate nature. Ideas are a product of reason and not experience. The empiricists, from Locke and Hume to the present, hold that man is a *tabula rasa*, and experience is the source of knowledge and ideas. From the rationalists came cognitive psychology, with an emphasis on the inner man and his mind. This is based on a mind-matter dualism, with the mind controlling the body. Internal non-physical processes are emphasized, and psychology is separated from biology and neurology. We can never get "inside the skin" to observe these mental processes, so we introspect and we observe behavior; and from these observations, we infer internal mental states that underlie behavior.

Freudian psychoanalysis is often interpreted as introspective or cognitive psychology, although Freud, originally a neurologist, argued that the id, ego, and superego had neurological foundations which would someday be understood.

Behaviorism

Behaviorism, as developed by Pavlov, Watson, and others, attempted to limit the science of behavior to observable events. Internal mental processes were denied, as were the effects of genetics and the makings of the brain. This is referred to as an "empty organism" or "black box" psychology in which experience determines behavior and the stimulus determines the response. This is pure environmentalism.

Psychobiology

Following the union of biochemistry and biology in the work of Watson and Crick on DNA and RNA, psychology rapidly joined with biology in the form of behavioral genetics and psychobiology. Although studies of the brain and behavior can be traced back to the 19th century, the role of the brain in behavior gained great importance only recently, and today many books are in print concerning psychobiology or physiological psychology.

An important aspect of the newer psychobiology is the joining of traditional American learning theory with European ethology or animal behavior studies. The environmentalism of the American learning theorists and the innate structure of behavior as found in ethology can be joined in an effort to understand learning as the interaction of brain and environment. It is not a stimulus-response (S-R) psychology, but a stimulus-organism-response (S-O-R) psychology, with the organism acting on experience through the brain and nervous system. The stimulus must be transmitted to the muscles (behavior) by means of neurons. This is a stimulus-brain-response model of behavior. The new biological psychology is a systems model of behavior based on the interactions of organisms and environment, heredity and environment, and brain and environment (Barnett, 1981; Dewsbury, 1978; Ginsburg, 1979; Hilgard & Bower, 1975; Hinde, 1974; Miller, Galanter, & Pribram, 1960; Pribram, 1971; Seligman & Hager, 1973).

Biological Psychiatry

Biological psychiatry emerged from 1950 on, built on the neurological model put forth but never completed by Freud, and based on the new genetics and new neurological sciences. The development of antipsychotic drugs, antidepressant drugs, and other biochemical means of treating behavioral disorders moved psychiatry from couch therapy to organic therapy. A major focus of modern biological psychiatry is on the neurotransmitters and on the relationship between the neurotransmitters and such mental disorders as schizophrenia, depression, and antisocial behavior.

New technologies are now available to study the brain, what goes on "inside the skin." The organism is no longer a black box. The internal processes related to behavior can now be studied through technologies which include brain imaging techniques such as the Computerized Axial Tomography (CAT scan), Positron Emission Tomography (PET scan), Nuclear Magnetic Resonance (NMR scan), evoked potentials and electroencephalograms (EEG's), hair analysis, and other means of looking at internal biochemical processes. Psychoanalysis was never a part of medicine or neurology. The new biological psychiatry is very much a part of neurology, biochemistry, and genetics. These biochemical events in the brain can be produced by experience and learning, and they can be controlled and altered by diet and drug therapies (Curzon, 1980; Jacobs & Gelperin, 1981; Lickey & Gordon, 1983; Reinis & Goldman, 1983; Restak, 1983; Snyder, 1980; Usdin, 1980; Usdin, Hamburg, & Barchas, 1977; van Praag, 1978; Wender & Klein, 1981; Wynne, Cromwell, & Matthysse, 1978).

Biology and Criminology

Although the origins of criminology were in biology (e.g., Lombroso, Freud, and the early geneticists, as well as Sheldon and the body-type anthropologists), since 1920 criminology has systematically ignored biology and psychology. However, in recent years there have been a number of studies relating criminal behavior to genetic processes and neurological and hormonal defects. Some of the disorders discussed in the literature include sociopathy, epilepsy, brain dysfunction, left hemisphere dysfunction, head trauma, alcoholism and drug abuse, hormonal defects (including testosterone defects in males and premenstrual syndrome in females), nutritional and dietary problems (including lead and cadmium in the brain), hypoglycemia, and other biochemical disturbances of the brain. Hair analysis can inferentially detect brain damage from lead and cadmium as well as nutritional defects, and hair analysis costs about $30 per person. Some criminal and non-criminal subpopulations have been differentiated as to concentrations of lead, cadmium, iron, sodium, potassium, copper, and zinc in the brain. The study of the criminal mind has shifted to the study of the biochemistry of the criminal brain (Fishbein & Thatcher, 1982; Hare & Schalling, 1978; Hays, Roberts, & Solway, 1981; Jeffery, 1979; Lewis, 1981; Mednick & Christiansen, 1977; Monroe, 1978; Raloff, 1983; Reed, 1983; Schauss, 1981; Wolfgang & Weiner, 1982).

CRIMINAL LAW AND BIOLOGICAL DISEASES OF THE BRAIN

The Insanity Defense

The law recognizes insanity as a defense to criminal responsibility because insanity negates the required *mens rea*. Insanity is a legal concept based on prescientific notions of mind and human nature. The insanity defense usually involves the issue of cognition, or the M'Naghten Rules, the right and wrong test. Another less popular concept of insanity is the irresistible impulse test which involves the issue of the ability of the defendant to control his/her behavior. The Model Penal Code of the American Law Institute (ALI) combines the cognitive and the volitional tests into one definition of insanity.

The insanity defense has created a major conflict between law and psychiatry. Insanity cannot be scientifically or medically defined, and there is no indisputable way to prove the existence of insanity. Questions of insanity are settled within an adversarial system, wherein psychiatrists on the opposing sides examining the same individual provide contradictory "expert" testimony regarding whether a particular defendant knew right from wrong. The conflict between law and psychiatry is beautifully illustrated by Gaylin (1982) in *The Killing of Bonnie Garland.*

The *U.S. v. Durham* (1954, 214 F. 2nd 862) decision attempted to redefine insanity in terms of mental illness and mental defect. Once again, there is no acceptable way to define mental illness and mental defect. The *Durham* decision also required a causal link between the mental illness and the criminal behavior, but again, there is no scientific way to relate mental illness to criminal behavior. Mental illness, in this context, connotes an illness of the mind without consideration of the brain. If one cannot study the mind, there is no way to show that the mind is diseased.

The free will and the punishment hypotheses of the criminal law conflict with the positivist position of causation and treatment. There are no indisputable scientific tests for insanity or mental illness. There is little evidence that psychoanalytic treatment is successful for serious biological disorders. Psychoanalytic treatment of criminals was judged to be a failure in a 1978 report by the National Academy of Sciences (Sechrest, White, & Brown, 1979), which concluded that there were not at that time any effective methods for rehabilitating offenders.

(For a discussion of law and psychiatry, see American Bar Association, 1983; Bromberg, 1979; Brooks, 1974; Jeffery, 1967, 1985; Robinson, 1980; Roche, 1958; Ziskin, 1975.)

Law and Biological Psychiatry: A New Model

With the emergence of psychobiology and biological psychiatry, there is a need and an opportunity for a new relationship between law and psychiatry. In this new relationship, *mens rea* and punishment would be replaced with concepts of brain function and treatments for brain disorders. A medical model would be put forth based on the right to treatment, the right to medical treatment, no right to refuse competent treatment when administered with a therapeutic bill of rights, and a limited notion of informed consent. Antisocial behavior would be defined and identified in terms of biological assessments such as the CAT scan, the PET scan, or hair analysis. In court, the psychiatrist would be asked to testify as to the nature of the physical impairments of the defendant's brain rather than to whether or not the defendant knew right from wrong. Evidence of brain disorders must be of a physical and neurological nature in order to be admitted into court.

The definition of insanity which I would put forth (Jeffery, 1985) would be: An abnormal condition of the brain or neurological system which affects the cortex and other higher thought processes, and/or which affects the limbic system and related emotional areas of the brain, when such neurological conditions impair behavior control due to these defects in the brain.

An example of this type of trial is found in the book *The Crocodile Man* (Mayer & Wheeler, 1982). A young college student had assaulted and almost killed two women after ingesting a small amount of beer. The defense attorney was able to secure a complete medical and neurological examination of the defendant where it was revealed that he had an enzyme deficiency in the brain which made the normal metabolism of alcohol impossible. The result was sudden and violent rage. Medical treatment rather than a prison term was the outcome of this unusual criminal trial, which could become a classic in the annals of biological psychiatry and criminal law.

A complete neurological examination of major felons and those on death row could be made in order to determine the neurological state of our criminal population. At this time, we do not know the nature of the brain damage of those we put in prison. A good example is the case of Charles Whitman, who climbed to the top of the library tower on the University of Texas campus and shot 26 people. Whitman had a tumor in the amygdaloid area of the brain, the area controlling violence. We also have the cases of Dr. Jeffrey MacDonald, Kenneth Bianchi, Christopher Wilder, Charles Manson, Henry Lee Lucas, and Ted Bundy (Jeffery, 1985).

The Current Legal Status of Biological Brain Disorders

The law under the right and wrong rule requires cognition or knowledge of right and wrong. Courts typically have held that cognition is not impaired by most biological brain disorders (Jeffery, 1985). Epilepsy and episodic brain dysfunction have been variously defined as insanity or as automatism and involuntary behavior. Hypoglycemia and other nutritional disorders are not a defense under the M'Naghten Rules, but they can be a mitigating circumstance as in the Dan White case in San Francisco. Dan White was a San Francisco supervisor who in 1978 shot and killed Mayor George Moscone and Supervisor Harvey Milk while under the influence of candy bars, cupcakes, and Twinkees. White was given an 8-year sentence based on the defense of hypoglycemia. The Dan White story was presented on public television on October 17, 1984 as "The People vs. Dan White." Post-trauma stress syndrome is also not a defense under M'Naghten, but can be under the ALI rule. Such a defense can be used to mitigate the sentence. The ALI Model Penal Code, Section 4:1, Part 2, places psychopathy outside the definition of insanity when it states that "mental disease or defect does not include any abnormality manifested only by repeated criminal or otherwise anti-social conduct." Psychiatrists are divided as to whether psychopathy is a mental illness or not (Jeffery, 1985). Alcoholism, if involuntary and/or if there is an unanticipated reaction to alcohol or other drugs so as to make *mens rea* impossible, is a defense to a criminal charge (e.g., the *Crocodile Man* case).

Where a biological condition is introduced as a defense, the usual legal response is one of shortening the sentence. The defendant goes to prison, is not treated, and is released earlier than usual because he has a biological defect. Defense attorneys appear to be playing games with biological disorders by introducing them in such a way as to get their clients released without treatment. If we are going to introduce biological testimony into our criminal trials, we must see to it that mandatory treatment is required and release from an institution is contingent upon a neurological evaluation which is capable of predicting future dangerousness. On the basis of the prevailing mind-brain distinction, biological defects of the brain are neither insanity nor mental illness. Nevertheless, the only way criminal law can relate to such conditions is to label them "insanity." The only realistic solution would be to recognize that the brain exists, that neurological disorders also exist, and that behavior is often a result of such neurological disorders. We could then start to put forth treatment programs for individuals with such disorders. It should be obvious that one would not have to be labeled a criminal in order to receive treatment, nor should the label criminal necessarily mean punishment, retribution, and imprisonment.

Premenstrual Syndrome as a Legal Defense

PMS is associated with tension and aggression, and the observation has been made that 49 percent of the females in prison committed their crimes during the premenstrual period (Dalton, 1964). Earlier, Morton, Addison, Addison, Hunt, and Sullivan (1953) found that 62 percent of violent crimes by females were committed during the premenstrual period. Because of the methodological difficulties of determining the date of menstruation in relation to the crime, which probably occurred months or years earlier, there have been serious reservations concerning PMS and crime (Bowker, 1978). However, in recent years, major research has been carried out on PMS, and over 350 clinics have been established in the United States for the diagnosis and treatment of PMS. The next step is to do better research as to the relationship between PMS and criminal violence. The relationship is apparently there, but the exact nature of this relationship is yet to be determined.

Dalton (1980) discusses three cases in Great Britain where PMS was introduced as a defense. It is particularly significant that all three defendants were successfully given progesterone treatment. (In the present volume, 11 relevant cases are described by Dalton.) Brahams (1981) discusses two of these cases in some detail. In *R. v. Craddock*, the defendant had 30 prior convictions for violent behavior. She had a long history of uncontrollable rage during the premenstrual period. In this particular instance, she was on trial for the murder of a barmaid. Nevertheless, Dalton successfully treated her with progesterone, and she was placed on probation. In the case of *R. v. English*, the court reduced a murder charge to manslaughter, and the defendant was given probation with the provision that she receive hormonal therapy. In another British case, *R. v. Smith* (1982), the court reduced a murder charge to manslaughter (Mulligan, 1983).

Caryl-Thomas (1982) discusses the British case of a female who was on trial for threatening to kill someone. The defendant had been under treatment for PMS at the time of the crime. The court held that PMS did not constitute a defense under the automatism rule, and neither was there authority for a defense under the irresistible impulse rule. The court stated the purpose of the law is to protect society. The court further stated that under a guilty verdict she could be placed on probation and treated, whereas if acquitted she would be free to return to the streets. Several comments can be made about the logic of this ruling. The court held that PMS is not automatism or irresistible impulse, when from a biological point of view, it constitutes both automatism and an irresistible impulse. The statement that the defendant had to be found guilty in order to be treated is a reflection of the legal position on law and insanity. A person can be placed in treatment under a finding of not guilty by reason of insanity, or a person can be found in need of treatment quite separate from a determination of guilt or innocence of a crime. The statement that society can only be protected by finding the defendant guilty of a crime is to totally ignore the possibility of treatment through non-criminal procedures.

PMS has been successfully introduced in Britain, Canada, and France as a legal defense, usually under the guise of insanity (which it is not). In a discussion of the PMS defense, Press (1983) notes that there is no evidence that PMS produces psychosis, and therefore PMS is not legal insanity. This approach defines insanity as psychosis, where there is no psychological or psychiatric reason for using the term "insanity" in this way. This is the M'Naghten defense. Press does note that PMS can be used as a mitigating circumstance to reduce the charges to a lesser offense. Press also raised the issue of standards for expert testimony in PMS cases. He asks, "Who are the experts on PMS: neurologists, psychiatrists, endocrinologists, or gynecologists?" The general medical practitioner is not an expert on PMS, and therefore most physicians are not expert witnesses on the issue. The answer to this issue is that anyone present in court as an expert witness should be an expert on the topic to be reviewed. In the case of PMS, the best type of expert testimony would be interdisciplinary in nature and would include all of the disciplines referred to by Press in his question.

In a highly publicized United States case (*Newsweek*, November 8, 1982), Shirley Santos was charged with assault on her daughter. She was prosecuted by former Congresswoman Elizabeth Holtzman and defended by Attorney Stephanie Benson, who raised the issue of PMS. The Santos case did not go to trial. The charges were reduced to harassment, and the defendant was discharged on the condition that she seek medical treatment (Mulligan, 1983).

According to Mulligan (1983), no American court has dealt with the issue of PMS as such. Where the issue is raised, it has been as a mitigating circumstance and used to reduce the charge and/or sentence. Mulligan is concerned that PMS might be used to harm women's rights; that is, any woman could be regarded as potentially insane, and therefore dangerous, but she agrees that PMS can be used as a mitigating circumstance. This would be a compromise between total acceptance and total rejection of PMS as a legal defense.

It must be pointed out that regardless of future research findings on PMS, the condition is *not* found in *all* women; and when present, the condition does not necessarily result in criminal acts. There are too many other intervening variables involved in behavior to draw any simple conclusions from relating any single condition to criminal behavior. At the same time, we cannot rule it out simply because not all crimes committed by women involve PMS. What we can do is treat those cases of PMS known to medical authorities and observe whether the behavior of the women changes dramatically after treatment. Based on the limited reports now available, it seems that appropriate treatment for PMS has produced dramatic changes in women suffering from this condition.

It is highly likely that PMS will be even better understood and more successfully treated in the future, and it is to be hoped that the legal system will be more responsive to medical research and will make the results of this research a part of the decision-making process, since PMS is now regarded as a real and serious medical condition.

The Philadelphia Conference, Premenstrual Syndrome, and the Criminal Law

The objective of the Philadelphia Conference was to focus on legal and ethical implications of the biobehavioral sciences in relation to the premenstrual syndrome. Preliminary drafts from each of the participants were circulated, presented, and discussed in plenary session. An evaluative consensus was attempted by assigning the conferees to post-plenary committees based on the major disciplines represented at the Conference (see Committee Reports). The Committee on Legal Ethics [Sadoff (Chair), Benson, Houlgate, and Jeffery] took a *status quo* position over my objection. The majority members argued that the major issues should be framed in terms of *mens rea*, or the voluntary nature of the behavior. This represents current legal dogma and does not deal with the implications of the biobehavioral information presented at the Conference. The difficulties in establishing *mens rea*, or of automatism, considered at the Conference also were not addressed, nor was the fact that *mens rea* is a legal and not a medical term. For these reasons, I must dissent from the Committee's statement, which, in my opinion, could have been written without ever attending the Conference.

The members of this Committee did not address the need to bridge the gap between law and biology. In contrast, the Committee statement refers to the fact that law and medicine approach their objectives from different perspectives, and thus the defense attorney is obliged to use PMS as a defense even where there are no scientific studies to support the notion that PMS causes violence, or even that PMS exists as a biological entity.

In dissenting from those views, this writer contends, along with some of the clinicians and biologists, that PMS is real and is involved in some instances of criminal activity (see chapter by Dalton, this volume). I also feel that biological knowledge must be integrated into legal procedures through serious interdisciplinary work. I do not feel that PMS can be integrated into the criminal justice system only by references to *mens rea* and automatism. It must be regretted that the participants did not adequately relate the major issues involving biological illnesses and criminal law. The lawyer cannot continue to use concepts that are meaningless to the scientist and expect the scientific community to be part of the legal process or to aid the criminal justice system in its attempt to solve the crime problem.

Criminal Law and the Medical Model

The medical model is based on preventing crime before it occurs, or treating criminal behavior after the fact by therapeutic means. In either instance, criminal behavior is seen as a medical problem and not as a legal problem. The medical model is based upon the sciences of biology, neurology, psychology, and associated disciplines. The hospital and the research center are the heart of such an approach, not the prison and the electric chair.

Several legal doctrines must be considered if we are to develop a medical model for the criminal justice system. Some of these doctrines support the medical model, some of them oppose the medical model. These doctrines concern the right to treatment, the right to medical treatment, the right to refuse treatment, the right to rehabilitation, the doctrine of informed consent, and the prediction of future dangerousness and future criminal activity.

The Right to Treatment. The right to treatment doctrine has been developed in mental health law for those confined to mental institutions. A person in such an institution must be either treated or released. Mandatory treatment is required for the mentally ill, but not for criminals. Here again, we differentiate the mad from the bad. For the mad, we have mental hospitals; and for the bad, we have prisons. If the arguments developed above concerning the neurological basis for mental illness and criminal behavior have any merit, then we must conclude that it is not possible on a neurological basis to differentiate the mad from the bad.

The Right to Medical Treatment. The right to medical treatment doctrine is by now well established legal doctrine (Krantz, 1981: 380 ff). Courts have held that inmates are entitled to adequate medical care, including psychiatric care. The major issue remaining is: Does the right to medical treatment extend to the newer concepts found in biological psychiatry? For example, does an inmate have a right to a CAT scan, PET scan, NMR, EEG, or a test for hypoglycemia, hormonal defects, PMS, or other detectable neurological and biochemical disorders? In the Dan White case mentioned above, does the hypoglycemic inmate have a right to a special diet?

The Right to Refuse Treatment. The right to treatment doctrine has as its counterpart the right to refuse treatment. The right to refuse treatment has arisen as an issue in cases involving drug therapies, lobotomies, electroconvulsive therapies, behavior modification programs, and psychosurgery (Brooks, 1974: 886-889). In *Kaimowitz v. Michigan Department of Mental Health* (Circuit Court of Wayne County, Michigan, 1973), the court held that the defendant could not give informed consent to experimental surgery. Psychosurgery and related legal and moral issues raised a major debate in the 1970's (Gaylin, Meister, & Neville, 1975; Institute of Society, Ethics, and the Life Sciences, 1973; National Institute of Mental Health, 1973; Valenstein, 1973, 1980).

In two recent cases, *Rennie v. Klein* (1978, 462 F. Suppl. 1131) and *Rogers v. Okin* (1979, 478 F. Suppl. 1342), courts have held that mental patients have a right to refuse medical treatment in the form of psychotropic drugs. This raised the issue of how one can commit a person to a mental institution for treatment if the patient can refuse treatment (Brooks, 1980).

The issues of right to refuse treatment and the right to refuse to participate as a research subject involve several serious moral and legal desiderata (Gaylin et al., 1975; Macklin, 1982). As a result of such legal and ethical concerns, several major research endeavors were terminated in the 1970's, including the XYY program at Harvard University, the behavioral modification project within the federal prison system, and the Center for the Study of Violence at the University of California at Los Angeles (Gaylin, Macklin, & Powledge, 1981).

It has been pointed out (Weinstein, 1982) that there must be legal ways in which to treat individuals for conditions which endanger their lives or the lives of others. Wilkinson (1979), a lawyer, has written that "unless modern psychiatry is allowed to explore new methods of treatment, the future growth of the profession and discovery of new cures will be greatly inhibited." In commenting on the intrusiveness of modern therapies, Judge Bazelon wrote in *U.S. v. Alexander* (1973, 471 F. 2d 923) at footnote 120:

"On the whole, distinctions based on 'coerciveness' or 'intrusiveness' seem unhelpful, since virtually every technique would be extremely coercive if it could be made to work perfectly. It may be that the techniques such as psychotherapy and psychodrama are thought to raise fewer moral questions than lobotomies, shock treatment and the like, because of the widely held assumption that the former are far less likely than the latter to effect any significant, long-lasting alteration in the subject's behavior or physical condition, especially where the subject is uncooperative. If that theory, and the assumption on which it rests, are valid, then a very difficult question arises: If we can tolerate the use of only those techniques that are unlikely to 'work,' in the sense of altering behavior or physical condition, how can we continue to justify involuntary hospitalization on the grounds that it permits us to use those very techniques in the 'treatment' of mental illness?"

The basis issue is, as Bazelon summarized it, "Can we refuse to use treatments which work and allow treatments which do not work?"

The Right to Rehabilitation. Another important approach concerns prison conditions which are so vile as to constitute cruel or unusual punishment under the Eighth and Fourteenth Amendments (Krantz, 1981, 347 ff.). In *Holt v. Sarver* (1970, 309 F. Suppl. 362), the court held that:

"The absence of an affirmative program of training and rehabilitation may have constitutional significance where in the absence of such a program conditions and practices exist which actually mitigate against reform and rehabilitation... The absence of rehabilitative services and facilities of which the Petitioners complain remains a factor in the overall constitutional equation before the court."

In *James v. Wallace* (1976, 1406 F. Suppl. 318), Judge Johnson said:

"The evidence in these cases also established that prison conditions are so dehabilitating that they necessarily deprive inmates of any opportunity to rehabilitate themselves, or even to maintain skills already possessed. While courts have thus far declined to elevate a positive rehabilitation program to the level of a constitutional right, it is clear that a penal system cannot be operated in such a manner that it impedes an inmate's ability to attempt rehabilitation, or simply to avoid physical, mental, and social deterioration... Not only is it cruel and unusual punishment to confine a person in an institution under circumstances which increase the likelihood of future confinement, but these conditions defeat the goals of rehabilitation which prison officials have set for their institutions."

While I would not claim that the view of Judge Johnson in *James v. Wallace* will act as a mandate to the legal system to require a right to treatment doctrine for criminals as well as the mentally ill, this statement is by far the most supportive of rehabilitation to be found, and one that suggests that an absence of rehabilitation facilities may constitute cruel and unusual punishment.

The Doctrine of Informed Consent. The doctrine of informed consent is often involved in the right to refuse treatment and the right to refuse to participate in research projects. Such a doctrine holds that a person should realize the conditions and consequences of treatment and/or research, and should have the capacity to consent to such procedures. The doctrine has meaning and applicability in the area of civil law and voluntary proceedings. A person can make decisions concerning the right to life or the right to death, refuse or elect open-heart surgery, or make other private and personal decisions. However, the real issue here is, "Can a criminal refuse treatment if it is competently administered with legal safeguards?" What if we make the purpose of criminal law the treatment and rehabilitation of criminals? Under such a doctrine, can a criminal refuse treatment? What do we do with those criminals who refuse to be treated? The problem is that the lawyer must then take a concept from civil law and apply it to criminal law where it has no present applicability. A criminal has no right to consent to punishment under the present criminal law. A criminal is not asked if he wants to be sent to prison or to be executed. How can we apply the voluntary consent doctrine of the civil law to the involuntary doctrine of punishment of the criminal law? The criminal law is based on force and coercion, and as such does not involve the concept of informed consent.

If we want to establish the right to medical treatment doctrine within the criminal justice system, we must first and foremost resolve the issues of informed consent and the right to refuse treatment. We cannot allow a criminal to refuse treatment if he does not have the right to refuse punishment. If the political state has the power to punish, it has the power to rehabilitate. Under our present system of justice, we can use coercive punishment without consent, but we cannot use coercive treatment without consent. Ethically, it does not make sense.

The Prediction of Future Dangerousness. If we are to establish a model which prevents future criminal behavior, we must first deal with the issue of prediction of such future behavior. As a result of a series of lawsuits which released mentally ill criminals from institutions, such as *Baxtrom v. Herold* (1966, 80 S. Ct. 760), it was discovered that few of these individuals were dangerous after their release (Brooks, 1974: 323 ff.). It is often stated that only one of three predicted to be dangerous is really dangerous. This is an error rate of two out of three. The two out of three "false positives" would be institutionalized under our present system for predicting dangerousness (Crain, 1982; Monahan, 1981). The libertarian view holds that we cannot accurately predict future behavior, and to hold individuals in custody for acts which they have not as yet committed is a violation of their civil liberties. As they say, we cannot detain two people in order to prevent one from committing murder or rape (Gross, 1979: 45-49; Hinton, 1983: 9 ff.).

Several problems are subsumed in the statements that we cannot predict future dangerousness. Although the false positive is usually viewed as the major issue, particularly from an ethical point of view (e.g., the person predicted to be dangerous but who is not dangerous), the more serious issue is that of the false negative (e.g., the person predicted to be non-dangerous, who upon release from prison or a mental institution kills four people). Such cases are familiar to us (Diamond, 1974).

Another issue concerns the way in which such predictions are made. We are inaccurate in our efforts to predict violence because of our sloppy prediction methods. We use verbal interviews and paper-and-pencil tests. If we used neurological measures, evidence suggests that we would obtain more accurate results. For example, Tong (Hinton, 1983: 59) successfully identified 95 percent of a mentally abnormal offender population who would recidivate, based on studies of their autonomic nervous system. Perkins (Hinton, 1983: 71) reported that the best prediction of dangerousness for sex offenders was a physiological measure of penile responses. Woodman (Hinton, 1983: 103) concluded that aggressive individuals can be diagnosed through their high norepinephrine levels. We can accurately predict the dangerous offender if we know what to look for.

A further issue pertains to the fact that we act on our prediction of dangerousness by punishing people and putting them in institutions. If we used predictive methods in order to help people and to prevent future antisocial behavior, such as what is done in the prediction and prevention of future heart attacks or immunization against small pox, then, if we are wrong, the results are not the same as putting people falsely identified as potential criminals into institutions.

Lawyers, judges, parole boards, and psychiatrists are called upon every day to make predictions about future behaviors in decisions concerning bail, sentencing, mental health assignments, prison assignments, and other criminal justice procedures. In *Tarasoff v. Board of Regents of the University of California* (1976, 551 P. 2d 334), the court held that psychiatrists must predict future dangerousness and warn third parties of the future dangerousness of certain individuals. In *Barefoot v. Estelle* (1983, 51 U.S.L.W. 5189), the Supreme Court held that a psychiatrist could testify as to future dangerousness in a case involving the death penalty.

In the light of the contradictory opinions concerning the prediction of future violence and dangerousness, and the many contradictory legal opinions concerning the legality of predicting future criminality and dangerousness, it is somewhat amazing to find the U.S. Supreme Court on June 4, 1984 declaring that juveniles may be placed in jails prior to trial and prior to conviction of a crime if the judge predicts that the juvenile is likely to commit a crime in the future if released from jail. One judge is quoted as saying, "You don't have to be a fortuneteller to determine that certain kids that come into court are dangerous," and Justice Rehnquist stated, "From a legal point of view there is nothing inherently unattainable about the prediction of future criminal conduct" (*Newsweek*, June 18, 1984, page 84).

The lawyer is willing to substitute his judgment and training for that of the behavioral science expert. What this Supreme Court decision says, in effect, is that lawyers are capable of predicting future dangerousness and criminality whereas psychologists, psychiatrists, and biologists are not. The finding that psychiatrists attempting such predictions have been wrong two out of three times (Crain, 1982; Monahan, 1981) should cast doubt on the accuracy of their present methods. What confidence may we have, then, in the predictions lawyers make about future criminality and dangerousness, where we do not have comparable research data?

CRIME PREVENTION AND CRIME CONTROL

The Criminal Justice System

The criminal justice system is a total failure. We know that 5-10 times as many crimes are committed as are known to the police. Of those crimes known to the police, 15-20 percent result in an arrest. Uniform Crime Statistics indicate that of 23,300,000 index crimes, 103,000 individuals are committed to prison. Of those arrested, approximately 25 percent are charged with a crime; and of those, 85-90 percent plead guilty to a lesser charge and receive a reduced sentence. Few of those committing crimes ever end up in prison; and of those who do, 65-80 percent recidivate (Jeffery, 1985: 146-147).

Even with these figures, we have overcrowded courtrooms, overcrowded prisons, and long delays of one year or more in bringing a case to trial. The present system does not deter nor rehabilitate, and we cannot continue to send people to prison just to see them return to the community more vicious and dangerous than ever. Yet the retributive justice people argue we should increase prison sentences. It has been estimated that an increase in the sentencing pattern for violent offenders from 1.5 years to 5 years would increase the prison population by 150 percent while reducing the rate of violent crimes by 6 percent (Wolfgang & Weiner, 1980: 339).

Crime Prevention

A crime prevention model has been developed in recent years by a small group of criminologists, geographers, and urban planners (Brantingham & Brantingham, 1981; Clarke & Mayhew, 1980; Georges-Abeyie & Harries, 1980; Harries, 1980; Jeffery, 1971, 1977, 1983; Newman, 1972). As yet, there is little public or political support for such a model. Our politicians want prisons and executions and not crime prevention. It is easy for politicians to get a $20 million grant for a new prison facility, while they do not ask for or receive $1 million for behavioral research on criminal behavior. We see major benefit performances by Hollywood personalities to fight various diseases, but we do not see similar benefits to build a new multi-million dollar research center for crime and criminal behavior research.

A major difficulty in developing a crime prevention model is that the criminal law is designed to wait until the crime has occurred before taking action. In fact, it is impossible to take action before a crime has been committed. If I report to the police that I know a dangerous person who is headed for trouble, I will be told that I must wait until he has committed a crime (perhaps even murder or rape) before they can intervene. Under the present structure of the criminal law, it is impossible to take many measures which would prevent crime before it occurs.

A prevention model is based on the public health model for preventing disease by taking action before the disease has struck. We can prevent heart attacks by actions taken to control diet, exercise, smoking, and other such preventive measures. We can use secondary prevention techniques such as stress tests, angiograms, and by-pass surgery. The incidence of cancer can be reduced by controlling diet, environmental pollution, and related causal agents. In the case of crime, we wait until the individual is a third-time loser. He has already been in juvenile court and adult court six or more times. Only the very worst offenders are funneled into the criminal justice system.

Crime Prevention: The Individual

A crime prevention program can be at the individual level or at the environmental level. At the individual level, crime prevention means identifying those individuals who show signs of behavioral disorders. We know that a small proportion of the population commits most of the crimes. The best estimates are that 6 percent of the population commits 50 percent of the crimes (Wolfgang & Weiner, 1982: 339). We must focus on this hard core group.

As mentioned, biochemical and neurological tests could be run on our potential offender populations. Hair analyses and PET scans could be used to diagnose potential behavioral problems and pre-delinquency conditions. Drug therapies are available for schizophrenia, depression, sociopathy, and alcoholism. Depo-Provera (an anti-androgen) is being used for the treatment of sex offenders, and progesterone therapy is being used for PMS offenders. Hypoglycemia, hyperactivity, alcoholism, and learning disabilities are among the behavioral disorders which can be treated. Excessive dosages of lead and cadmium can be reduced both by individual therapies and by antipollution measures which clean up the environment. Early diagnosis and treatment of these disorders of the brain would help to prevent many of our major behavioral problems.

As the law now stands, we cannot take blood from an inmate in order to detect hypoglycemia or psychopathology, but we can insert a needle into the arm for execution. The former is regarded as an unlawful intrusion into the body and into the mental processes; but at the same time, it is not an unlawful intrusion into the body to place the individual in prison or in the electric chair. The State of Texas is now being sued by an inmate because he is not afforded the proper diet for hypoglycemia (personal communication). Several major projects are now underway using diet and nutrition as means of controlling antisocial behaviors, and it is a very cheap and effective way to accomplish this end.

Special clinics could be established for adolescents with behavioral problems where they could have a complete neurological examination and evaluation. Referrals to such clinics could be made by parents, teachers, police, courts, pediatricians, and others who have contact with adolescent populations.

Crime Prevention: The Environment

Crime prevention through environmental design is also possible through the design of streets, parks, buildings, terminals, and other man-made features of the environment. About 25 percent of the environment is crime-prone. We can focus on high-risk environments as we can focus on high-risk individuals. One study showed that computer analysis could predict 90 percent of the rapes that occur in public places, thereby providing a basis for potential prevention by altering high-risk environments (Stoks, 1982).

Demographic and ecological changes produce new crime patterns. Major crime areas are created by our interstate highway system and our ecological patterns of urban development. Through environmental psychology, urban design, and computer analysis, we can locate those environments where crimes are likely to occur. Through environmental design, we can reduce crime.

Programs and Policies for the Future

In order to put into place a crime prevention program based on a medical model, we would need a major center or centers for research and training in criminal law and criminology. Mention has already been made of the failures of past research efforts in criminology and the opposition which exists in legal circles to research criminal behavior. An Institute for the Study of Criminal Law and Criminology has been recommended by Michael and Adler (1933), Radzinowicz (1965), and Hall (1982). Such an institute must be attached to a major medical center and law school, and must be interdisciplinary in nature, including biologists, psychologists, psychiatrists, criminologists, lawyers, philosophers, urban planners, and systems analysts. Such an institute could train lawyers, psychiatrists, and criminologists in the problems involved in integrating law and the behavioral sciences. Lawyers would be exposed to neurology, to the CAT scan and PET scan, and to the nature of antisocial behavior, while the psychiatrist would be exposed to legal doctrines concerning the insanity defense, the right to treatment, the right to medical treatment, and the right to refuse treatment. Legal and medical issues could be addressed outside the adversarial system in a scientific manner.

Another major component of such an institute would be a major research center for the study of criminal behavior. Violent and aggressive criminals such as Kenneth Bianchi, Ted Bundy, and Henry Lee Lucas would be scientifically studied over a period of five or ten years by an interdisciplinary team composed of geneticists, biochemists, neurologists, endocrinologists, psychiatrists, psychopharmacologists, criminologists, and lawyers. At the end of such a major research project, we would know a great deal about criminal and antisocial behavior and how to prevent it. This would constitute a far lesser invasion of their rights than the restrictions on their freedom imposed upon them under the present system — which includes the use of the death penalty.

It has been argued that such a research project would be expensive. Yet we do such research in other areas such as heart disease, cancer, and space flight. It seems we can create a National Institute for Cancer Research or NASA, but we cannot do the same for a major social issue. It costs $30,000 a year to keep an inmate in prison, another $60,000 to build the cell, and an indeterminate amount to arrest and convict a criminal. In the case of Ted Bundy, it has cost the State of Florida over $2 million to date, and Bundy is still in court contesting his death sentence. The State of Florida will spend that kind of money to execute Bundy, but not to understand the nature of his brain and his behavior.

Law and science must be united in the 1980's if we expect to be able to make progress in controlling crime in our nation.

REFERENCES

American Bar Association, 1983. *First Tentative Draft: Criminal Justice Mental Health Standards*. American Bar Association, Washington, D.C.

Barnett, S. A., 1981. *Modern Ethology*. Oxford University Press, New York, NY.

Bowker, L., 1978. Menstruation and female criminality. Paper presented at the annual meeting of the American Society of Criminology, Dallas, TX.

Brahams, D., 1981. Premenstrual syndrome: A disease of the mind? *The Lancet 2:* 1238-1239.
Brantingham, P. J. and P. L. Brantingham, 1981. *Environmental Criminology.* Sage Publications, Beverly Hills, CA.
Bromberg, W., 1979. *The Uses of Psychiatry in the Law.* Quorum Books, Westport, CT.
Brooks, A. D., 1974. *Law, Psychiatry, and the Mental Health System.* Little, Brown, and Co., Boston, MA.
Brooks, A. D., 1980. The constitutional right to refuse antipsychotic medications. *Bulletin of the Academy of Psychiatry and the Law 2:* 179-221.
Caryl-Thomas, E., 1982. Premenstrual syndrome — whether a defense. *Criminal Law Review,* August, pp. 531-532.
Clarke, R.V.G. and P. Mayhew, 1980. *Designing Out Crime.* Her Majesty's Stationery Office, London.
Crain, P., 1982. Assessing dangerousness. In: R. Rosner (Ed.), *Critical Issues in American Psychiatry and the Law.* Charles C. Thomas, Springfield, IL.
Curzon, G. (Ed.), 1980. *Biochemistry of Psychiatric Disturbances.* John Wiley and Sons, New York, NY.
Dalton, K., 1964. *The Premenstrual Syndrome.* William Heineman Medical Books, Ltd., London.
Dalton, K., 1980. Cyclical criminal acts in the premenstrual syndrome. *The Lancet 2:* 1070-1071.
Dewsbury, D., 1978. *Comparative Animal Behavior.* McGraw-Hill, New York, NY.
Diamond, B., 1974. The psychiatric prediction of dangerousness. *University of Pennsylvania Law Review 123:* 439-452.
Ehrlich, I., 1975. The deterrent effect of captial punishment: A question of life and death. *American Economic Review,* June, pp. 397-417.
Feinberg, J. and H. Gross, 1980. *Philosophy of Law* (second edition). Wadsworth, Belmont, CA.
Ferri, E., 1967. *Criminal Sociology.* Agathon Press, New York, NY.
Fishbein, D. and R. W. Thatcher, 1982. Nutritional and electrophysiological indices of maladaptive behavior. Paper presented at the annual meeting of the American Society of Criminology, Toronto, Ontario, Canada, November.
Fogel, D., 1975. *We Are the Living Proof.* Anderson Co., Cincinnati, OH.
Gaylin, W., 1982. *The Killing of Bonnie Garland.* Simon and Schuster, New York, NY.
Gaylin, W., R. Macklin, and T. M. Powledge (Eds.), 1982. *Violence and the Politics of Research.* Plenum Press, New York, NY.
Gaylin, W., J. S. Meister, and R. C. Neville, 1975. *Operating On the Mind.* Basic Books, New York, NY.
Georges-Abeyie, D. E. and K. D. Harries (Eds.), 1980. *Crime: A Spatial Perspective.* Columbia University Press, New York, NY.
Ginsburg, B. E., 1979. The violent brain: Is it everyone's brain? In: C. R. Jeffery (Ed.), *Biology and Crime.* Sage Publications, Beverly Hills, CA, pp. 47-64.
Gross, H., 1979. *A Theory of Criminal Justice.* Oxford University Press, New York, NY.
Hall, J., 1982. *Law, Social Science, and Criminal Theory.* Fred B. Rothman and Co., Littleton, OH.
Hare, R. D. and D. Schalling, 1978. *Psychopathic Behavior.* John Wiley and Sons, New York, NY.
Harries, K. D., 1980. *Crime and the Environment.* Charles C. Thomas, Springfield, IL.
Hart, H.L.A., 1968. *Punishment and Responsibility.* Oxford University Press, New York, NY.
Hays, J. R., T. K. Roberts, and K. S. Solway, 1981. *Violence and the Violent Individual.* SP Medical and Scientific Books, New York, NY.

Hilgard, E. R. and G. H. Bower, 1975. *Theories of Learning.* Prentice-Hall, Englewood Cliffs, NJ.

Hinde, R. A., 1974. *Biological Bases for Human Social Behavior.* McGraw-Hill, New York, NY.

Hinton, J. W., 1983. *Dangerousness: Problems of Assessment and Prediction.* George Allen and Unwin, London.

Institute of Society, Ethics and the Life Sciences, 1973. *Physical Manipulation of the Brain.* Hastings Center, Hastings-on-Hudson, NY.

Jacobs, B. L. and J. Gelperin, 1981. *Serotonin, Neurotransmission and Behavior.* M.I.T. Press, Cambridge, MA.

Jeffery, C. R., 1967. *Criminal Responsibility and Mental Disease.* Charles C. Thomas, Springfield, IL.

Jeffery, C. R., 1971. *Crime Prevention Through Environmental Design.* Sage Publications, Beverly Hills, CA.

Jeffery, C. R., 1977. *Crime Prevention Through Environmental Design* (revised). Sage Publications, Beverly Hills, CA.

Jeffery, C. R. (Ed.), 1979. *Biology and Crime.* Sage Publications, Beverly Hills, CA.

Jeffery, C. R., 1983. Crime prevention: environmental and technological strategies. In: S. H. Kadish (Ed.), *Encyclopedia of Crime and Justice.* Free Press, New York, NY, p. 362.

Jeffery, C. R., 1985. *Attacks on the Insanity Defense: Biological Psychiatry and New Perspectives on Criminal Behavior.* Charles C. Thomas, Springfield, IL.

Kittrie, N., 1971. *The Right To Be Different.* Johns Hopkins Press, Baltimore, MD.

Krantz, S., 1981. *The Law of Corrections and Prisoners' Rights* (second edition). West, St. Paul, MN.

Lewis, D. O. (Ed.), 1981. *Vulnerabilities to Delinquency.* SP Medical and Scientific Books, New York, NY.

Lickey, M. E. and B. Gordon, 1983. *Drugs for Mental Illness.* W. H. Freeman, San Francisco, CA.

Lipton, D., R. Martinson, and J. Wilks, 1975. *The Effectiveness of Correctional Treatment.* Holt, Rinehart, and Winston, New York, NY.

Low, P. W., J. C. Jeffries, and R. J. Bonnie, 1981. *Criminal Law.* Foundation Press, Mineola, NY.

Macklin, R., 1982. *Man, Mind, and Morality: The Ethics of Behavior Control.* Prentice-Hall, Englewood Cliffs, NJ.

Mannheim, H. (Ed.), 1970. *Pioneers in Criminology.* Fred B. Rotham, Montclair, NJ.

Mayer, A. and M. Wheeler, 1982. *The Crocodile Man.* Houghton-Mifflin, Boston, MA.

Mednick, S. and K. O. Christiansen, 1977. *Biosocial Bases of Criminal Behavior.* Gardner Press, New York, NY.

Menninger, K., 1968. *The Crime of Punishment.* Viking Press, New York, NY.

Michael, J. and M. Adler, 1933. *Crime, Law and Social Science.* Harcourt, Brace and Company, New York, NY.

Miller, G. A., E. Galanter, and K. W. Pribram, 1960. *Plans and the Structure of Behavior.* Holt and Company, New York, NY.

Monahan, J., 1981. *Predicting Violent Behavior.* Sage Publications, Beverly Hills, CA.

Monroe, R. B., 1978. *Brain Dysfunction in Aggressive Criminals.* D.C. Heath and Company, Lexington, MA.

Morris, N., 1974. *The Future of Imprisonment.* University of Chicago Press, Chicago, IL.

Morton, J. H., H. Addison, R. G. Addison, I. Hunt, and J. J. Sullivan, 1953. A clinical study of premenstrual tension. *American Journal of Obstetrics and Gynecology 65:* 1182-1191.

Mulligan, N., 1983. The premenstrual syndrome. *Harvard Women's Law Journal 6:* 219-227.
National Institute of Mental Health, 1973. *Psychosurgery.* National Institute of Mental Health, Washington, D.C.
Newman, O., 1972. *Defensible Space.* Macmillan, New York, NY.
Press, M., 1983. Premenstrual stress syndrome as a defense in criminal cases. *Duke Law Journal 1:* 176-195.
Pribram, K. H., 1971. *Languages of the Brain.* Prentice-Hall, Englewood Cliffs, NJ.
Radzinowicz, L., 1965. *The Need for Criminology.* William Heinemann Medical Books, Ltd., London.
Raloff, J., 1983. Locks — a key to violence? *Science News,* August 20, pp. 122-125.
Reed, B., 1983. *Food, Teens and Behavior.* Natural Press, Division of Contemporary Books, Chicago, IL.
Reid, S. T., 1985. *Crime and Criminology.* Holt, Rinehart, and Winston, New York, NY.
Reinis, S. and J. M. Goldman, 1983. *The Chemistry of Behavior.* Plenum Press, New York, NY.
Restak, R. M., 1983. Psychiatry in America. *The Wilson Quarterly,* Fall, pp. 80-115.
Robinson, D. N., 1980. *Psychology and Law.* Oxford University Press, New York, NY.
Roche, P. Q., 1958. *The Criminal Mind.* Farrar, Straus, and Cudahy, New York, NY.
Schauss, A., 1981. *Diet, Crime and Delinquency.* Parker House, Berkeley, CA.
Sechrest, L., S. O. White, and E. D. Brown (Eds.), 1979. *The Rehabilitation of Criminal Offenders: Problems and Prospects.* National Academy of Sciences, Washington, D.C.
Seligman, M.E.P. and J. Hager, 1973. *Biological Boundaries of Learning.* Appleton-Century-Crofts, New York, NY.
Snyder, S. H., 1980. *Biological Aspects of Mental Disorders.* Oxford University Press, New York, NY.
Stoks, F.G.G., 1982. Assessing urban public space environments for danger of violent crime — especially rape. Ph.D. Dissertation, University of Washington, Seattle, WA.
Usdin, E., 1980. *Enzymes and Neurotransmitters in Mental Disease.* John Wiley and Sons, New York, NY.
Usdin, E., D. A. Hamburg, and J. D. Barchas (Eds.), 1977. *Neuroregulators and Psychiatric Disorders.* Oxford University Press, New York, NY.
Valenstein, E. S., 1973. *Brain Control.* John Wiley and Sons, New York, NY.
Valenstein, E. S., 1980. *The Psychosurgery Debate.* W. H. Freeman, San Francisco, CA.
van den Haag, E., 1975. *Punishing Criminals.* Basic Books, New York, NY.
van Praag, H. M., 1978. *Psychotropic Drugs.* Brunner/Mazel, New York, NY.
von Hirsch, A., 1976. *Doing Justice.* Hill and Wang, New York, NY.
von Hirsch, A., 1983. Commensurability and crime prevention: evaluating formal sentencing structures and their rationale. *Journal of Criminal Law and Criminology 74:* 209-248.
Weinstein, H., 1982. Legal activism — the right to refuse treatment. In: R. Rosner (Ed.), *Critical Issues in American Psychiatry and the Law.* Charles C. Thomas, Springfield, IL, pp. 23-42.
Wender, P. W. and D. F. Klein, 1981. *Mind, Mood, and Medicine.* Father-Straus-Gireau, New York, NY.
Wilkinson, A. P., 1979. Psychiatric malpractice: identifying areas of liability. *Trial,* October, pp. 73-77.

Wilson, J. Q., 1975. *Thinking About Crime.* Basic Books, New York, NY.
Wolfgang, M. E. and N. A. Weiner (Eds.), 1982. *Criminal Violence.* Sage Publications, Beverly Hills, CA.
Wootton, B., 1963. *Crime and the Criminal Law.* Stevens and Sons, London.
Wynne, L. C., R. L. Cromwell, and S. Matthysse, 1978. *The Nature of Schizophrenia.* John Wiley and Sons, New York, NY.
Ziskin, J., 1975. *Coping With Psychiatric and Psychological Testimony* (second edition). Law and Psychology Press, Beverly Hills, CA.

SOCIAL ISSUES

PREMENSTRUAL SYNDROME AND THE MEDICALIZATION OF MENOPAUSE: A SOCIOLOGICAL PERSPECTIVE

Susan E. Bell, Ph.D.

Department of Sociology and Anthropology
Bowdoin College
Brunswick, Maine

INTRODUCTION

> "For countless generations, women have suffered the distressing mental and physical symptoms of premenstrual tension, and its role as a disruptive force in the harmony of the home and community has been well-known. But the economic factor as a problem of decreased productiveness and absenteeism in industry has only gradually, in the past decade or two, come to the fore."
>
> — J. H. Morton (1953a: 463)

> "Distressing premenstrual symptoms afflict a major proportion of the female population. In a significant percentage of these women the cluster of symptoms is severe enough to cause temporary disruption of interpersonal relationships and on-the-job effectiveness."
>
> — R. L. Reid and S.S.C. Yen (1981: 96-97)

More than 50 years ago, Robert T. Frank (1931: 1053-1054), an eminent medical scientist, gave the name of Premenstrual Tension to the "minor disturbances," including "increased fatigability, irritability, lack of concentration and attacks of pain," as well as to the "indescribable tension" experienced by some women premenstrually. These physical disturbances, he believed, led to disruptions in the social fabric; he cited instances of patients' complaints of interference in their family lives and in their employment. Implicit in this formulation of the problem was a belief that relief of women's physical distress would lead to social order, and that the proper role of medicine was to intervene. These assumptions about the connection between physical and social disorder and about the role of medicine in treating these disorders are mirrored by many others in medical publications since the 1950's (Morton, 1953a; Reid & Yen, 1981).

In studies of the medical profession, sociologists have pointed out that these connections were not inevitable; instead, they were forged by institutions and individuals in an historical process of struggle which can be uncovered and examined critically. Paul Starr (1982: 13), for example, traces how the medical profession was able to assert its "cultural authority," ensuring that its "particular definitions of reality and judgments of meaning and value [would] prevail as valid and true." Conrad and Schneider (1980: 17) examine how certain categories of deviant behavior have become defined as medical problems instead of moral problems and "how medicine, rather than, for example, the family, church, or state, has become the dominant agent of social control for those so identified." Conrad and Schneider (1980: 242) also trace the consequences of medical social control: "the ways in which medicine functions (wittingly or unwittingly) to secure adherence to social norms — specifically, by using medical means to minimize, eliminate, or normalize deviant behavior." Frank's statements, in sum, can be viewed as part of a process of the introduction of a "medical deviance designation" (Schneider & Conrad, 1980) to the premenstrual period. To understand how the medical profession is achieving "cultural authority" over this phase of the menstrual cycle, we must examine the verbal expressions of the medical point of view within an historical context.

The phenomenon to which Frank gave the name "Premenstrual Tension" is currently known as "Premenstrual Syndrome" or "PMS." The actual prevalence of PMS has been a matter of dispute. In the 1940's, Greenhill and Freed (Freed, 1953: 466) contended that although it "was relatively rare, more moderate degrees of premenstrual tension were very common" and called these episodes "premenstrual distress." In their view, up to half of all menstruating women suffered from premenstrual distress. By the early 1950's, however, Freed (1953: 466) remarked that what he and Greenhill had "termed premenstrual distress [was] now known as premenstrual tension." Today, Reid and Yen (1981: 86) estimate that 20 to 40 percent of the female population experience "some degree of temporary mental or physical incapacitation," that is premenstrual tension, and 70 to 90 percent of the population "will admit to recurrent premenstrual symptoms," or premenstrual distress.

The "nature" of PMS is also a contested matter. Medical scientists have no clear consensus regarding premenstrual symptoms as these may define or constitute a syndrome. By the late 1960's, more than 150 premenstrual symptoms had been identified (Rubinow & Roy-Byrne, 1984). Recent reviews of the literature (Reid & Yen, 1981; Rubinow & Roy-Byrne, 1984) list somatic symptoms such as headache, breast tenderness and swelling, bloating, edema, acne, constipation, increased thirst or appetite, and craving for sweet or salty foods, in addition to affective changes such as fatigue, depression, irritability, and tension (see also chapter by O'Brien, this volume).

Questions about the role of physiological, psychological, and environmental factors in the etiology and treatment of premenstrual symptoms continue to plague research in psychiatry (Rubinow & Roy-Byrne, 1984), as well as gynecology (Reid & Yen, 1981). Studies are, in the words of two reviewers (Rubinow & Roy-Byrne, 1984: 163), riddled with "serious errors in. . . design," compounding medical uncertainty further. So many treatments have been recommended that Steiner and Carroll (1977: 330) concluded that the "outstanding feature" of all treatments was introduction "with enthusiasm on the basis of uncontrolled studies" and then failure to survive "rigorous testing in controlled clinical trials" (see chapters by Reid, and Steiner & Haskett, this volume).

Although the focus of this paper is the transformation of medical ideas, medicine is not alone in its interest in PMS. Psychologists have begun to consider the relationship between physiology, behavior, and emotions in menstruating women. Attorneys have explored the use of PMS as a defense in criminal cases, and women's groups have drawn attention to PMS by forming self-help groups to distribute information and provide support to women who suffer physically and/or emotionally before their menstrual periods. PMS has become the object of interest in professional and public arenas. The transformation in medical thinking is embedded in these arenas; these arenas are shaping and shaped by changing medical ideas. More research is needed to explore the relationship between them.

In this paper, I develop a theoretical framework for analyzing how medical professionals are coming to define and understand PMS, as well as an evaluation of the likely outcome of their work. I will pursue a critique of medical perspectives on PMS and show how they can serve to perpetuate sexist beliefs about the effect of menstruation on women's behavior, reinforce women's structural subordination to men, and increase the power of medicine over human experiences. To do this, I first introduce the concept of "medicalization," which refers to the process and product of defining and treating human experiences as medical problems. Next, I argue that PMS is becoming medicalized. Following this, I consider the medicalization of menopause, another phase in the life cycle of women, which occurred in the 1930's and 1940's. Finally, I show how the menopause example can shed light on the consequences of the medicalization of PMS.

MEDICALIZATION: A SOCIOLOGICAL FOCUS

Since the late 19th century, modern medicine has been based on the biomedical model (Mishler, 1981a). The biomedical model defines disease as a deviation from normal biological functioning and describes each disease as having a distinctive pathogenesis, pathology, and set of symptoms. The biomedical model is so deeply ingrained in modern medicine "that health professionals tend to forget that it is a conceptual model, a way of thinking about the world" and not the only "representation or picture of reality" (Mishler, 1981a: 1). This model focuses the medical gaze on the bodies of individuals, abstracting them from their social environments (Bologh, 1981). It leads medicine to select only certain problems to study, to choose specific research designs that focus attention on a limited number of aspects of a problem, and to organize and interpret only some of the data. The biomedical model, in other words, is a paradigm that guides how physicians see and solve problems.

Critics of the biomedical model (Conrad & Kern, 1986; Freidson, 1970; Koeske, 1982, 1983; Mishler, AmaraSingham, Hauser, Liem, Osherson, and Waxler, 1981) have shown that it masks the social and political processes of medicine and obscures the social roots and consequences of the expansion of medical control. In his now classic study of the medical profession, sociologist Eliot Freidson (1970: 205) concluded that medicine has won a "well-nigh exclusive jurisdiction over determining what illness is and therefore how people must act in order to be treated as ill." Medicine, in other words, does not only diagnose and treat disease but *creates* illness as a social state. Medicine, according to the critique of the biomedical model, is a "social practice" involving "active interpretive work through which a particular social reality is constructed, a 'reality' constituted by diagnosed illnesses and prescribed treatments" (Mishler, 1981b: 162).

Beginning with the work of Freidson (1970) and Zola (1972), a number of sociologists (Conrad, 1975; Conrad & Schneider, 1980) have explored the origins and consequences of "medicalization," the expansion of medical jurisdiction over human life. In the process of medicalization, certain behaviors or conditions are given medical meaning, and medical practice is given the task of eliminating or controlling them (Conrad, 1975). Through medicalization, physicians have increased their power over human experiences. The meaning of this power and the scope of medical authority are matters which, according to Schneider and Conrad (1980: 40), "are negotiated and renegotiated regularly." Although the profession of medicine may *invoke* the biomedical model to justify the expansion of its jurisdiction, its ability to *assert* the "medical deviance designation" (Schneider & Conrad, 1980) rests on political and social grounds as well.

There are two kinds of medicalization. The first kind consists of defining deviant behaviors such as alcoholism, homosexuality, child abuse, and hyperactivity as medical problems with medical solutions (that is, in terms of health and illness); "badness" becomes reclassified as "sickness" (Conrad & Schneider, 1980). The second kind consists of defining normal life events, such as pregnancy, childbirth, and menopause, as diseases; natural biological processes become illnesses. In each of these instances, medicalization is not an inevitable outcome of advances in medical knowledge, but comes about through the imposition of medical control, supported by intellectual and social forces.

Women's experiences are particularly vulnerable to medicalization for a variety of biological, social, and psychological reasons, including the fit between women's biology and medicine's biomedical orientation, women's structural subordination to men (which is replicated in relations between male physicians and female patients), and women's patterns of dealing with their own symptoms as well as their social roles as mothers and kin (which bring them into contact with medicine more often than men)(Riessman, 1983). But women have not been simply passive victims of medicalization. The medicalization of women's problems has resulted from a fit between women's class-specific needs and the medical profession's interests and beliefs. As Riessman (1983) has argued, some upper-class women found medicalization to be useful in retaining class privileges.

The consequences of medicalization for women have been paradoxical. On the one hand, women's experiences are acknowledged as real and not "figments of their imagination" (Posner, 1979), and some of women's suffering has been relieved. On the other hand, medicalization stigmatizes women further by reinforcing traditional stereotypes of the relationship between female biology and behavior. It also categorizes women's problems as individual biological or personal deficits, thereby removing them from their social context and treating them on an individual basis, one after another (Riessman, 1983; Rome, 1986). More generally, medicalization preserves the structures and categories of sexist society.

Schneider and Conrad (1980) characterize medicalization as occurring in five stages in five different arenas of contest. They caution that while separable for analytic purposes, the stages and arenas are interconnected in a complicated interacting whole. The stages are: First, the prior designation of deviance to the behavior in question; second, medical discovery of etiology and/or treatment; third, claimsmaking and counter-claimsmaking by professionals and nonprofessionals about the proposed medical definitions of the behavior; fourth, a struggle for "ownership" of the problem; and fifth, the institutionalization of the problem. The arenas of contest in which medicalization comes about include intraprofessional and interprofessional disputes, lay and public challenge to or support of medical definitions of a problem, and legislative politicking and court cases. This model can be used to discern some of the patterns at work in the case of PMS.

PREMENSTRUAL SYNDROME: STAGES OF MEDICALIZATION

PMS is becoming medicalized. It is being defined as a medical problem, and medical personnel are being given the responsibility for treating it. In the process, behaviors that previously were identified as the symptoms of neurosis or criminality or the products of women's imaginations are coming to be seen as manifestations of a biological imbalance that can be diagnosed and treated by medical professionals. One way that this process can be discerned is by discussing PMS in terms of the stages of medicalization outlined by Schneider and Conrad (1980). First, in the United States, behaviors assumed to be associated with the menstrual cycle have been designated as deviant, both historically (Smith-Rosenberg, 1973) and today. In a review of popular and scientific articles, Ruble and Brooks-Gunn (1979: 172) discovered a number of persistent assumptions about the impact of menstruation on women's behavior, including the beliefs that women experience "fluctuations in somatic, emotional, and behavioral characteristics across phases of the menstrual cycle," and that these fluctuations are "severe and possibly debilitating." According to Koeske (1976: 12), most of the behaviors associated with the menstrual cycle "are thought of as negative and implicitly, unusual, for women."

The discovery of a medical etiology of PMS, the second stage of medicalization, can be traced to the 1930's, when Frank (1931: 1056) proposed that "the continued circulation of an excessive amount of female sex hormone in the blood" could "produce serious symptoms." Consistent with Schneider and Conrad's model of the stages of medicalization, which lists as the third stage claimsmaking and counter-claimsmaking, subsequent medical and scientific research has challenged Frank's theory of an excessive amount of female sex hormones. To date, there is no agreement about the etiology of PMS.

Use of progesterone replacement therapy to treat PMS began in the 1940's in England, became popular in the 1950's, and remains the most publicized medical intervention, despite negative results in controlled, double-blind clinical trials of efficacy and the lack of long-term studies of safety (Harrison, 1984; Reid & Yen, 1981; Rubinow & Roy-Byrne, 1984). Progesterone treatment for PMS has been prescribed by American physicians since June 1981, although it has not been approved by the Food and Drug Administration for this purpose (Harrison, 1984).

Since the late 1940's, Dr. Katharina Dalton, a British physician, has championed the medical orientation to PMS (see chapter by Dalton, this volume). She has consistently advocated treating sufferers with progesterone and is presently the Director of the Premenstrual Syndrome Clinic at the University College Hospital in London. Dalton's work has been sharply criticized as methodologically unsound (Reid & Yen, 1981; Rubinow & Roy-Byrne, 1984). PMS Action, an advocacy group, has praised her work, and has actively sought to make progesterone treatment available in the United States (PMS Action, 1983).

Currently, there is contest over ownership of PMS, the fourth stage of medicalization. At this stage, according to Schneider and Conrad (1980: 16), "One is likely to find appeals to the ultimate arbiter of power and legitimacy, the state, to recognize and officially endorse the medical designation." Significant arenas of contest at this stage are courts, legislative committees, and other committees "called either by the state or its representatives." This contest is especially clear in the discussions over whether women committing crimes during the premenstrual phase of the menstrual cycle are responsible for their behavior (criminals) or not (victims of diminished capacity attributable to PMS). For example, in a bankruptcy case involving a personal injury judgment based on a stabbing incident (*Lovato v. Irvin*, 1983: 258), the debtor claimed that "her actions were not deliberate or intentional and thus not 'willful' because she was allegedly suffering from premenstrual syndrome." In his judgment for the creditor, Judge Jay Gueck (*Lovato v. Irvin*, 1983: 259) wrote, "The scientific evidence relating PMS and its application here is too sketchy, inconclusive, and unreliable to be accepted as an explanation for otherwise willful and malicious conduct." In part, this was because "too much uncertainty" still surrounded the studies of PMS "for it to be considered a generally accepted theory" in the medical community (*Lovato v. Irvin*, 1983: 260).

PMS is also becoming institutionalized — the fifth stage in Schneider and Conrad's model of medicalization. PMS has provided the impetus for the growth of clinics in the United States and England. It has been successfully used as a defense in British and French courts. It is not a psychiatric diagnostic category in the *Diagnostic and Statistical Manual of Mental Disorders* (DSM-III), but it has been proposed for inclusion in the revised *Manual* (DSM-III-R) as "premenstrual dysphoric disorder" (Holden, 1986).[1] Finally, the experience of PMS has led American women to form a non-profit organization, PMS Action, to support sufferers of the condition and to crusade for the medical deviance designation. In sum, the phenomenon of medicalization is taking place.

PREMENSTRUAL SYNDROME: ARENAS OF CONTEST

The process of medicalization is complex, and the stages are contained in a number of different arenas of contest. First, there are intraprofessional and interprofessional disputes over the etiology and treatment of PMS. In addition to controversy within and between gynecology and psychiatry, there is controversy in psychology and the law.

Social scientists, primarily psychologists (Koeske, 1976; Parlee, 1973), have also turned their attention to examining the relationship between biology and culture in women's experience of premenstrual symptoms. They, too, remain uncertain of this relationship, although they generally emphasize the role of the environment, arguing that "cultural beliefs about menstruation exist and may influence women's menstrual experiences" (Ruble, Boggiano, & Brooks-Gunn, 1982: 626; see also chapters by Ruble & Brooks-Gunn, and by Ericksen, this volume). Koeske (1982, 1983) is particularly interested in interactions among biology, psychology, and the environment, and has proposed that a new perspective is needed to study how they interrelate in women's experiences.

At the same time, the role of premenstrual symptoms in criminal behavior has become a topic of interest to legal scholars, exploring the possibility of identifying "avenues by which female criminal defendants suffering from the premenstrual syndrome may take advantage of existing legal doctrines" (Wallach & Rubin, 1971: 215). While some American

---

[1] This proposal has been sharply criticized by some mental health professionals who contend that this would contribute "to the stigmatization of normal women" (Holden, 1986: 327).

legal scholars (Wallach & Rubin, 1971) argue in favor of using PMS as a defense for women accused of crimes, others (Horney, 1978: 34) warn, "It would seem unwise to further cloud the already difficult issues of criminal responsibility with an expanded insanity defense based on premenstrual tension." In this arena, the dispute centers on the scientific validity of PMS studies as well as on the social implications of legal "recognition of the lack of control concept" (Horney, 1978: 34). [See also Wallach & Rubin (1971) on this point.] Despite the lack of general acceptance among medical scientists about the causes and consequences of premenstrual symptoms, British courts have accepted the argument that "severe premenstrual syndrome" is a factor in manslaughter, arson, and assault; and French courts have recognized premenstrual syndrome as a cause of temporary insanity (Dalton, 1980: 1070).

Surrounding the inter- and intra-professional contests over the meaning, causes, and consequences of premenstrual symptoms is an expanding public awareness of and interest in the issues. A spate of articles about PMS appeared from 1981 to 1984 in major American women's magazines *(Glamour, Mademoiselle, McCalls, Ms.)*, as well as in *Essence, Newsweek,* and *Reader's Digest.* *The New York Times* ran a series of stories in 1982 about the case of Shirley Santos, a New York woman accused of assaulting her daughter. According to these articles, she maintained a defense of diminished capacity, arguing that premenstrual stress caused her to act irrationally. During this same general period, two women suffering from premenstrual symptoms founded PMS Action in 1980 "to help women become informed, active, health care consumers" (PMS Action, 1983: 2; see also Cassara, this volume). They sought recognition for the biological basis of premenstrual symptoms, contending that "sufferers of PMS are neither neurotics nor hypochondriacs, but women with a hormonal imbalance that can be treated" (PMS Action, 1983: 2). A more cautionary approach has been taken by the Boston Women's Health Book Collective, authors of *Our Bodies, Ourselves,* who warn of the dangers of labeling premenstrual behaviors as hormonally based, arguing that to call them "symptoms of disease" is a way of keeping women in their place (Rome, 1986: 146).

The "medicalization" of PMS is fraught with paradoxes. On the one hand, it can explain the experiences of individual women. On the other hand, it carries with it the likelihood of reinforcing the belief that women are controlled by their hormones. As two participants (Wallach & Rubin, 1971: 216) wrote over a decade ago, showing a connection between the menstrual cycle and women's behavior means taking the risk that this information could be seized "as the long-awaited documentation of the claim that women are biologically unable to competently perform in responsible occupations."

THE MEDICALIZATION OF MENOPAUSE[2]

A sociological analysis of the transformation in medical thinking about PMS is enhanced by comparing it to the transformation in medical thinking about menopause. Both cases exemplify how women's experiences are vulnerable to medicalization. The medicalization of menopause has had mixed effects for women, such as (positively) relieving hot flushes and sweats with estrogen replacement therapy, yet (negatively) contributing to an increased incidence of endometrial cancer associated with this treatment and reinforcing traditional social roles for aging women.

[2] This section is a summary of my analysis of the medicalization of menopause (Bell, 1985).

This historical example can illuminate some of the pitfalls of medicalizing PMS.

The medicalization of menopause exemplifies how medical theory is embedded in social and historical circumstances. It points to the need for locating discussions of medical theories within an historical context in order to distinguish the ways in which these ideas are both made possible and bound by these circumstances (Bell, 1985, 1986). I have argued elsewhere that the medicalization of menopause by medical specialists reflected and reinforced stereotypical views of aging women, but was not determined by these views. Further, broad political and economic transformations were occurring during the New Deal, which framed and influenced the medical profession as it rapidly created models for understanding and treating problems associated with menopause. Today, as we consider the medical, social, and legal ramifications of defining PMS as a disease, we can reflect back on and benefit from analyzing circumstances surrounding the medicalization of menopause. Menopause (the cessation of menstruation) is a biological and social phase in the female life cycle which became medicalized in the 20th century. This process was not the inexorable result of discoveries made by members of the medical profession, but the outcome of struggle between the profession and other institutional actors as they negotiated and renegotiated the meaning of menopause and the role of medicine in diagnosing and treating it. Although science and humanitarian values were elements in the medicalization of menopause, as in medicalization generally, these ideas and values alone did not "cause" this changed orientation (Schneider & Conrad, 1980). The medicalization of menopause depended upon a theory linking together women's emotions, behaviors, and physiological changes; a treatment for menopausal symptoms; legitimation of medical control over this treatment by the state; and the possibility of a receptive patient population. These elements merged together in the late 1930's and 1940's. First, sex endocrinology offered medical specialists a new way of seeing and explaining "the form, function and behavior of the sexes" (Hall, 1977: 18). This paradigm enabled them to construct a theory. Second, the pharmaceutical industry began to distribute a synthetic estrogen substitute, which was cheap, potent orally, and easily synthesized (the substance was diethylstilbestrol, commonly known as DES) (Bell, 1986). Third, the Food and Drug Administration (FDA) gave medicine control over distributing DES. When it released DES for sale in 1941, the FDA restricted it for use upon the advice of a physician only (Bell, 1986). Finally, all women who live long enough experience menopause, and in the United States, menopausal women were already stigmatized at this time, ensuring a receptive patient population (Bart & Grossman, 1978; Perlmutter & Bart, 1982).

In the section that follows, I consider how medical specialists forged a new way of thinking about menopause. A comprehensive analysis of the medicalization of menopause would include an examination of multiple layers of social and intellectual life. This analysis would range from the contest within specialist medicine over how to set standards for medical practice in the era of miracle drugs, and the relative merits of laboratory tests versus clinical judgment in medical research, to the struggle between the American Medical Association and the Food and Drug Administration over the relative autonomy of medicine in light of federal legislation giving the state the right to determine which drugs could be safely prescribed. An analysis such as this is beyond the scope of this essay. Elsewhere (Bell, 1985, 1986), I identify these multiple layers and consider how they contributed to the medicalization of menopause. Here, I elucidate the transformation of medical ideas. The data for this are drawn from the published works of a group of 37 prominent medical specialists.[3] As a group, the specialists were at the top of the medical profession; most were full-time specialists; and close to half of them had teaching appointments at medical schools. Their professional status and identities meant that their perspectives about menopause were more likely to gain acceptance (Schneider & Conrad, 1980).

Medical specialists recognized a number of different types of changes during menopause: biological, psychological, and environmental.[4] The paradigm of endocrinology enabled them to distinguish biologically-caused changes from those "caused" psychologically or environmentally. As we shall see, each model considered separately — the biological, psychological, and environmental — highlights an aspect of the problem at the same time that it limits and restricts the field of vision by excluding the others. For rarely did medical professionals include in the perspective a dynamic understanding of how a woman's biology and her psyche and her environmental circumstances might combine to make the transition into menopause a difficult one, especially in the context of a culture which valued youth.

Most commonly, specialists focused on the biological changes and described menopause as a physiological process caused by cessation of ovarian function. This focus was an advance over the "traditional concept of menopause as an aberration of somatic function, predominantly psychogenic in origin and requiring only sedation or psychotherapy" (Salmon, Geist, & Walter, 1941: 1843). According to this biological view, the reduction of estrogen caused physical and hormonal changes outside of a person's control. If a specialist believed that a woman's symptoms were caused by a lack of estrogen, estrogen replacement therapy would supply "the patient with the hormone she [lacked]" (Salmon et al., 1941: 1843).

In contrast to earlier generations of medical professionals, and to many of their contemporaries, medical specialists in the 1930's believed that menopause constituted a normal, biological phase in the lives of most women, not just a few (Novak, 1940; Pratt, 1939; Shorr, 1940). For 85 percent of the female population, they argued, menopause was physiological, not pathological.

Secondary effects of the loss of estrogen could also occur. According to these specialists, estrogen deficiency could cause hot flushes and sweats which could awaken "the patient at night and [cause] her to catch cold" or "produce a feeling of insecurity, in extreme cases

---

[3] The 37 physicians comprise a sample of the 178 physicians investigating the drug DES. Only these 37 physicians published papers about menopause in medical journals and were interested in using DES to treat menopausal symptoms. The other 141 physicians either were not interested in using DES in menopause or had not published papers about menopause. The 178 physicians consist of all the individuals contributing evidence to the Food and Drug Administration about the safety of DES in applications submitted by 14 pharmaceutical manufacturers in May 1941. For a fuller discussion of the ideas of the 37 physicians, see Bell (1986). For a discussion of their role in the production of DES, see Bell (1984, 1985).

[4] Typologies described by Koeske (1982) and Perlmutter and Bart (1982) in their analyses of attitudes towards menopause today helped me to see these three themes in physicians' work in the 1930's and 1940's.

inducing the patient to stay at home and lead a hermit existence (Frank, 1941: 856).

The focus on biological changes acknowledged and explained the presence of menopausal symptoms in all women and the particularly uncomfortable experiences of some women. It then provided a simple solution for relieving a woman's symptoms: Estrogen replacement therapy. However, when used as the sole explanatory model of menopausal symptoms, it risked reducing the problems faced by aging women to biologically-determined ones, and reinforcing the traditional view of women as biologically different and inferior. Further, the biological model located the problem and solution in the individual. At the same time a biological model released individual women from responsibility for their distress, it made them individually responsible for effecting a cure. Thus, it relieved society from responsibility for menopausal women's distress.

Specialists also recognized that psychic and emotional disturbances formed an "important part of the menopausal syndrome" (Pratt, 1938: 567). According to the psychological model, the symptoms of menopause were "most stormy in nervous, neurotic and unbalanced women and less marked in the well-poised and stable individual" (Frank, 1941: 856). In other words, a woman's personality pattern could be the underlying cause of symptoms, instead of estrogen withdrawal. If this was the case, psychotherapy, not estrogen therapy, was warranted.

The focus on psychological symptoms continued a long tradition of attributing women's experiences during menopause to their previous behavior (Smith-Rosenberg, 1973), but used new psychiatric concepts and terminology to do so. When used as the only explanation for women's menopausal symptoms, it blamed women and placed responsibility for alleviating symptoms on them; an individual woman's symptoms would disappear along with her neuroses. This model could lead physicians to overlook the biological nature of menopausal symptoms and to treat women improperly with psychotherapy alone. However, this model potentially offered a corrective to the narrow biological one by suggesting that gynecologists should not diagnose and treat ovarian failure alone, and that, in the words of one, "the menopause is neither psychic nor organic but a combination of the two" (Pratt, 1938: 567). Nevertheless, the predominant tendency of the psychological model was to assert that women's complaints were "all in their heads" (Posner, 1979).

Infrequently, specialists identified environmental factors underlying menopausal symptoms. For example, in his contribution to a special issue of the *American Journal of Obstetrics and Gynecology*, commemorating the 20th anniversary of its founding, gynecologist Emil Novak (1940: 589) warned against "the easy assumption of menopausal etiology of symptoms in women of the fifth decade." He argued that often these symptoms were "explainable more rationally as the result of the stress and strain resulting from the rearing of large families of children, or because of domestic, economic, or marital problems. . ." than as the result of hormonal changes. For these women, he recommended "reassurance" as well as "correcting so far as possible any detrimental environmental factors which may exist" (Novak, 1940: 592). J.P. Greenhill (1940: 535), an editor of the *Year Book of Obstetrics and Gynecology*, pointed out that menopause was a time of transition out of childbearing and childrearing, which many women dreaded. To women who feared that they would be "unattractive and perhaps repulsive to their husbands," he advised his colleagues, a good tactic would be to disabuse them of these fears and then to remind women of the "importance of a proper mode of living, including sufficient rest, sleep, some exercise, fresh air, reading of good books and other activities to occupy [their] time."

The environmental model widened the vision of medicine to include more than a woman's personality and physiology in diagnosing and treating menopausal symptoms. It acknowledged the social and cultural aspects of the passage into menopause for women in American society, and the attendant stresses and strains of their new status. Women's complaints, according to this model, were the manifestations of changing circumstances in their social lives, not the results of estrogen deficiency; and women were responding to real events, not imagined ones. Most often, however, specialists recommended changing individual habits (reading, sleeping, and exercising) instead of the environment. While they might identify the problem as external, in contrast to the biological and psychological models which discovered internal sources of the symptoms, they identified the solution as internal. At the same time the environmental model created the possibility of social change, it turned away from this solution.

Gynecology transformed menopause, defining it as a medical problem and labeling it as a deficiency disease. In their urge to help patients in distress, specialists' underlying message was that all menopausal women should see physicians, who could prescribe estrogen replacement therapy, psychotherapy and/or talking and reassurance. In recommending that even talking to a physician could be therapeutic and that all menopausal women should seek medical advice, they were defining menopause as a medical problem.

Specialists invoked the biomedical model to justify the application of the medical deviance designation to menopause. They attributed their findings to their ability to discover "facts" about it with methods that were objective and value neutral; that it was caused by the decrease in estrogen and that accompanying symptoms could be treated hormonally; that it was universal to the human female; that hormonal symptoms and signs could be distinguished from environmental and psychological ones. They believed that their conclusions were entirely the products of "good science." In reality, their science directed them to ask particular questions in specific ways and to see particular data; it limited their gaze at the same time that it sharpened its focus. Their work was also shaped, however, as all medicine is, by social and political factors, and, in turn, had social and political implications.

Ironically, the disease orientation to menopause was introduced by medical specialists who intended to reassure women that most often menopause was a normal physiological event. While they succeeded in demonstrating the biological basis of this event, this had social and sexist implications. Unwittingly, they promoted a new view of menopause as pathological and abnormal, and reinforced the stereotypical picture of women already in existence.

The medicalization of menopause reflected and reinforced traditional views about the role of hormones in women's behavior [see Kaufert (1982) on this point]. Specialists were members of a culture that stigmatized menopause (Perlmutter & Bart, 1982). This stigma was expressed in their published papers. For example, two gynecologists at the Lying-In Hospital at the University of Chicago (Davis & Boynton, 1941: 341) wrote, ". . . the cessation of ovarian function brings in its wake a bizarre train of symptoms which may completely upset the normal equilibrium of even the well-balanced individual."

Cultural norms about the "proper" role of aging women were also reflected in and reinforced by the medicalization of menopause (Bart & Grossman, 1978; Smith-Rosenberg, 1973). Specialists' prescriptions for their menopausal patients, such as reading, resting, and engaging in social and helpful activities, encouraged menopausal women to act in socially appropriate ways (Greenhill, 1940; Pratt, 1938). In their role as counselor and advisor to women, (male) physicians replicated their dominant social status at the same time as they replicated the subordination of women — giving expert advice about how to grow old gracefully.

Medical ideas — the development of three conceptual models and the connection between these models and the notions and categories of sexist society — cannot entirely account for the medicalization of menopause. The availability of a "cure" for the "disease" was also a prerequisite; so was a convergence between the needs of women and physicians. Moreover, institutional settings conditioned and shaped the timing and course of this process. Medical specialists could not have been successful in achieving social control over menopause without the pharmaceutical industry (which provided a drug which could be used to treat as many patients as needed it) and the state (which, through the Food and Drug Administration, gave physicians control over prescribing the new drug). (For more on these points, see Bell, 1986.)

Physicians' ideas fitted with the needs of their married middle- and upper-class female patients in the 1930's. First, women's complaints of hot flushes and sweats were no longer dismissed by medical specialists. The biological model legitimated their complaints, attributed them to hormonal (not behavioral or psychological) causes, and provided a cure for them. Medicine's "cultural authority" derived in part because of the scientific basis upon which the specialists constructed the three models of menopausal changes. The paradigm of sex endocrinology enabled them to describe and explain the etiology of menopause and also to design a simple treatment for the discomfort associated with it.

Second, the environmental model acknowledged the difficulty of passing into old age for these women. These women may have believed that their happiness depended on their ability to bear and raise children and to serve the needs of their husbands. They had lost their children and feared the loss of sexual attractiveness, and believed their lives would therefore become meaningless. Medicine served the interests of these women by legitimating their depression.

IMPLICATIONS OF THE MEDICALIZATION OF MENOPAUSE

The consequences for women of the medicalization of menopause have been paradoxical. While their complaints have been recognized and in some cases successfully treated by medicine, there have also been serious medical and social implications. Here, I will point out just a few relevant ones. First, the medicalization of menopause ignores the ways that social characteristics and social relationships influence health and illness, even though the psychological and environmental models explicitly acknowledge this. By superimposing science onto medicine, physicians have tended to look for universal physical and psychological signs and symptoms of menopause in their patients. Put simply, according to this view, the social and cultural context surrounding women is irrelevant to diagnosis and treatment; the reduction of estrogen produces the same symptoms regardless of a woman's race or social class. Simultaneously, women's experiences are acknowledged and treated medically while the social roots of their problems are ignored.

However, recent cross-cultural studies of menopause have shown that the experiences of menopausal women are not universal, and that social and cultural contexts have an effect on how women interpret and respond to the physical signs and symptoms of menopause (Voda, Dinnerstein, & O'Donnell, 1982).

Second, the medical perspective implicitly assumes that all menopausal women live in similar social circumstances (Kaufert, 1982). According to medical specialists in the 1930's and 1940's, menopausal women were married, had stayed at home raising children who had since left home, and had the economic resources and leisure time to rest, relax, and do good works; they were not in the labor force (Greenhill, 1940; Novak, 1940). Although most women did marry and have children, a look at United States census figures for this same period shows that the lives of many American women passing into menopause did not fit this narrow view. For example, in 1940, roughly 24 percent of women aged 45-54 were in the labor force (Blau, 1978: 51). For black women, the percentage was higher than this. Furthermore, assuming that a man and woman married when they were ages 25 and 22, 71 percent of marriages beginning in 1900 would have been disrupted due to death or divorce by 1940 (Uhlenberg, 1983: 174). Specialists' prescriptions for their patients were based on a narrow and biased view of the lives of aging women.

Third, instead of drawing from the environmental, psychological, and biological models to treat patients, physicians have tended to rely on the biological one and prescribed estrogen replacement therapy indiscriminately (Bart & Grossman, 1976; McKinlay & McKinlay, 1973). As Kaufert and McKinlay (1985: 129) observe, "Once menopause was defined as a deficiency condition, its treatment with estrogen was not only legitimate, but became an obligation." In their review of the controversy over estrogen replacement therapy which took place from 1970 to 1980, they write that by the 1970's, estrogen had become one of the five most frequently prescribed drugs in the United States (Kaufert & McKinlay, 1985: 114). Endometrial cancer rates rose sharply during this same period; a number of studies, published in the *New England Journal of Medicine* and the *Journal of the American Medical Association*, triggered debate over the safety of estrogen therapy (Kaufert & McKinlay, 1985: 117). By 1976, researchers "had linked estrogen therapy with gall bladder disease, endometrial and breast cancers and with higher levels of the risk factors for coronary disease, but not with myocardial infarction" (Kaufert & McKinlay, 1985: 119-120). The medicalization of menopause, in other words, has had serious negative effects on women's health.

Fourth, the medicalization of menopause has attributed the problems of aging women to individual causes, with individual solutions (McCrea, 1983). At the same time it has absolved women from responsibility, it has held them responsible for their plight; and excused sexist society from any responsibility for complaints voiced by menopausal women. This mitigates against the possibility that women will recognize and protest against oppressive social circumstances. It preserves the status quo by encouraging women to conform to their traditional social roles as wives, mothers, and community members, and delegates responsibility for this restoration to physicians.

In summary, the transformation in medical thinking was embedded in social and historical circumstances. These circumstances shaped but did not determine the content, direction, and timing of this change. In turn, the transformation in medical thinking was an important factor in the medicalization of menopause.

MEDICAL MODELS OF PREMENSTRUAL SYNDROME

The transformation in medical thinking about menopause can be compared with its transformation in the case of PMS. At the outset of this discussion, I must caution that my assessment of the PMS case is speculative and represents my initial and tentative review of the process of medicalization. Nevertheless, it is instructive to compare the two, as Greene and Dalton (1953) recognized more than 30 years ago.

The medicalization of PMS, like the medicalization of menopause, depends upon a theory linking together women's emotions, behaviors, and physiological changes, as well as a treatment, legitimation of medical control, and a receptive patient population. Earlier, I sketched out how these elements can be fit into a sequence proposed by sociologists Joseph Schneider and Peter Conrad (1980). Here, I will consider how three models (biological, psychological, and environmental) are being advanced to explain PMS.

The material used in this section is drawn primarily from review articles which have summarized the medical literature about PMS (Friedman, Hurt, Arnoff, & Clarkin, 1980; Reid & Yen, 1981; Rubinow & Roy-Byrne, 1984; Steiner & Carroll, 1977), from contributions to a symposium on PMS (*International Record of Medicine*, Volume 166, 1953), and from articles such as those by Frank (1931) and Dalton (Dalton, 1964; Greene & Dalton, 1953), which are widely cited in the literature about PMS. Future sociological analyses of PMS could profitably examine the ways in which the models themselves have changed and overlapped since first advanced, and consider the social and intellectual roots and consequences of these changes.

Dalton (1964: 18) stated the biological model clearly: "Menstruation is a normal physiological function, and many are unaware of the influence of the menstrual hormones on different aspects of a woman's life, especially in circumstances common to men and women." Frank (1931) was the first to propose a biological explanation for women's premenstrual behavior. He reasoned that estrogen excess caused women to behave aberrantly, and thus women were not responsible for these behaviors. Although Frank's theory has been disputed, the biological model has itself been retained. As Morton (1953b: 505) observed 20 years later, this was considered an advance over earlier theories, which attributed symptoms to "'nerves' or imagination" and which recommended "reassurance and mild sedation" for the milder forms of PMS and referral to a psychiatrist in more severe cases.

The biological model has been modified in recent years. Researchers have recognized the complexity of biological factors, prompting some (Rubinow, Roy-Byrne, Hoban, Gold, & Post, 1984: 684) to posit the existence of "at least several overlapping syndromes rather than a single syndrome." They have also acknowledged that "nonhormonal events," such as "environmental events, attitudes about menstruation, and personality traits" (Friedman et al., 1980: 722) play a role in the experience of premenstrual symptoms. As in the case of menopause, the biological model serves to legitimate women's experiences by attributing them to hormones instead of hysteria. Similarly, the biological model describes these "symptoms" as normal for most women, and attempts to explain the especially difficult experiences of some.

Frank (1931: 1056) proposed a treatment (radiating the ovaries or prescribing substances to induce "excretion of the female sex hormone" such as calcium lactate, caffeine, or saline laxatives) on the basis of his biological theory. Subsequently, other treatments have been proposed, each of them relying on a theory of the etiology of PMS. According to Morton (1953b: 505), "Practically every commercially available hormone has been used by the various investigators. . ." The most popular of the treatments has been progesterone, although like all the others, it has not been proven effective, both because the etiology of PMS remains obscure (Rubinow & Roy-Byrne, 1984) and because treatment response studies have suffered from methodological problems (Morton, 1953b; Rubinow & Roy-Byrne, 1984; Steiner & Carroll, 1977).

The psychological model, too, can be discerned in medical studies of PMS. Suarez-Murias (1953: 475) wrote that the "incidence" of PMS was higher in patients with neurotic and psychotic disorders, and lower in those considered psychologically normal. This expression of the psychological model is reminiscent of the pronouncements made by specialists concerning their menopausal patients, and implies that a woman's personality pattern, not her biology, could be the real "cause" of her symptoms. Psychotherapy, according to this reductionist view, would resolve women's premenstrual complaints.

However, most of the discussions about the role of women's personality and emotions in their experience of premenstrual symptoms are more sophisticated than this. These discussions are similar to the view of at least one medical specialist (Pratt, 1938: 567) involved in the medicalization of menopause, who noted that there is a combination of "psychic" and "organic" factors underlying women's experiences. For example, Morton (1953a: 463) observed that "the emotional components do play a role in premenstrual tension." However, he cautioned that "while emotional disturbances can and often do alter the functions of the endocrine glands, the converse also holds true. Endocrine dysfunction can definitely influence the psychogenic factors and produce mental symptoms." Morton, and others subsequently, observed that there could be a reciprocal relationship between psychology and biology.

Today, the importance of psychological factors in PMS is disputed. Friedman et al. (1980: 736), for example, suggest that while for most women "*the fact* that fluctuation in the intensity of affect states occur is a direct result of primary (although unknown) biological determinants . . . , the psychosocial and intrapsychic consequences of such fluctuations all depend on cognitive state, itself a product of social context and psychobiographical determinants." In contrast, Steiner and Carroll (1977: 322) argue that psychological and psychosocial factors appear to account for only a minor part of the symptoms, and Rubinow and Roy-Byrne (1984: 166), citing Gannon (1981), argue that "evidence in support of a psychological basis for menstrually related mood disorders is currently lacking."

The environment has also been identified as having a role in the etiology of PMS, although not very frequently. Billig (1953: 490) wrote, "In industry there must be taken into account the many sensory stimuli (including emotional) to which the female worker is exposed, since they all must bear their share of responsibility in the breakdown of the individual to the point where the terminal functioning glands become deficient and symptoms of failure supervene. . ." Coppen and Kessel (1964: 718) acknowledged that social class and marital status can be factors in the experience of premenstrual symptoms. More recently, in a review of the literature on the relationship between behavior and the menstrual cycle, Friedman et al. (1980) noted that external events have been shown to have an effect on a person's interpretation of physiological change; a woman's mood can fluctuate in response to the presence of stressful external events irregardless of the phase of her menstrual cycle.

The environmental model of PMS acknowledges that women's symptoms might be attributable to difficult circumstances in their lives, such as ongoing problems associated with their roles as workers and wives. External events, not physiology or psychology, could account for their premenstrual distress, according to this view. This model legitimates women's experiences by explaining their symptoms as responses to real events, not imagined ones.

Although at best suggestive (since it was published in 1953 and I do not have more recent treatments proposed by adherents of the environmental model), a look at one of the treatments that was recommended in light of the environmental model is of interest. Billig (1953: 490) proposed "dietary management" as a solution to PMS. He believed that if women followed diets that were high in protein and low in carbohydrates, they would feel better. In turn, if women felt better, they would take off less time from work and be more productive when they labored. As expressed by Billig, the environmental model discovers external causes of women's symptoms, but then proposes an internal solution to them. In this respect, it serves to individualize and privatize women's problems.

To summarize, in the case of PMS, three models are being advanced by the medical community to explain the etiology of symptoms and to lead to recommendations for treatment.

CONCLUSIONS

There are similarities between the transformation in medical thinking about PMS and menopause. In both cases, three models have been developed — biological, psychological, and environmental. Initially in each case, the medical community argues that while most women have symptoms, few women need medical treatment. Further, in both cases it is assumed that medical professionals should determine the cause and treatment for an individual woman's symptoms.

The historical case of the transformation of menopause into a medical problem can be used to illuminate some of the tendencies in the events surrounding PMS today. One way in which medical discussions of PMS and menopause are similar is that they are both based on the biomedical model. Since the 1930's, members of the medical profession have attempted to describe, explain, and treat symptoms associated with the premenstrual phase of the menstrual cycle, and have conducted their work within the framework of the biomedical model. They, like their predecessors in the medicalization of menopause, have assumed that if they use objective and value neutral methods they can discover the etiology of PMS, distinguishing more than one variation of the syndrome if more than one pathogenesis and pathology exist. Yet, as in the case of menopause, the connections between their work and a broader social, political, and historical context can be discerned.

In an early and significant paper, Greene and Dalton (1953: 4818) drew a connection between PMS and menopause: "Just as, before the days of stilboestrol [DES], women in general accepted the unpleasant symptoms of 'the change of life' as a necessary part of the business of being a woman, so still they pass through one week of discomfort in every month, usually without complaining to their doctors but not necessarily without disturbing the tranquillity of their homes." Their discussion reveals some of the ways in which the intellectual work of physicians is embedded in the broader context. Implicit in their brief description of the parallels between premenstrual and menopausal experiences are a number of assumptions. A look at each of them in turn can be useful as a way of thinking about the role of the social and historical context in the transformation of medical knowledge about PMS.

The medicalization of PMS, like the medicalization of menopause, is, to some extent, an attempt to improve women's experiences by using modern medical theories, methods, and tools. Hitherto, women had accepted cyclical discomfort. Modern medicine would, Greene and Dalton implied, show women that this was not "a necessary part of being a woman." Their vision was shared by American medical specialists. In a symposium on PMS, published the same year, Freed (1953: 467) observed that "regardless of the disagreements among the various investigators, it is gratifying to see that the syndrome of premenstrual tension has been recognized by the medical profession as an important condition which interferes with the health and happiness of women and which can be treated readily."

Medical knowledge, like all knowledge, reflects cultural norms. In the earlier discussion about menopause, it was revealed that social and cultural factors influenced the construction of a medical deviance designation. There, specialists' self-concept of objectivity and scientific neutrality was not an accurate reflection of their theories and practices with regard to menopause: For example, sexism and cultural norms about suitable activities for aging women also influenced their work. Although a number of cultural norms are exhibited in the literature about PMS, only two of them are considered here: the role of women in the family and their role in the labor force.

In their article published in 1953, Greene and Dalton refer to "the tranquillity of their homes" which women disturb each month. Medicine, according to them, can find a solution to these disturbances and restore harmony along with women's health. Guiding their discussion are norms about the "proper" role of adult women. According to these norms, women should have homes with husbands and children living in them, and are responsible for maintaining a happy and harmonious home life (Skolnick & Skolnick, 1983). As Frank (1931: 1054) wrote in his pioneering work, not only do women who have PMS "realize their own suffering, but they feel conscience-stricken toward their husbands and families, knowing well that they are unbearable in their attitude and reactions." References such as these about the effect of the menstrual cycle on home life can be found today in the medical literature. Reid and Yen (1981: 85), for example, refer to Greene and Dalton's work and write of "a temporary deterioration" in women's "interpersonal relationships which frequently develops" in the premenstrual week. When they become irritable, tense, or depressed during the premenstrual week, marital discord and even baby battering can occur (Reid & Yen, 1981). This perspective assumes that "normal" families are happy and that women are responsible for preserving happiness of the individual family members. In this respect, the medical literature attributes problems in families (unhappiness, arguments, and violence) to women in general and PMS in particular, and recommends that they can be solved medically. This locates the problems and solutions within the family. A specific individual — the woman — is then identified as the source of the problem, and her menstrual cycle is discovered as the cause of her behavior. This kind of reasoning mitigates against the possibility of exploring men's contributions or other social roots and social solutions to these problems.

In the past, occupational segregation and pay differentials for men and women were rationalized on the basis that women's performance is inferior to men's. Women's inferiority, according to this rationalization, results from their biology; specifically, their reproductive systems. The medical literature about PMS reflects and reinforces these sexist assumptions about women's performance in the labor force. Beginning with Frank's (1931: 1053) reference to "employers of labor" who "take cognizance" of premenstrual disturbances "and make provision for the temporary care of their employees," discussions in the medical community have consistently referred to an association between PMS and reduced productivity. Billig (1953: 487), for instance, wrote that "entry into the secretarial, communication, stenographic, etc., fields has been followed by an industrial invasion. World War II hastened this widening of the horizon for feminine employment, bringing with it the necessity for dealing with the symptomology of the menstrual cycle." Not surprisingly, he conducted a survey of plants employing more than 500 women and discovered that absenteeism and inefficiency could be "markedly" reduced with adequate treatment for PMS. One study (cited in Reid & Yen, 1981) estimated that in 1969, absenteeism due to PMS cost industry $5 billion, and a recent editorial in the *New England Journal of Medicine* (Vaitukaitis, 1984: 1372–1373) identified PMS as a "serious public health problem, which results in decreased productivity and increased absenteeism among women with severe premenstrual syndrome." Not only is medicine expressing the notions and categories of sexist society — that their biology determines women's performance — but in these discussions, medicine is claiming that this performance can be controlled by medicine and that medicine can do this on an individual basis by diagnosing and treating individual women. Implicitly, these discussions assume that the problems are individual, and that they can be solved individually; the biomedical model underlies medical opinion about productivity. Further, these discussions give scientific credibility to sexist notions about differences between men and women.

In each role — women's role in the family and in the factory — medicine claims control over deviant behavior as its proper jurisdiction. However, a closer look at the kinds of deviant behavior that medicine is claiming as its jurisdiction shows some differences between the cases of PMS and menopause. In the case of menopause, social disruptions described by physicians included fears of loss of sexual attractiveness, anxiety about an "empty nest," and leading a "hermit existence." In contrast, social disruptions described with regard to PMS were/are decreased productivity and absenteeism in industry (Bickers & Woods, 1951; Frank, 1931; Reid & Yen, 1981) and marital or family discord (Frank, 1931; Greene & Dalton, 1953; Reid & Yen, 1981). Although in each instance one of the symptoms of the problem was failure to fulfill a routine social role, the identified behaviors are different. This may reflect both the different prescribed social activities of women before and after menopause and different historical periods in which the medical discussions occur. That is, women's participation in the industrial labor force has increased, especially since World War II; the literature on PMS, written after the 1940's, may reflect this social change as well as differences in life cycle activities for women. In any case, the literature about both PMS and menopause assumes that by controlling women medically, family and social life and industrial production will be maintained. Physicians, instead of priests, family counselors, or management, will control deviant behavior.

However much the medical profession may wish to be the appointed authority in matters such as these, medical dominance depends not only on intellectual forces, but on the ability of medicine to convince potential patients and significant others, such as employers and judges, that it is most qualified to do so. Medicalization, in other words, depends on a fit between the ideas of the medical profession in combination with the perceived needs of women and legitimation by the state. The changing status of adult women, increasing involvement by consumers in the organization and provision of medical care, shifting interests and analytic frameworks in legal theory, as well as changing medical theory and practice must all be considered in understanding the emergence and implications of the medicalization of PMS. A comprehensive analysis would necessarily elaborate and connect the threads in each of these groups in turn. Furthermore, not all groups support the medical deviance definition of the premenstrual period of the menstrual cycle. Psychologists (Parlee, 1973; Ruble, 1977; Ruble & Brooks-Gunn, 1979), as well as some feminist health advocates (Rome, 1986), disagree with this definition, criticizing it both because of the tenuous theoretical and methodological basis on which it rests and because of its social and physical implications for women. A comprehensive account of the process of medicalization would need to identify and explain the existence of contrary ways of defining and understanding emotions, behaviors, and physical changes which medicine labels "PMS."

In addition to shedding light on the ways in which the transformation in medical ideas about PMS are shaped by social forces, the historical case of the medicalization of menopause can point out some of the social consequences of the medicalization of PMS. For example, the historical case warns of the implications of diagnosing and treating some women with specific medical therapies for PMS. The use of estrogens to treat menopause has had serious negative health effects; prescription of remedies for PMS, which would presumably be used regularly until menopause, could also have deleterious consequences. Additionally, the medical tendency to expand its purview, alongside of sexist views of the hormonal basis of women's behavior and their "proper" role in the family and the workplace, tends to define all premenstrual women as diseased, thereby strengthening medical control over women and reinforcing sexist stereotypes and practices. In the case of menopause, this led to the recommendation that since menopause is an estrogen deficiency disease, all menopausal women should be treated with estrogen replacement therapy. Some of the current literature on PMS suggests that the theoretical groundwork for this already exists; for example, Vaitukaitis (1984: 1372) notes, "In some studies, essentially all women had one or more of the symptoms, whereas in other studies only 20 to 40 percent were considered to have the syndrome."

In addition to reinforcing sexist stereotypes about the relationship between hormones and female behavior, the effect of medicalizing PMS is to individualize and privatize women's experiences, making diagnosis and treatment a topic of discussion between each woman and her doctor, serving to ignore the role of the social environment in both symptoms and treatment. It may, in other words, serve to discourage married women from seeking changes in their relationships with their spouses and other members of their families, or to dissuade them from consideration of divorce. Alternatively, it may encourage them to seek medical solutions to problems with their employers, rather than looking for ways to change their daily activities in the workplace. In each of these spheres of social life, medicalization mitigates against change of the environment in favor of change in the individual.

The medicalization of PMS, like the medicalization of menopause, will be the construction of professionals and other individuals in institutional settings, along with women. This construction, despite the best of intentions, may have negative consequences for the status of all women, even though it improves the lot of some. For this reason, we all stand to benefit by learning from the past, and from recognizing the ways in which the process of medicalization is socially embedded. As critics and scholars, now is the time to stand aside from and examine these circumstances so that we may enter into and influence the direction they take in such a way that helps women, instead of unwittingly harming them.

ACKNOWLEDGMENTS

Phil Brown, Catherine Kohler Riessman, Diane N. Ruble, Rosemary C.R. Taylor, and Irving Kenneth Zola read and commented on a draft of this chapter. Their assistance is gratefully acknowledged.

REFERENCES

Bart, P. B. and M. Grossman, 1976. Menopause. *Women and Health 1:* 3-11.

Bart, P. B. and M. Grossman, 1978. Menopause. In: M. T. Notman and C. C. Nadelson (Eds.), *The Woman Patient: Medical and Psychological Interfaces.* Plenum Press, New York, NY, pp. 337-354.

Bell, S. E., 1984. Medical perspectives on gender and science: The case of DES. Paper presented at the Sixth Berkshire Conference, Smith College, Northampton, MA, June.

Bell, S. E., 1985. Changing ideas: The medicalization of menopause. Unpublished manuscript.

Bell, S. E., 1986. A new model of medical technology development: A case study of DES. In: J. Roth and S. Ruzek (Eds.), *Research in the Sociology of Health Care, Volume 4.* JAI Press, Greenwich, CT, pp. 1-32.

Bickers, W. and M. Woods, 1951. Premenstrual tension — rational treatment. *Texas Report on Biology and Medicine 9:* 406-419.

Billig, H. E., 1953. The role of premenstrual tension in industry. *International Record of Medicine 166:* 487-491.

Blau, F. D., 1978. The data on women workers, past, present, and future. In: A. H. Stromberg and S. Harkess (Eds.), *Women Working.* Mayfield Publishing, Palo Alto, CA, pp. 29-62.

Bologh, R. W., 1981. Grounding the alienation of self and body: A critical, phenomenological analysis of the patient in western medicine. *Sociology of Health and Illness 3:* 188-206.

Conrad, P., 1975. The discovery of hyperkinesis: Notes on the medicalization of deviant behavior. *Social Problems 23:* 15-21.

Conrad, P. and R. Kern (Eds.), 1986. *The Sociology of Health and Illness: Critical Perspectives.* Second Edition. St. Martin's, New York, NY.

Conrad, P. and J. W. Schneider, 1980. *Deviance and Medicalization: From Badness to Sickness.* C. V. Mosby, St. Louis, MO.

Coppen, A. and N. Kessel, 1964. Menstruation and personality. *British Journal of Psychiatry 109:* 711-721.

Dalton, K., 1964. The influence of menstruation on health and disease. *Proceedings of the Royal Society of Medicine 57:* 18-20.

Dalton, K., 1980. Cyclical criminal acts in premenstrual syndrome. *The Lancet 2:* 1070-1071.

Davis, M. E. and M. W. Boynton, 1941. Indications, clinical use and toxicity of 4'4' Dihydroxy-diethyl Stilbene. *Journal of Clinical Endocrinology 1:* 339-345.

Frank, R. T., 1931. The hormonal causes of premenstrual tension. *Archives of Neurology and Psychiatry 26:* 1053-1057.

Frank, R. T., 1941. Treatment of disorders of the menopause. *Bulletin of the New York Academy of Medicine 17:* 854-863.

Freed, S. C., 1953. History and causation of premenstrual tension. *International Record of Medicine 166:* 465-468.

Freidson, E., 1970. *Profession of Medicine*. Dodd, Mead, New York, NY.
Friedman, R. C., S. W. Hurt, M. S. Arnoff, and J. Clarkin, 1980. Behavior and the menstrual cycle. *Signs 5:* 719-738.
Gannon, L., 1981. Evidence for a psychological etiology of menstrual disorders: A critical review. *Psychological Reports 48:* 287-294.
Greene, R. and K. Dalton, 1953. The premenstrual syndrome. *British Medical Journal 1:* 1007-1014.
Greenhill, J. P., 1940. Gynecology. In: J. DeLee and J. P. Greenhill (Eds.), *Year Book of Obstetrics and Gynecology*. Year Book Publishers, New York, NY.
Hall, D. L., 1977. The social implications of the scientific study of sex. Paper presented at the symposium on Scholar and the Feminist IV: Connecting Theory, Practice, and Values, Barnard College, April, pp. 11-20.
Harrison, M., 1984. *Self-Help for Premenstrual Syndrome*. Matrix Press, Cambridge, MA.
Holden, C., 1986. Proposed new psychiatric diagnoses raise charges of gender bias. *Science 231:* 327-328.
Horney, J., 1978. Menstrual cycles and criminal responsibility. *Law and Human Behavior 2:* 25-36.
Kaufert, P. A., 1982. Myth and the menopause. *Sociology of Health and Illness 4:* 141-166.
Kaufert, P. A. and S. M. McKinlay, 1985. Estrogen-replacement therapy: The production of medical knowledge and the emergence of policy. In: E. Lewin and V. Olesen (Eds.), *Women, Health, and Healing*. Tavistock, New York, NY, pp. 113-138.
Koeske, R. D., 1976. Premenstrual emotionality: Is biology destiny? *Women and Health 1:* 11-14.
Koeske, R. D., 1982. Toward a biosocial paradigm for menopause research: Lessons and contributions from the behavioral sciences. In: A. M. Voda, M. Dinnerstein, and S. R. O'Donnell (Eds.), *Changing Perspectives on Menopause*. University of Texas Press, Austin, TX, pp. 3-23.
Koeske, R. D., 1983. Lifting the curse of menstruation: Toward a feminist perspective on the menstrual cycle. *Women and Health 8:* 1-16.
Lovato v. Irvin, 1983. In re Irvin. *Bankruptcy Reporter*, pp. 251-262.
McCrea, F. B., 1983. The politics of menopause: The "discovery" of a deficiency disease. *Social Problems 31:* 111-123.
McKinlay, S. M. and J. B. McKinlay, 1973. Selected studies of the menopause. *Journal of Biosocial Sciences 5:* 533-555.
Mishler, E. G., 1981a. Viewpoint: Critical perspectives on the biomedical model. In: E. G. Mishler, L. R. AmaraSingham, S. T. Hauser, R. Liem, S. D. Osherson, and N. E. Waxler, *Social Contexts of Health, Illness, and Patient Care*. Cambridge University Press, New York, NY, pp. 1-23.
Mishler, E. G., 1981b. The social construction of illness. In: E. G. Mishler, L. R. AmaraSingham, S. T. Hauser, R. Liem, S. D. Osherson, and N. E. Waxler, *Social Contexts of Health, Illness, and Patient Care*. Cambridge University Press, New York, NY, pp. 141-168.
Mishler, E. G., L. R. AmaraSingham, S. T. Hauser, R. Liem, S. D. Osherson, and N. E. Waxler, 1981. *Social Contexts of Health, Illness, and Patient Care*. Cambridge University Press, New York, NY.
Morton, J. H., 1953a. Editorial. *International Record of Medicine 166:* 463-464.
Morton, J. H., 1953b. Treatment of premenstrual tension. *International Record of Medicine 166:* 505-510.
Novak, E., 1940. The management of the menopause. *American Journal of Obstetrics and Gynecology 40:* 589-595.

Parlee, M. B., 1973. The premenstrual syndrome. *Psychological Bulletin 80:* 454-465.
Perlmutter, E. and P. B. Bart, 1982. Changing views of "the change:" A critical review and suggestions for an attributional approach. In: A. M. Voda, M. Dinnerstein, and S. R. O'Donnell (Eds.), *Changing Perspectives on Menopause.* University of Texas Press, Austin, TX, pp. 187-199.
PMS Action, 1983. *The PMS Connection, Volume 1.*
Posner, J., 1979. It's all in your head: Feminist and medical models of menopause (strange bedfellows). *Sex Roles 5:* 179-189.
Pratt, J. P., 1938. Treatment of the menopause. *Southern Medical Journal 31:* 562-567.
Pratt, J. P., 1939. Sex functions in man. In: E. Allen, C. H. Danforth, and E. A. Doisy (Eds.), *Sex and Internal Secretions.* Williams & Wilkins, Baltimore, MD, pp. 1263-1334.
Reid, R. L. and S.S.C. Yen, 1981. Premenstrual syndrome. *American Journal of Obstetrics and Gynecology 139:* 85-104.
Riessman, C. K., 1983. Women and medicalization: A new perspective. *Social Policy 14:* 3-18.
Rome, E., 1986. Premenstrual syndrome (PMS) examined through a feminist lens. *Health Care for Women International 7:* 145-151.
Rubinow, D. R. and P. Roy-Byrne, 1984. Premenstrual syndromes: Overview from a methodologic perspective. *American Journal of Psychiatry 141:* 163-172.
Rubinow, D. R., P. Roy-Byrne, M. C. Hoban, P. W. Gold, and R. M. Post, 1984. Prospective assessment of menstrually related mood disorders. *American Journal of Psychiatry 141:* 684-686.
Ruble, D. N., 1977. Premenstrual symptoms: A reinterpretation. *Science 197:* 291-292.
Ruble, D. N. and J. Brooks-Gunn, 1979. Menstrual symptoms: A social cognition analysis. *Journal of Behavioral Medicine 2:* 171-194.
Ruble, D. N., A. K. Boggiano, and J. Brooks-Gunn, 1982. Men's and women's evaluations of menstrual-related excuses. *Sex Roles 8:* 625-638.
Salmon, U. J., S. H. Geist, and R. I. Walter, 1941. Treatment of the menopause: Evaluation of estrogen implantation. *Journal of the American Medical Association 117:* 1843-1849.
Schneider, J. W. and P. Conrad, 1980. The medical control of deviance: Contests and consequences. In: J. Roth (Ed.), *Research in the Sociology of Health Care, Volume 1.* JAI Press, Greenwich, CT, pp. 1-53.
Shorr, E., 1940. The menopause. *Bulletin of the New York Academy of Medicine 16:* 453-474.
Skolnick, A. S. and J. H. Skolnick (Eds.), 1983. *Family in Transition: Rethinking Marriage, Sexuality, Child Rearing, and Family Organization.* Fourth edition. Little, Brown and Co., Boston, MA.
Smith-Rosenberg, C., 1973. Puberty to menopause: The cycle of femininity in nineteenth-century America. *Feminist Studies 1:* 58-72.
Starr, P., 1982. *The Social Transformation of American Medicine.* Basic Books, New York, NY.
Steiner, M. and B. J. Carroll, 1977. The psychobiology of premenstrual dysphoria: Review of theories and treatments. *Psychoneuroendocrinology 2:* 321-335.
Suarez-Murias, E. L., 1953. The psychophysiological syndrome of premenstrual tension with emphasis on the psychiatric aspect. *International Record of Medicine 166:* 475-486.
Uhlenberg, P., 1983. Death and the family. In: M. Gordon (Ed.), *The American Family in Social-Historical Perspective.* Third edition. St. Martins, New York, NY, pp. 169-177.

Vaitukaitis, J. L., 1984. Premenstrual syndrome. *New England Journal of Medicine 311:* 1371-1373.
Voda, A., M. Dinnerstein, and S. O'Donnell (Eds.), 1982. *Changing Perspectives on Menopause.* University of Texas Press, Austin, TX.
Wallach, A. and L. Rubin, 1971. The premenstrual syndrome and criminal responsibility. *U.C.L.A. Law Review 19:* 210-312.
Zola, I. K., 1972. Medicine as an institution of social control. *Sociological Review 20:* 487-504.

MENSTRUAL SYMPTOMS AND MENSTRUAL BELIEFS: NATIONAL AND CROSS-NATIONAL PATTERNS

Karen Paige Ericksen , Ph.D.

Department of Psychology
University of California, Davis
Davis, California

INTRODUCTION

The purpose of this paper is to provide a broad comparative perspective within which menstrual beliefs and menstrual-related symptoms may be considered. Until very recently, there has been a serious bias in the kinds of questions researchers asked about the event of menstruation in Western countries compared to non-Western cultures. In the West, the focus has been almost completely on the psychological and biomedical aspects of the menstrual cycle, most notably the variety of symptoms reported just prior to and during the menses. In non-Western cultures, however, researchers customarily document beliefs and practices pertaining to menstruating women.

The national and cross-national patterns described below should help correct this bias by demonstrating, first, that the beliefs about menstruating women in our own society share important similarities to the beliefs held in other cultures; and second, that the menstrual-related symptoms most commonly reported in Western societies are also prevalent in other cultures. I will begin by discussing the prevalence of menstrual beliefs among men and women in the United States. The prevalence of menstrual-related symptoms among American women will then be described, as well as the demographic and physical characteristics that best predict these symptoms. Following this analysis is a summary of cross-cultural and cross-national studies of menstrual beliefs and practices and a discussion of menstrual symptoms in ten Third World nations.

AMERICAN BELIEFS AND SYMPTOMS

Prevalence of Menstrual Beliefs

Let us first examine the national prevalence of the most ancient practice in the world — the taboo of sex during a woman's menstrual period. In a recent nationwide survey (Ruder & Finn, 1981), 51% of men and 56% of women agreed that women should not have intercourse while menstruating. When married men and women in a representative household survey were asked if they had *ever* had sexual relations during the woman's menstruation, half of each sex indicated they had not (Paige, 1977). When a sample of 628 white, educated couples in Detroit were asked a similar question, the majority of each sex indicated they either had never had sex with their spouse during the menses, or felt menstrual sex was less enjoyable. Only about a third of the wives and less than half of the husbands ignored the menstrual sex taboo and felt sex during menstruation was no different than sex during any other time of the month. Studies monitoring the daily sexual activity of women over the menstrual cycle (Udry & Morris, 1968, 1970) have found that by the fifth day of the cycle between 55% and 70% of women in three different samples had still not engaged in sexual relations, compared with a range of 30% to 45% reporting sex for any given day between menstrual periods.

When men and women are asked directly about their attitudes about menstruation, their responses appear to reflect an underlying belief about women's inferiority as persons. In a nationwide survey of menstrual attitudes (Ruder & Finn, 1981), virtually all of the men and women agreed that women were more emotional during menstruation, while 39% of men and 25% of women agreed that menstruation affects a woman's ability to think, and 20% of men and 24% of women agreed that menstrual pain is psychological rather than physical. In this same survey, two-thirds of each sex thought that women should conceal the fact that they are menstruating in a social situation, and about one-quarter agreed that women look different when menstruating. A little more than half agreed that menstruating women have a different scent; 24% of men and 18% of women thought it harmful to bathe or swim while menstruating; and 34% of men and 24% of women believed menstruating women should restrict their physical activities. Men, however, are much more likely than women to say that menstruating women do not function well at work (89% vs. 66%), and there are even some who believe that women should stay away from people while menstruating (12% of men and 5% of women).

"Sexual pollution," as analyzed by Douglas (1966), implies that male contact with women's sexual organs will lead to grave physical danger, moral contamination, and supernatural sanctions. The extent to which the menstrual beliefs and practices of Americans are embedded in this underlying cultural notion was studied by examining the kinds of attitudes and practices most highly correlated with adherence to the menstrual sex taboo (Paige, 1977). The menstrual taboo was not only associated with adherence to sex taboos during pregnancy and the postpartum, but with other attitudes reflecting a supernatural fear of sexual practices; attitudes about sexual fluids; and the adherence of certain hygienic practices (e.g., douching, vaginal deodorant, fellatio). These attitudes comprised a statistical index quite distinct from other attitudes about sexual behavior or about women's role.

Social Antecedents of Menstrual Beliefs and Practices

Men's and women's adherence to menstrual social and sexual prohibitions in this society do, however, show considerable variation. Not all men and women express strong negative beliefs about menstruation, not all sexually experienced adults adhere to the menstrual sex taboo, and not all women observe customary prohibitions on swimming, bathing, social interactions, and the like. The United States is, after all, one of the most culturally diverse nations in the world. Is it possible, then, that social and ideological antecedents can be identified that distinguish between individuals who continue to adhere to traditional beliefs and those who have abandoned or ignored them?

An analysis of a representative household survey of nearly 1,000 married people revealed three important predictors of adherence to traditional menstrual practices: Age, strength of the beliefs in "patriarchal familism," and religious fundamentalism (Paige, 1977). The joint effects of these predictors accounted for 24% of the variability in adherence to the menstrual taboo. Adherence to the sex taboo, then, and, by implication, the pollution beliefs this taboo expresses, is much more likely among Americans who are older, hold strong values about the traditional family, and attend more fundamentalist churches. Those who have abandoned or rejected the menstrual sex taboo are likely to be young, reject beliefs about the traditional family, and either attend liberal churches or express no religious identification. When the effects of additional variables were taken into account, such as attitudes about the women's movement, educational attainment, and attitudes about sexuality, none increased the explanation of variability in taboo adherence beyond the 24% already described.

An extension of this analysis was completed on data collected from a large household sample of Detroit couples (Paige, 1983). Additional measures of traditional values about women were considered, such as the belief in the importance of sexual chastity, and whether or not the wife was a mother. The analysis of particular interest showed how important a husband's own values were in determining a wife's adherence to the traditional menstrual sex taboo.

For wives, adherence is best accounted for by three variables: (1) their motherhood status; (2) their own beliefs in the importance of patriarchal familism and sexual chastity for women; and (3) their husband's beliefs in patriarchal familism. Since these variables were highly intercorrelated, their effects on taboo adherence independent of each other were examined. The regression analysis showed, first, that motherhood had an independent effect on the taboo, with mothers more likely to adhere to it than childless women, regardless of beliefs. Second, once her husband's set of beliefs are considered, a wife's beliefs in either patriarchal familism or sexual chastity had no effect on taboo adherence. It is also noteworthy that religious fundamentalism plays a somewhat different role in this analysis than in the previous one. A wife's religious fundamentalism has a strong zero-order correlation with her beliefs about the family and about sexual chastity, but only a weak association with the menstrual sex taboo. The regression analysis showed, however, that it is again the husband's religious fundamentalism, not the wife's, that best predicts the wife's own beliefs regarding family and chastity.

Quite a different pattern of results is observed for a husband's menstrual sex taboo. First of all, none of his wife's beliefs or her religious fundamentalism have any association with his taboo adherence. Second, men with children are more likely to adhere to the taboo than those without children — a finding similar to that for wives. Third, examination of the relative effects of a husband's and his wife's familism and chastity beliefs show that only his own familism beliefs affect his taboo adherence. His wife's beliefs had no effect. Finally, a husband's social class background has a significant effect on his adherence to the taboo, an effect not observed among wives. For husbands, then, the best predictors of the adherence to the menstrual sex taboo were his beliefs in patriarchal familism and his social class background; the other variables were less strongly associated.

These findings suggest quite different antecedents of the menstrual sex taboo among men and women. It seems that a wife's adherence depends to a large extent on her husband's beliefs about women's chastity and men's authority over women in the family, and on her husband's fundamentalism and social class background. A husband's adherence is determined by his social class background and his own beliefs about the family.

In summary, the empirical research described above demonstrates the significance of menstrual beliefs and practices among contemporary Americans. The national attitude survey shows that American men and women share beliefs about menstruating women that have important similarities to the beliefs expressed in non-Western cultures. Further analysis provided evidence that practices and the beliefs they express are linked to an American value system emphasizing the importance of women's traditional role in the family and a religious ideology that upholds this role. When antecedents of the menstrual sex taboo were examined separately for men and women, the most interesting finding was the importance of the husband's attitudes and his social class background in determining the taboo adherence of his wife as well as himself. This suggests that while roughly the same proportion of men and women in the population hold to traditional menstrual beliefs and practices, it is men's (not women's) notions about chastity and family authority relations that seem to be the significant force in their maintenance.

Menstrual Symptoms and Their Antecedents

Let us now turn to that aspect of menstruation that has received the most attention by Western researchers — the emotional and physical symptoms experienced just prior to and during the menstrual period. There has been considerable psychological and biomedical research on these symptoms during the last decade, although there is still no clear perception of the proportions of adult women in the general population who experience them. Most estimates are based on convenience samples, such as clinic patients, students, or self-selected female groups.

Like the research on menstrual beliefs and practices, the single national survey provides data on the prevalence of symptoms, but little understanding of the causes of variation in symptom experience among women (or the perception of female symptoms among men). Analyses of the correlates of symptom reports are based on smaller household surveys of specific geographic regions, although the method of selection of respondents allows us to make generalizations about national trends.

The nationwide survey about menstruation conducted in 1981 asked approximately 1,000 men and women over 18 years old about the severity of physical discomfort and the experience of mood changes just prior to the last menstrual period. Overall, 56% of the respondents associated at least some physical discomfort with the premenses and 58% reported the perception of at least some changes in moods. The physical discomfort was reported as severe ("a lot") among 18%, and 13% reported "a lot" of moodiness (Ruder & Finn, 1981).

Ruder and Finn (1981) do not report the responses to these questions separately for men and women, although they do describe a substantial sex difference in the response to an attitude item about whether they believe menstruation is painful. Compared to only 39% of men who believe it is painful, 56% of the women associated pain with menstruation. Sex differences were examined, however, in the sample of 314 Detroit couples (Paige, 1983) who were asked about menstrual symptoms perceived during the last period. There was high agreement between husbands and wives about the presence of physical discomfort, its severity, and the specific kinds of pain (e.g., cramps, aches and pains), with husbands only slightly overestimating the intensity of the pain. 15.3% of the husbands believed their wives experienced "a lot" of physical pain, compared to 13% of the wives themselves. The sex differences were more pronounced for the perception of mood changes, especially severe mood changes. Compared to nearly a quarter of wives (23.3%) who associated "a lot" of moodiness with their last menstruation, only 8.6% of the husbands perceived their wives as having such intense mood changes. Husbands, more than wives, tended to perceive menstrual-related mood changes as relatively moderate or absent, although the kinds of moods reported were the same as those described by wives.

In another regionally-based household survey, Woods, Most, and Dery (1982) analyzed both the prevalence and severity of specific symptoms, as well as the pattern of correlates of those symptoms. They report, first, that physical symptoms were more prevalent than emotional ones. Over 30% of the sample reported experiencing varying degrees of weight gain, headaches, skin disorders, cramps, fatigue, and painful breasts. The only two emotional changes reported by over 30% of the women were anxiety and irritability. Only a few, however, perceived these symptoms as intense (i.e., as either "severe" or "disabling"). Between 2% and 8% reported any symptoms as severe, with two exceptions: Cramps were reported as severe by 17% and irritability was intense among 12%.

The prevalence rates reported in each of these household survey studies do not resolve the problem of whether or not the menstrual cycle actually produces physical and/or emotional side effects in a sizable proportion of the female population. These rates do, however, give us the only good estimates of the proportion of the population who associate increased physical discomfort (especially cramps) and moodiness with the premenstrual and menstrual phases of the cycle. Unlike "convenience samples," the individuals included in these samples are not self-selected on the basis of characteristics that could bias the reports of symptoms; they were included in the samples because they represented either the nation or particular geographic regions within the nation. Equally important, the very heterogeneity of the samples allows the examination of possible sources of variation among women (and men) in the perception of menstrual-related symptoms.

In the analysis of Woods et al. (1982), three important sets of correlates of symptom severity were found: Contraceptive use (oral, intrauterine), menstrual bleeding (length, amount), and social demographic characteristics (age, income, education, race). Women using oral contraceptives reported a significant decrease in menstrual-related cramps and skin disorders, and women using intrauterine devices (IUD) reported a significant increase in premenstrual cramps. The use of these contraceptives, however, had no effect on the severity of other common symptoms. Women with longer menstrual periods and with heavier bleeding whatever the length were significantly more likely to report cramps and other symptoms than women with shorter periods and with lighter bleeding. Other examined characteristics of the menstrual cycle had little or no effect on symptoms. Although women reporting longer cycles also reported greater moodiness and physical swelling, the the woman's own report of cycle length was found to be relatively unreliable; only 51% were able to predict accurately their next menstrual period.

The finding that symptoms, especially cramps and moods, are negatively correlated with increased age is of particular interest since, as is discussed below, this trend is found in many other countries as well. Better educated women, those who were employed, and particularly those with higher income, had significantly lower prevalence of symptoms than women with less education or income, or those unemployed. Since these variables are commonly used as representations of one's social status, the findings of Woods et al. (1982) suggest sociocultural variation in the perception of menstrual-related symptoms in this country. Further support for this interpretation is the significant race difference in symptomatology independent of social status. Black women have lower rates of cramps and emotional symptoms than white women, even when income and education levels are controlled.

The national patterns of menstrual beliefs and symptoms reviewed in this section demonstrate the need to consider internal social and cultural variation in the United States in future research. Since menstrual-related symptom experiences are necessarily derived from women's own reports, it is possible that a woman's social and cultural context influences those reports — contexts that affect beliefs about menstruation, about women's role, and about the sexual body, as well as affecting norms about expressing emotions and physical discomfort.

CROSS-CULTURAL AND CROSS-NATIONAL PATTERNS

Menstrual Customs in Tribal Societies

Probably the best known aspects of menstruation in the non-Western context are the variety of customary social restrictions observed by women in tribal and band societies. Until recently, our knowledge of the beliefs and symptoms of Third World nations was limited to anecdotes and case studies of individual communities. In this section, the tribal customs will be briefly summarized, followed by a review of beliefs, practices, and symptoms in a survey of Third World nations.

The numerous ethnographic studies conducted over the decades describe an immense variety of special menstrual restrictions and observances throughout the world. Cross-cultural surveys show a consistent ordering of these menstrual customs from the most pervasive (sex taboo) to the less prevalent, but seemingly most restrictive (physical segregation). In fact, these studies have classified menstrual customs into four major categories and have shown that they can be ordered along a Guttman-type scale (Paige & Paige, 1981; Schlegel, 1972; Stephens, 1961; White & Saltz, 1967; Young & Bacdayan, 1971). Based on representative samples of societies, empirical analyses rank the practice of secluding women in menstrual huts as the most elaborate custom, followed by cooking prohibitions, "other" social restrictions, personal restrictions, and, finally, the menstrual sex taboo. For example, societies in which menstruating women are physically segregated are very likely to observe all the other menstrual customs as well; those in which menstruating women are prohibited from cooking do not usually segregate them, but usually do observe other social restrictions, personal restrictions, and the sex taboo.

The worldwide patterns of menstrual customs have been interpreted from many different theoretical perspectives. It has been proposed that the elaborateness of the restrictions imposed on women is an expression of underlying psychodynamic conflicts in the menfolk, specifically the severity of the castration complex (Stephens, 1961). Others argue that they are expressions of the intensity of sexual antagonism generally (Douglas, 1966; Schlegel, 1972), or the degree of social rigidity and male dominance (Young & Bacdayan, 1971). Paige and Paige (1981) propose that menstrual restrictions should be seen as one of two major forms of sex segregation; the other form restricts men to men's clubs, or separate living quarters in which special instruments (e.g., flutes or bull roarers) are guarded from women. Menstrual restrictions and male segregation are interpreted as ritual forms of political bargaining. As Paige and Paige demonstrate in detail, these rituals are implicit mechanisms by which political claims over women and other men may be demonstrated. Menstrual segregation and the pollution beliefs they express are interpreted as demonstrations of "ritual disinterest" in a man's most valuable asset — a woman's demonstrated ability to continue reproducing offspring which will add to his own prestige, wealth, and power.

While theorists differ in their interpretations of the menstrual customs, there is general agreement that they are closely linked with the ideological notion of women's "pollution." In fact, the ethnographic case studies make this linkage clear by data collected from informants in the society studied.

Menstrual Beliefs and Practices in Third World Nations

The most extensive examination of worldwide patterns of beliefs, practices, and symptoms associated with menstruation was recently completed by the World Health Organization (W.H.O.)(Snowden & Christian, 1984). A collaboration of European and American consultants and principal investigators from ten different nations produced a detailed statistical portrait of both within-nation and between-nation variations among women of reproductive age. A minimum of 500 women (parous, non-lactating, premenopausal) were interviewed in each nation who represented the major sociocultural group or groups in both urban and rural areas, and from both high and low socioeconomic classes. Data on women's beliefs, practices, and symptoms were obtained from verbal interviews in the local dialect as part of a general social survey. The preliminary statistical analyses summarized here were based on English translations of all interviews.

The nations comprising the sample represented five world regions: Mexico and Jamaica (North America); Egypt (Middle East); Philippines, Korea, and Indonesia (East Asia); India and Pakistan (South Asia); and Yugoslavia and United Kingdom (Europe). Nations from South America and Africa were originally included, but were excluded prior to data collection for administrative reasons.

The survey included items about menstrual-related practices that are analogous to those comprising the Guttman-type scale used in cross-cultural surveys of tribal societies: Restrictions on cooking, social restrictions (visiting friends and relatives), changes in personal behavior (bathing, washing hair), and avoidance of sexual intercourse. They were also asked about many menstrual attitudes and beliefs that are similar to those asked of Americans on recent household surveys. Therefore, the similarities between tribal cultural norms and Western beliefs and attitudes may be examined among women in nation states that are largely kin-based and agrarian. The inclusion of the United Kingdom in the survey allows for direct comparisons of all responses with a representative Western industrialized nation.

Less than 10% of women in most surveyed nations believed that *cooking* should be avoided during menstruation. However, there were two important exceptions. The vast majority of both high caste and low caste women in India and two-thirds of women in the Philippines thought cooking should be avoided. The prohibition against cooking was also customary among the Ancient Hebrews, according to the Old Testament (e.g., Leviticus *15:* 19-33), and is still observed among Orthodox Jews. Again, the popularity of this custom among some cultures (Hindu, Muslim, and Jewish) but not others should be examined.

The practice of *restricting one's social contacts* during menstruation is a cultural expectation among many tribal societies. In the W.H.O. sample, there was considerable internal variation in adherence to this norm within each country, with roughly half of the women in Egypt and India avoiding social contacts, a third of those in Jamaica, and a quarter of those in the Philippines and non-Muslim Yogoslavia. A little over 10% of women in Muslim Yugoslvaia, the Sind of Pakistan, and Mexico reduced social contacts, and the proportions were less than 10% in Indonesia, Korea, and the Punjab of Pakistan. Such explanations of this cross-national variability in proportions cannot be explained by geographic (or cultural) region, religion, or level of socioeconomic development. The reason why social restrictions are more common in some nations than in others must await further statistical analysis. For our purposes, it is interesting to note that the notion of social segregation during menstruation is shared by at least some women in widely different cultures, including the 5% of women (and 12% of men) in the national United States survey (Ruder & Finn, 1981) who believed menstruating women should "stay away from other people."

Changes in *personal habits* during menstruation, such as avoiding washing hair and bathing, were more common cross-nationally than the cooking and social restrictions. Washing hair is avoided by the large majority of women in the Philippines and Indonesia, and by about a third of those in Yugoslavia and in the Sind of Pakistan. Between 10% to 20% of those in Egypt, high caste India, Jamaica, Korea, Mexico, and the Punjab of Pakistan also avoid washing hair. Even 5% of the women in the United Kingdom and, according to folk wisdom, some women in the United States, postpone hair washing. Avoiding baths tends to be more common than the avoidance of hair washing, since larger proportions of women in each nation in the sample agreed with this cultural restriction. The vast majority (nearly 75%) of women in Korea and the Philippines avoided bathing, and between one-quarter to one-half of those in Egypt, Pakistan, and Yugoslavia. Between 10% and 20% in Jamaica, Mexico, and the United Kingdom avoided bathing, but only very few (less than 10%) in Indonesia and low caste India. According to the W.H.O. report (1981), open-ended responses from women indicated a variety of rationales of this practice, such as bathing causing increased menstrual pain, affecting the character of menstrual bleeding, and affecting the quality of health generally.

By far the most prevalent menstrual practice is the *sex taboo.* Virtually all women in the cross-national study indicated sex should be avoided during menstruation. The exception was the United Kingdom, where about half of the women adhered to the menstrual sex taboo, the same proportion as reported in various American samples. Clearly, the sex taboo is the one menstrual practice that is shared by tribal cultures, Third World nations, and a substantial proportion of Western industrialized nations.

Like the menstrual sex taboo, there was substantial cross-national agreement about two beliefs about menstruation: that it is necessary for femininity and that it is "dirty." Most women in each country studied associated menstruation with femininity, except in the United Kingdom, where this belief was held by 42%. Virtually all women (over 90%) in Egypt, India, and the Philippines held this belief, and over three-fourths of those in Korea, the Punjab of Pakistan, and the

Sundanese of Indonesia. The lower agreement among women in the United Kingdom was also shared by the Javanese of Indonesia, Mexicans, and non-Muslim Yugoslavs. Although women believe menstruation is part of being feminine, they also believe that it is "dirty." This belief is especially pervasive in Egypt (88%), Indonesia (82% among the Javanese and 93% among the Sundanese), Muslim Yugoslavia (68%), and high caste India (69%). With the exception of the United Kingdom (in which only 7% believed it was "dirty"), in the remaining nations between one-third to one-half held this belief. Anecdotal data showed that women usually associated the concept of "dirty" (in the various languages) with the notion of sexual pollution described in the ethnographic and general theoretical literature.

Menstrual Symptoms in Third World Nations

Included on the general survey questionnaire was a list of physical and emotional symptoms used in studies of menstruation among American women. This makes it possible for the first time to see if women in non-Western nations experience the same kinds of menstrual-related discomfort and emotional changes reported in the West. The inclusion of the United Kingdom in the cross-national study makes direct comparisons possible, although the prevalence rates can also be compared to those reported on United States household surveys discussed earlier. The extent to which many of the social and biomedical variables correlate with American symptom reports analyzed by Woods et al. (1982) can also be compared, since similar analyses for each of the ten nations were conducted in the W.H.O. study (Snowden & Christian, 1984; W.H.O., 1981).

Menstrual Pain. Women were asked if they experienced such menstrual-related physical discomforts as backaches, cramps, headaches, breast swelling, and general aches and pains. The most common symptoms were backaches and cramps. Cross-national comparisons can be made for the presence of any of these physical symptoms.

In the United Kingdom, 57% of the women reported at least some physical discomfort. This rate is comparable to the 48% of wives in Detroit reporting either "a little" or "a lot" of pain, and the 53.1% of women in the survey of Woods et al. (1982) reporting cramps. (Woods et al. did not present a summary index of menstrual-related pain.) The prevalence rates in the Third World nations are not dramatically different from these Western rates, although they reach as high as 65% to 70% in Indonesia, the Sind of Pakistan, and Muslim Yugoslavia. In the remaining nations, the prevalence is comparable to the United Kingdom.

Within each nation, examination of internal variation in reports of discomfort suggest that "traditional" women (i.e., rural, low status, or non-literate) perceive more pain than "more modern" women (i.e., urban, high status, or literate). The trend was most apparent in Egypt, low caste India, and Yugoslavia. Among women in high caste India, Java (Indonesia), Korea, and the Punjab of Pakistan, however, discomfort tended to be associated with at least one indicator of "modernity." In the remaining nations, there were no differences in reports of discomfort by locale, status, or literacy. It should be noted, however, that the association in some Third World nations between reports of menstrual discomfort and "traditionalism" is similar to findings reported on American samples discussed earlier.

The most important determinants of internal variation were the same as those found by Woods et al. in the American sample: age, contraceptive use, and menstrual bleeding length and amount. With only three exceptions, older women were more likely to report physical discomfort than younger women, especially those under 24 years of age. (The opposite age trend is found in high caste India, Muslim Yugoslavia, and Korea. No consistent age trend is observed in low caste India and Javanese Indonesia.) As reported for the United States, the women using oral contraceptives either experience a reduction in physical symptoms or no change in discomfort; in no nation is an appreciable increase (i.e., over 3%) in discomfort observed. In only one case, Javanese Indonesia, did the IUD users report less physical symptoms than other women. Unlike findings for women in the United States or in the United Kingdom (where IUD users reported significantly greater discomfort), the data indicate that this method of birth control does not increase menstrual-related pain.

It is the length and amount of menstrual bleeding that has the greatest effect on physical discomfort among women in almost all nations; and in most cases, this effect is substantial. The relationship between menstrual bleeding characteristics and discomfort is particularly strong in the United Kingdom. Only in Javanese Indonesia and Pakistan is the relationship weak.

Menstrual Mood Changes. The cross-national trends for menstrual-related mood changes show important differences from the well known Western pattern. American samples and the European women in the United Kingdom and Yugoslavia participating in the W.H.O. survey show the large increase in mood shifts reported premenstrually (e.g., irritability, mood swings, and depression) and very low rates intermenstrually (between menses and ovulation). For example, Woods et al. report from their American sample that one-third to one-half report irritability, depression, or mood swings during the premenstrual and menstrual phases, but only about one-fifth experience any of these moods intermenstrually. The United Kingdom pattern shows about three-fourths of women with these mood changes premenstrually, nearly half during the menses, but only one-third intermenstrually. In Yugoslavia, between two-thirds and three-fourths report mood changes both premenstrually and menstrually, but only about one-quarter intermenstrually.

In most other nations, the biggest shift in moods corresponds to the onset of menstrual bleeding, not during the premenstruum. After bleeding subsides, negative moods decrease substantially. However, in both Egypt and the Philippines, no menstrual cycle shift in moods is reported: women in these two nations report high levels of negative moods throughout the cycle (i.e., between one-third and one-half at the premenstrual, menstrual, and intermenstrual phases).

It is not surprising, then, that data from all Third World nations indicate substantially lower rates of premenstrual mood changes than do data from the United Kingdom (and, to a lesser extent, Yugoslavia). If mood shifts occur, they are observed during menstrual bleeding. Even during the menses, however, fewer women in each nation experience negative moods than in Western societies.

For mood changes, as with physical symptoms, the possible effects of age, contraceptive used, length and amount of menstrual bleeding, and social characteristics were examined. Of these, the two variables that affect moods are the use of the IUD and the length and amount of menstrual bleeding. Women in Javanese Indonesia, Jamaica, Korea, the Philippines, and Yugoslavia are more likely to report negative menstrual moods while using the IUD than women using oral contraception or neither. This relationship was not observed in any other nation, including the United Kingdom; Woods et al. (1982) also found no IUD effect on moods among American women.

With the exception of the Philippines and Muslim Yugoslavia, women in each nation who experience heavy menstrual bleeding also report more mood changes than those who experience lighter bleeding. Number of days of bleeding has a similar relationship to moodiness, with more women reporting mood changes the longer the menstrual period. It is important to note that in virtually all nations, women with heavier and/or longer menstrual bleeding are significantly more likely to report mood shifts only during the menses; premenstrual moods are not affected. The relationship between menstrual flow and moods was also found in Woods et al.'s American sample, although bleeding characteristics affected both premenstrual and menstrual mood swings.

CONCLUSIONS

What conclusions may be drawn about the similarities in beliefs and practices in Western and non-Western societies? First, it seems that the idea that menstruation is central to femininity in women, and the notion that both menstruation and femininity are associated with the concept of "pollution" is widespread in world societies. An important expression of this linkage is the pervasive practice of avoiding sex during the menstrual period. Although the concept of pollution is never measured directly, numerous case studies of individual societies and indirect empirical measures of the concept in the United States strongly suggest a cultural logic that classifies women as a "polluted" class and the periodic event of menstruation as an expression of that pollution. As Max Weber (1978) describes in his analysis of the untouchables in India, the concept of pollution implies the belief in the necessity of keeping one group separate from another "in the interest of maintaining purity of blood and prestige" of the unpolluted. That this notion of pollution is important in the analysis of menstrual beliefs is indicated by the American data showing the importance of a man's beliefs about traditional gender relations in the family in explaining the adherence to menstrual sex taboos by both himself and his wife. Menstrual taboos and associated practices could be a metaphor by which traditional hierarchical relations between the sexes are maintained.

Second, customary menstrual practices, such as social, cooking, and personal restrictions, show important cross-cultural and cross-national variations. These variations have been shown to be quite systematic among tribal and band societies, in which four classes of practices form a Guttman scale. The variations in the W.H.O. (1981) survey of Third World nations have yet to be analyzed in depth, although differences in prevalence rates do show strong between-nation differences. For example, there appears to be a strong expectation that menstruating women restrict social contacts in Egypt and India, and a strong expectation that they not cook only in India. The bathing restriction is especially pronounced in Korea and the Philippines, and is a dominant practice in Egypt, Pakistan, and Yugoslavia. The avoidance of hair washing is pervasive in Indonesia, although this practice is not shared by any other nation in the sample. None of these practices are prevalent in Western cultural tradition, although the avoidance of hair washing, swimming, hair permanents, certain foods, and the like are part of the general folk wisdom of female culture. The national attitude survey also showed strong American expectations that menstruating women refrain from discussing the event, avoid social activities, refrain from swimming and bathing, and avoid men; a significant number of Americans also believe that menstruating women smell differently and look differently.

What conclusions can be drawn about the patterns of menstrual-related symptoms among women in non-Western nations? Based on the preliminary analyses of the W.H.O. survey, it appears that a large proportion of women in Third World nations in different world regions do experience the same kinds of physical and emotional symptoms as women in Western industrialized nations. Although the severity of these symptoms has not been ascertained, the data show clearly that the expression of symptoms is not a Western phenomenon. Symptoms most commonly reported by women in the United States and the United Kingdom are also the most common ones reported in the Third World — cramps, aches and pains, irritability, depression, and moodiness. The prevalence rates of physical symptoms are more similar cross-nationally than the rates for emotional changes. Roughly the same proportion of women in each nation report some menstrual-related physical discomfort, while the proportion reporting emotional changes varies more widely. As in the West, physical symptoms among women in Third World nations tend to decrease with age and, to some extent, with oral contraceptive use. Similarly, the Western pattern of increased pain and moodiness with increased menstrual flow is also observed. The major difference, however, is the relative uniqueness of the "premenstrual syndrome" in the West. Symptom reports throughout the non-Western nations surveyed are much more closely associated with the event of menstruation itself; while physical symptoms are reported during the premenstrual phase, they are just as likely to be reported at menstruation as well (W.H.O., 1981). The emotional symptoms are much more likely to be reported throughout the cycle or during the menstrual phase; only the two European nations showed the premenstrual increase in moods. As was found for physical symptoms, the length and amount of menstrual bleeding showed a strong and consistent effect on reports of menstrual phase emotional symptoms.

The difference in the cyclic timing of emotional changes between Western and non-Western women, as well as the absence of emotional shifts among some non-Westerners, has implications for the interpretation of menstrual cycle mood changes by researchers. Most obviously, the notion that "PMS" is a biologically-induced condition must be examined carefully. The biology of the menstrual cycle is the same for women regardless of culture, so that the absence of important premenstrual mood shifts among women in Third World nations must be accounted for by something other than biology. Emotions during the menstrual cycle occur in the larger context of a woman's daily emotional experiences. As Rossi (1980) has shown, emotional shifts occur during social cycles, such as the work week, as well as during biological cycles. It is possible that there are cultural differences in the centrality of the menstrual cycle in women's emotional lives. Among nations in which a large proportion of women do report negative moods (but report those moods consistently throughout the menstrual cycle), there are more important determinants of emotional shifts that could produce individual variation. The large number of nations in which there was an increased number of women reporting negative moods during the event of menstruation itself suggests that menstrual bleeding has important social and personal connotations not necessarily shared by many Western women. As we have described elsewhere (Paige & Paige, 1981), in most tribal and peasant societies a woman's social and economic security depends to a large extent on her ability to continue producing children. The event of menstruation is the clearest indication (other than pregnancy) that a woman remains fertile. As long as a woman continues menstruating after each pregnancy, her status is secure; once menopause begins, her status as a wife changes in many ways. In Western nations, child-bearing does not have the same critical implications for women's status that it has in non-Western societies. It is possible, then, that the psychological meaning of menstruation differs in the West. While it may remain a cultural symbol of women's "pollution," menstruation may have quite different emotional implications. These are simply a few of many possible interpretations of the data presented here. The similarities and differences in national and cross-national patterns of both beliefs and symptoms should make clear the necessity of a broad comparative approach in future research on the menstrual cycle.

ACKNOWLEDGMENTS

Original data described in this chapter were collected as part of a research project funded by NIMH Grant No. 32138. My analysis and interpretation of data collected by the World Health Organization are partly informed by consultation on the survey described.

REFERENCES

Douglas, M., 1966. *Purity and Danger.* Penguin, London.

Paige, K. E., 1977. Sexual pollution: Reproductive sex taboos in America. *Journal of Social Issues 33:* 144-165.

Paige, K. E., 1983. Social exchange and dilemmas of reproduction. Plenary Address to the American Sociological Association Convention, Detroit, MI, August.

Paige, K. E. and J. M. Paige, 1981. *Politics of Reproductive Ritual.* University of California Press, Berkeley, CA.

Rossi, A., 1980. Body time and social time: Mood patterns by menstrual cycle phase and day of the week. In: J. Parsons (Ed.), *The Psychobiology of Sex Differences and Sex Roles.* Hemisphere Press, New York, NY, pp. 269-303.

Ruder and Finn Associates, 1981. *The Tampax Report.* Research Forecasts Inc., New York, NY.

Schlegel, A., 1972. *Male Dominance and Female Autonomy.* HRAF Press, New Haven, CT.

Snowden, R. and B. Christian, 1984. *Patterns and Perceptions of Menstruation.* St. Martins Press, New York, NY.

Stephens, W., 1961. A cross-cultural study of menstrual taboos. *Genetic Psychology Monographs 72:* No. 11.

Udry, J. R. and N. Morris, 1968. Distribution of coitus in the menstrual cycle. *Nature 220:* 593-596.

Udry, J. R. and N. Morris, 1970. Effects of contraceptive pills on the distribution of sexual activity in the menstrual cycle. *Nature 227:* 502-503.

Weber, M., 1978. *Economy and Society, Vol. 2.* University of California Press, Berkeley, CA.

White, B. and E. Saltz, 1967. The measurement of reproduceability. In: D. Jackson and S. Messick (Eds.), *Problems on Human Assessment.* McGraw-Hill, New York, NY, pp. 241-257.

Woods, N. F., A. Most, and G. Dery, 1982. Prevalence of perimenstrual symptoms. *American Journal of Public Health 72:* 1257-1264.

World Health Organization Task Force on Psychosocial Research in Family Planning, 1981. A cross-cultural study of menstruation. *Studies in Family Planning 12:* 3-16.

Young, F. and A. Bacdayan, 1965. Menstrual taboos and social rigidity. *Ethnology 4:* 225-240.

MEDIA TREATMENT OF PREMENSTRUAL SYNDROME

Mary Brown Parlee, Ph.D.

Graduate School and University Center
City University of New York
New York, New York

INTRODUCTION

This topic was included in the Conference because, as the list of participants reflects, the phenomenon of premenstrual syndrome (PMS) and scientific knowledge about it bear on a wide range of clinical, social, and legal issues. Media coverage is one means by which the science-based knowledge about PMS is conveyed to the general public and to those non-scientific professionals for whom it is relevant. Research on the mass communication and the media has traditionally been conducted by sociologists, none of whom as yet has focused on contemporary media treatments of PMS or of women's reproductive functions more generally (e.g., Curran, Gurevitch, & Wollacott, 1979; Dexter & White, 1964). Because of the importance of the topic for PMS researchers, however, this paper attempts to bridge the gap between relatively technical scholarly treatments of the media by sociologists (see, for example, works cited in Gans, 1979) and the practical concerns of the working scientists dealing with the media. It draws, in part, on the author's experience as a full-time writer and editor for a monthly magazine covering social science, as chair of the Public Information Committee of the American Psychological Association during the time the Association was developing and testing strategies for promoting responsible media coverage of psychological research, and as a researcher who has often interacted with media representatives covering PMS and/or menstrual cycle research. As Dr. Halbreich suggested in discussion at the Conference, media coverage of PMS may represent a useful model for analysis of the complex issues arising in media treatment of medical subjects more generally (Dick, 1954). Systematic research of this sort is needed to bridge solidly the gap to which this paper is addressed in a necessarily preliminary way.

Media coverage of PMS and scientific knowledge about PMS are both produced by individuals working in socially organized professional communities defined by particular practices, values, and goals. The professional communities — journalism and science — are, in turn, part of a larger sociocultural system that both affects and is affected by the professions and individuals within it. These complex interrelationships are experienced by the working scientist or journalist in ways highly dependent on the particular scientific community or medium in which they work (Curtis & Petras, 1970; Mannheim, 1936, 1952).

This paper will briefly characterize media treatments of PMS and suggest some ways in which the social organization of science and of journalism may contribute to an apparent consistency of treatment despite diversity of media. Scientific investigations of PMS in the context of normal menstrual function will then be discussed in light of research on socially-shared beliefs about menstruation. Finally, the preliminary results of a study will be described which begin to uncover some of the interrelationships between socially-shared beliefs, media treatment of PMS, and scientific research on menstruation.

MEDIA TREATMENT OF PREMENSTRUAL SYNDROME

> "It has many names: period, monthly, that time, my friend. But for many women the most apt description is the curse. For about half of all women of child-bearing age, menstruation is a monthly misery that causes intense physical and mental discomfort. In the U.S. alone, menstrual problems result in the loss of 140 million hours of work a year. Menstrual pain, says Pathologist Laurence Demers of the Milton S. Hershey Medical Center in Hershey, PA, 'probably is the most common cause for absence of women from the work force.'"
>
> — *Time* Magazine, July 27, 1981

Following this introductory paragraph, the *Time* article describes what the reporters call the medical profession's previous neglect of menstrual distress, and the shift of medical attitude brought about by newly available drugs for treatment of menstrual cramps. Then premenstrual syndrome is introduced:

> "Less understood than menstrual cramps is the pre-menstrual syndrome. Days or even two weeks before menstrual bleeding begins, many women experience tenderness and swelling of the breasts, migraine headaches, abdominal bloating and acne. They become lethargic, irritable and depressed. Researchers contend that severely distressed women are apt to have accidents, abuse their children or commit suicide or violent crime."

The article continues with a summary of one of Katharina Dalton's studies in which she observed three female convicts whose law-breaking occurred "only in the days just before the period." One of these convicts was the woman charged (in a legal case widely publicized in England) with manslaughter rather than murder "on the grounds that she has committed a fatal stabbing when she was experiencing premenstrual syndrome." Dalton's advocacy of progesterone treatment for PMS is described, as are the treatments (mostly biological) offered by one of her "supporters" who operates a PMS clinic. A final paragraph describes the beneficial effects for many women of recognizing and labeling their complaints as menstrual-related.

Headlined "Coping with Eve's Curse: Doctors Are Finally Treating Menstrual Miseries," the article is accompanied by a cartoon-like drawing of a Victorian woman reclining on a couch with her hand on her forehead. In the foreground a young child whisperingly asks an adult man, "What makes Mama so cross?"

As a weekly newsmagazine with a readership of millions, *Time* Magazine represents only one of the media through which different segments of the American population receive information about menstruation in general and about PMS in particular. Reporters and editors for print media with weekly deadlines such as *Time's* operate under different temporal pressures and have slightly different goals as purveyers of news than do daily newspapers or monthly magazines. These publications also differ in their audiences: pieces written for mass audiences or for narrower groups of "opinion leaders" vary in tone and style, and some of these stylistic differences are related to the complexity of facts and ideas that can be included. Some writers and editors, regardless of audience or medium, are better than others at combining complexity and clarity in limited space and often under time pressures. For example, part of a *Harper's Bazaar* article entitled "Menstruation: How It Affects Working Women" contains material similar to that included in *Time's* opening paragraph. ". . . sociologists have begun to look at the amount of time lost from work because of symptoms apparently related to menstrual periods. . . And it has been discovered that much time has been lost from work reportedly because of these differences" (*Harper's Bazaar,* November, 1975). From the scientific point of view, the use here of "apparently" and "reportedly" are important qualifiers; they serve to keep the popular account closer to the scientific data.

Treatment of menstruation and PMS by electronic news media (TV, radio) is similar to that of print media in being shaped by varying types of deadline pressures, "space" (time) constraints, "news" orientation, and audience. Reports of PMS research on the *Today Show* and on *Nova,* for example, will necessarily differ in important respects because of differences on these as well as other dimensions.

While there are significant similarities, electronic and print media are obviously dissimilar in the relative importance they accord to certain production values. An experiment conducted in a laboratory bulging with equipment and computers offers more visual interest and is more readily accessible to the reporters and camera crews than research based on interviews, surveys, or questionnaires. In electronic media, as in print, there are, of course, differences in the quality of coverage within a particular format.

The relevance of all this to a discussion of media treatments of PMS is twofold: One is to underscore most researchers' experience-based recognition that "the media" are diverse on several dimensions. This means that research scientists, especially those whose work bears upon significant health and social issues, need a variety of skills to deal with this diversity effectively when their research is being reported to non-scientific audiences. Some professional associations have already begun to develop resources to guide their members in interactions with journalists from different media, and this seems a promising, small beginning toward clearer communication (American Psychological Association, 1981). Both the general public and the scientific community benefit when leading scientists have the skills — which can be learned — to communicate effectively with representatives of the media. Journalists can always find scientists who will talk to them and whom they can understand; if the best scientists do not or cannot do this, others will.

A second reason for discussing differences among media is to point to an apparent paradox. Despite their diversity, media treatments of menstruation and PMS seem to convey a relatively consistent image of PMS, an image presented implicitly or explicitly as representing the results of scientific research or a consensus among clinical practitioners. The following discussion is based on the supposition that the image of

PMS conveyed to popular audiences through mass media, despite their differences, is roughly similar in content to the one in the *Time* Magazine article. This supposition is based on an informal but fairly systematic tracking of media coverage of PMS and menstrual cycle research over the past decade. (Two clear exceptions to the otherwise relatively consistent treatment appeared in *Ms.* Magazine; Parlee, 1982a; Steinem, 1978). Quantitative research based on content analyses of a comprehensive survey of the coverage is badly needed. Characteristically, the media image of PMS involves the following: a focus on physical symptoms and negative moods, a discussion of associated undesirable or antisocial behaviors, and identification of biological causes and/or treatments of the negative moods and behaviors. In addition, media treatments of PMS are usually characterized either by extreme vagueness ("many," "some") about the proportion of women experiencing a specific cluster of symptoms, or by a pseudo-precision about the prevalence of PMS which does not represent a consensus among the scientific community. For example, a July 10, 1981 article in the *Washington Post* refers to "the estimated 40% of women who have PMS to one degree or another." Like careful scientists, many editors would have challenged the reporter with, "Whose estimates? How do they know?" and not have been satisfied until there was an answer. In many journalistic circles, a phrase like "to one degree or another" is called "fluffing it." It is a response — in this case to the question, "What does 'have PMS' mean, exactly?" — that becomes more acceptable as the deadline closes in.

Why does media coverage of PMS research emerge with this consistent image, given both the diversity among media and the relatively much greater diversity of scientific views than is reported? Part of the answer probably lies in the social organization of science (Halmos, 1972; Merton, 1973) and in the way this interacts with journalistic practices.

INTERACTION BETWEEN SCIENCE AND JOURNALISM

For every set of research problems, a certain relatively small group of investigators comes to be recognized by those in the field as eminent by virtue of the significance of their research contributions (Zuckerman & Merton, 1971). These leading researchers constitute what sociologists call the "invisible college" of the field or subfield in which they work (Crane, 1972). Invisible college members communicate with each other informally at conferences and elsewhere and more formally through exchange of preprints. The social networks that make up the invisible colleges serve a "gatekeeping" function: their members serve on editorial boards of the major journals in the field (Crane, 1967), and they play important roles in allocating desirable and prestigious jobs among newcomers (Caplow & McGee, 1965). The members of invisible colleges thus represent through their research what is acknowledged to be the leading edge of their field, and have the power and authority to shape the work of others in directions they believe to be promising.

Journalists working in media of all kinds are quick to tap into the invisible college in a field. That is how they do their research; a reporter for a prestigious publication or TV/radio show can almost always get to the leading scientists in a field with relatively few phone calls. As a result, journalists often gather information from a fairly small set of scientifically like-minded investigators. When a reporter moves beyond one network of individuals, as they endeavor to do, the result is that they tap into the invisible college of another field. In media coverage of PMS, this process means that journalists usually interview (more or less extensively) key individuals in networks of physicians who research and treat PMS as a clinical syndrome, social scientists whose research is on social processes shaping premenstrual experience, and biomedical and social science researchers who focus on biological causes of premenstrual symptomatology. Sometimes networks of self-help or feminist health organizations are also included.

Journalistic reasoning very often seems to be that for every viewpoint (as represented in one network) there is an "other (or opposite) side," and the truth lies halfway in between. This is referred to as an "on the one hand. . . on the other hand" approach, and is ridiculed if it actually appears with this phrase in the final piece. Nevertheless, the structure of the reasoning is pervasive in journalistic practice, and is believed to be fundamental to objective reporting. [For scholarly discussions of these issues, see Tuchman (1972, 1978) and Gans (1979, Chapter 6)].

The articles or reports that emerge from this journalistic research are shaped both in initial assignment and in subsequent editing by editorial focus (Sigelman, 1973; White, 1950). For the larger media, topics in science, medicine, health, and technology are frequently handled by different editors, each of whom has a somewhat different view about the focus and type of piece appropriate for his or her department. For example, research on menstrual-related problems and networks of clinical investigators are likely to be interviewed more extensively and featured more prominantly if the report is being handled by the editor in charge of medical coverage than if the editor covering health (nutrition, prevention, wellness) is in charge. From the perspective of the scientist interviewee, it is often fairly clear whether the journalist is eliciting views as part of the major focus of the piece or as a gesture to "on the other hand." In the latter case, it becomes evident fairly quickly in the interview that the piece has essentially been completed in the reporter's mind on the basis of interviews in another network, and a discussion of research from a different viewpoint will not affect the substance of the report.

The piece is also shaped in the editorial process for newsworthiness, a value whose definition and importance varies within the particular medium (Gans, 1979; Tuchman, 1978). Editorial judgments about what constitutes "news" are complex, and, despite the individual editor's sense of autonomy and decision-making power, appear to be largely determined by the implicit or explicit rules of the organizational system within which s/he works (Enzenberger, 1974). When applied to research on menstruation and PMS, the effect of such editorial judgments has been to emphasize illness and treatment (there was a problem and now there is a cure) and to imply that the phenomenon is a problem that affects many women in a socially disruptive way.

While individual scientists usually provide reporters with accurate and up-to-date information from their fields, it is clear that the results of the journalistic research and editorial process do not always accurately reflect either the specific facts or the general import of the scientific knowledge base. As in the article from *Time*, for example, media coverage of PMS very frequently mentions Katharina Dalton's reports of premenstrual increases in crimes, accidents, and the like, and also the variously attributed belief that women lose time from work because of menstrual problems. Estimates of the prevalence of PMS among women are often given. From a scientific point of view, however, a simple interpretation of Dalton's correlational data as resulting from PMS needs to be modified (Dalton, 1982; Parlee, 1982a), and the attribution of lost work time to menstruation can be very sharply challenged.

The fact is that, despite its consistent recurrence in journalistic (and in some scientific) accounts, scientific data have not until recently been reported in the professional literature to suggest that women lose time from work because of menstrual problems. For example, Andersch and Milson (1982) and Widholm (1985) both report such a finding, but neither provides sufficient information regarding procedures for the research to be replicated. Both use self-report questionnaires to assess absenteeism. It would appear from an extensive review of the literature that no observational or archival data have been reported on this issue. If reliable behavioral data showing an association between self-reported menstrual problems and absenteeism were available, scientists familiar with the research on the social and psychological functions of beliefs about menstruation would be likely to reject the causal interpretation suggested in the media accounts (Parlee, 1982a; Ruble & Brooks-Gunn, 1979). The reasoning would be that if "menstrual problems" are a more socially acceptable excuse for absence from work than are, for instance, child care problems, it is possible that women would offer the employer the more socially acceptable excuse. Since data on absences and menstrual problems would have to be based on reasons given by the employee (the employer would not know her menstrual status directly), the scientific meaning of the self-report data is unknown and alternative interpretations are possible (i.e., the women had menstrual problems *or* they were offering socially acceptable excuses). An interpretation in terms of a direct causal relationship between menstrual problems and absenteeism logically requires additional justification in light of at least one plausible alternative explanation.

However, the fact that scientists do not know what some particular set of data means is not as interesting from a journalistic perspective as the possibility that (as *Time* reports) "140 million hours of work a year are lost" because of menstrual problems. Sometimes the more newsworthy claim is simply reported with "fluffing" to obscure a crucial lack of specificity. (The 1975 article in *Harper's Bazaar* previously mentioned attributes it to "sociologists.") It is better from the editorial point of view, however, if the journalist can locate a scientist who will endorse the more newsworthy view. A direct quotation from that individual is then included and an appearance of scientific backing for the newsworthy "fact" is created. Thus, *Time* Magazine reporters quote a pathologist who claimed menstrual pain is "probably. . . the most common cause" of lost work time. When fact checkers go over the piece in the final stage of the editorial process, the "fact" checked is whether or not the individual was quoted correctly, not whether what he said can be supported by scientific data. Similarly, serious researchers are well aware of the complexity inherent in estimating the prevalence of PMS. They recognize, as the journalistic accounts do not, that such estimates are entirely dependent on how PMS is defined in a particular investigation and are therefore meaningful only relative to a specific definition of the syndrome. Again, however, this is not newsworthy from a journalistic perspective, and vagueness and/or pseudo-precision characterize media estimates of the prevalence of PMS.

The scientific community has both the knowledge and the professional motivation (science is supposed to be a self-corrective enterprise) to identify instances such as these where media treatments imply or invoke conclusions from research evidence that is weak or nonexistent, or where interpretations clearly need to be justified in light of empirically plausible alternatives. How or whether the scientific community as a whole or individual scientists in it can respond to what they see as inadequacies in media coverage remains problematic, since scientific concerns and views may genuinely conflict with journalistic goals and values. It may be useful, however, for individual scientists and journalists to recognize that difficulties they encounter at the interface of scientific research and reporting are likely to be the result of deeply ingrained professional norms rather than clashes between individual personalities. Some mutual education can productively occur at this interface if the journalist has the time and the scientists the patience (which often come to the same thing in the lives of professionals).

Given the social organization of science into networks of specialists with different views and emphases — sometimes on the same research topic — transactions at the interface between disciplines can sometimes seem almost as difficult as those between science and journalism (Merton, 1973). (A difficult issue at one of these interfaces, for example, has been the interpretation of self-report data in menstrual cycle and PMS research.) In both cross-professional and cross-disciplinary communication, difficulties are likely to arise not so much over specific facts (in this case, scientific data) as over the context which give the facts meaning, their salience *vis-à-vis* other facts, and their significance in other realms of activity (see L. Wirth's preface to Mannheim, 1936; Parlee, 1981a, 1982a). Such differences in interpretive view point (within science, they are related primarily to disciplinary training) are, in turn, related to different views about how scientists acquire knowledge about physical and social phenomena (such as PMS) and how journalists convey this knowledge to the general public. At their most fundamental, they are differences in views concerning the relationship between the knower and what is or can be known.

In one view, scientific research is seen as a cumulative, self-corrective activity which ultimately will reveal the properties of a more or less objectively known or knowable reality; support for this view comes in part from the successful applications of scientific knowledge in both engineering and medicine. The media, in turn, convey this knowledge with varying degrees of accuracy (which they also call objectivity) to different audiences. The methods and practices of science and of journalism operate to ensure that the outcome is an objective reflection of physical and social reality (in this case, PMS) insofar as this is possible. In this view, scientific research tends to focus on biological causes of negative premenstrual moods and behaviors because this is how the physical and psychological phenomena are in nature, and the journalistic image of PMS, while highly oversimplified and sometimes distorted, tends in general to report this scientific knowledge as it is.

In another view (the one outlined at the beginning of this discussion), emphasis is placed on the fact that both the journalist and the scientist are members of the society in which they live and work. This means not only that they as individuals hold assumptions and values characteristic of their culture and class, but also that the social institutions within which they work represent patterns of activities organized in ways that are compatible with and support other major institutions of society. The information and knowledge that journalism and science produce, in this view, can therefore be seen as social products which in part serve an ideological function; that is, they support the social order by rationalizing ("explaining" from the point of view of one social group) differences among groups, and by mystifying individuals whose experience does not accord with the ideology. This is not to say that individual scientists and journalists necessarily work with an ideological intent. In this view, the focus of scientific research on PMS as a biological condition afflicting many women both reflects and reinforces the interests of powerful social groups and institutions. Drug companies, many biomedically oriented researchers, physicians who are reimbursed by third party payments for treatment of specified diseases, and an increasing conservative political climate on issues related to women, work, and family — all function well with this definition of PMS, and less well with a focus that defines and locates PMS in a different context (for example, as a statistically unusual condition unrelated to normal menstruation and/or as a culturally transmitted set of beliefs and attitudes that significantly shape an individual's experience). In this view, one role of the media is to mediate conflict over control of the public discourse about PMS, a discourse that influences the way the reading public (and especially the "opinion leaders") perceives PMS and its significance. An illuminating example can be found in historical scholarship on a very different topic: the case of Jack the Ripper (Walkowitz, 1980). In that case, there were many rumors circulating about the identity of the murderer — each reflecting a different set of assumptions, a different world view. One was that the killer was a madman, that this was an aberrant, irrational act in an otherwise fairly stable and enduring social order. A competing view was that the murderer exemplified the moral deterioration of society, a deterioration consequent to the decline in religious influence and to be halted by its restoration. A third view was that the murderer was a man of noble birth, whose capture was being delayed or avoided because his rank protected him in a society where the rich and well born flourished at the expense of the poor. These rumors represented different ways of talking about the phenomenon, different discourses which embodied and perpetuated different world views. The way the press of the time reported/reflected these different discourses determined which would prevail in the ideology, and therefore which would have the opportunity to shape the consciousness of the reading public — not only on this particular issue, but also on the world view (rational, religious, class consciousness) embodied in the discourse. A contemporary example of the way the media have effectively controlled the discourse on a social issue, and thus the way the public thinks about it, is feminism. A similar situation exists in media coverage of PMS: the range of scientific views on the nature and causes of this entity is much broader than the media image, where it is the biological rather than social emphasis that is conveyed to the public.

The two general viewpoints outlined here are not entirely incompatible, despite failures of communication engendered when it is assumed they are. PMS could well be a clinical entity for which effective medical treatments need to be sought through research, while at the same time it could well be that most researchers do not differentiate PMS and menstrual problems from normal menstrual experience as carefully as they could or might if the topic were unrelated to significant social issues concerning the role of women. Some of the social structural issues involved have been described and analyzed by Merton (1972).

SCIENTIFIC RESEARCH ON PREMENSTRUAL SYNDROME: THE SIGNIFICANCE OF SOCIALLY-SHARED BELIEFS

Using a standard Menstrual Distress Questionnaire, social science researchers have shown that there are socially-shared beliefs about the existence and nature of psychological changes associated with the menstrual cycle (see review and discussion by Ruble & Brooks-Gunn, this volume). In general, the questionnaire data have been interpreted as suggesting that people believe the premenstrual phase of the cycle is a time of increased negative affect and other psychological and physical symptomatology (Brooks-Gunn & Ruble, 1982; Parlee, 1974). As documented in the research, such premenstrual changes appear to represent a mild form of premenstrual syndrome, either as a clinically-defined syndrome or as it is portrayed in media treatments. Since these beliefs about the nature of premenstrual psychological and physical changes have been reported not only by menstruating women but also by prepubertal girls and by men, it has been suggested that the socially-shared beliefs or expectations are not necessarily based on personal experiences of physiologically-induced psychological changes, but are or can be learned (Brooks-Gunn, Ruble, & Clark, 1977; Clark & Ruble, 1978; Paige, 1973; Parlee, 1974; Ruble & Brooks-Gunn, 1979).

The suggestion is that socially-shared beliefs about the nature of menstrual experience may be transmitted to the individual from a variety of sources and can serve as a basis by which she comes to interpret the psychological meaning of the bodily changes of her menstrual cycle (Ruble & Brooks-Gunn, this volume; see also Brooks-Gunn & Ruble, 1983). Cognitive information processing mechanisms potentially underlying the development and persistence of such beliefs have been described, and the function of the beliefs in the interpretation of the individual's own and others' behavior have been explored (Koeske & Koeske, 1975; Rodin, 1976; Ruble & Brooks-Gunn, 1979).

As the work of Ruble, Brooks-Gunn, and their colleagues indicates, such research points to a potentially fruitful line of theoretical and empirical work on the relationships among basic cognitive mechanisms, cultural sources of information, and physiological states of individuals. It should be noted that the emphasis in such work is on a conceptualization of patterns of responses on menstrual questionnaires as beliefs or expectations or perceptions about menstruation rather than as a form of self-reports, and on an exploration of the psychological and social processes with which they are associated. The researchers have not been primarily concerned in this work with whether or not, or in what ways, the content of the beliefs is true. ("True" is used here to mean that the phenomena would exist and could be measured in other ways regardless of whether or not the women cognitively believed in their existence.) The research is not designed at this stage to determine whether the pattern of responses given by menstruating women on a Menstrual Distress Questionnaire is, in fact, an accurate (in the sense just given) description of their personal experiences, verifiable through use of measurement techniques other than questionnaires. The beliefs or attitudes or perceptions about menstruation which are the object of research may indeed be what philosophers call justified, true beliefs; that is, they may accurately describe matters of empirical fact for which the holder of the beliefs has good, relevant, and sufficient evidence. Or they may be beliefs describing a particular social group which have little or no basis in empirical fact, but which appear to rationalize or to make sense of certain social relations or institutions. Without additional scientific evidence, we do not know where to locate popular beliefs regarding premenstrual changes on the dimension between these two possibilities.

Therefore, a second line of empirical work arising from research on menstrual beliefs (related to, but not the same as the one above) is to develop multimethod approaches to determine ways in which the content of the beliefs are or are not accurate descriptions of the menstrual experiences of most women or of particular groups of women when the experiences are measured in ways other than with retrospective questionnaires (e.g., Abraham, Mira, McNeil, Vizzard, Fraser, & Llewellyn-Jones, 1985; Parlee, 1982c; Rubinow, Roy-Byrne, & Hoban, 1985).

In addition to these programs of empirical research, however, there is also an important non-empirical outcome of the research on beliefs about menstruation, one which has significant implications for differentiating PMS from normal menstrual experience. The intellectual significance and the general scientific import of the demonstration that there are socially-shared beliefs about menstrual experience are not that symptoms of premenstrual tension and other negative affect are learned or that these phenomena are "all in the head" (or, more technically, "socially constructed" — Berger & Luckman, 1967). It is that the methodological and conceptual burden of proof is now shifted, in logical terms, to those who want to claim that a pattern of self-reported symptoms obtained on questionnaires is justified and true. In light of available evidence, researchers can no longer simply assume, for example, that non-cognitive (e.g., physiological) processes are significant causes of women's self-reports of premenstrual psychological changes; we know such reports could be acquired through learning from the sociocultural environment (as they are by men and prepubertal girls). If investigators wish to offer a biologically-based interpretation of questionnaire data, the logic of research questions as they have developed now requires that they justify such a conclusion by, for example, identifying specific physiological processes as potential determinants, by demonstrating the effectiveness of particular treatments or manipulations, and/or by specifying for which populations these are effective. This kind of argument is a statement about research strategies and about the kinds of evidence that are logically relevant to particular kinds of conclusions; it is not a statement about the determinants of menstrual experience (see also Rubinow & Roy-Byrne, 1984).

On the whole, the evidence seems clearly to indicate that biological processes play an overwhelmingly large role in causing certain premenstrual syndromes, well defined as clinical entities, in some women (Halbreich, Endicott, & Nee, 1983; Halbreich, Endicott, & Schacht, 1982). On such an interpretation, these women would have PMS regardless of whether or not there were cultural beliefs that ascribe a milder form of this syndrome to most women. The crucial question for both science and public policy is one of context. How should PMS be located and discussed in the context of normal menstrual experience? Is severe, socially-disabling, biologically-caused PMS as rare as a brain tumor, or is it a condition which afflicts some 80% of women at some time in their lives? Are any psychological changes that are empirically correlated with (for whatever reasons) different phases of the normal menstrual cycle most accurately described as changes in the premenstrual phase (Parlee, 1973)? Right now, given the variability of definitions and the limited range of psychological phenomena that have been explored, all that is known for certain is that for some — perhaps many — women, biological processes appear to have significant influences on symptoms, personality, and behavior. On the other hand, research on beliefs suggests that some — perhaps many — women have absorbed the messages of their culture regarding menstrual experience and have constructed their self-descriptions from their socially-acquired beliefs. The empirically correct apportionment of "some" and "many" between these two possibilities and the elaboration of other possibilities is crucial to the question of context. Clarification of at least some important aspects of this problem may depend, in part, on developing, through the three approaches indicated above, a more precise understanding of the nature and significance of socially-shared beliefs about menstrual experience.

Media treatments of PMS, as shapers of public consciousness, are for a number of complex reasons even less likely to distinguish carefully between clinical syndromes and normal experiences. If "women [are] unfit for top jobs" because of the "raging hormonal influences of the menstrual cycle" — as a July 26, 1970, article in the *New York Times* claimed — then social and legal issues surrounding the role of women at work (like affirmative action, comparable worth, day care) seem beside the point. This is an example of what is meant by the ideological function of the media. It is somehow more disturbing, however, when scientists put forward a similar view in more subtle form by failing to apply rigorous standards of scientific method and reasoning to their work. For example:

> "It is estimated that more than 50% of menstruating women are affected by dysmenorrhea, and 10% of them have severe dysmenorrhea which incapacitates them for 1-3 days each month (Ylikorkala & Dawood, 1978). Since women constitute 42% of the adult work force in the United States of America (Waite, 1981), about 600 million working hours will be lost annually because of incapacitating dysmenorrhea if adequate relief is not provided."
>
> — M. Y. Dawood, 1985, p. 177

This line of reasoning from what are presumably self-report data on incapacitating dysmenorrhea to conclusions about 600 million working hours lost annually contains several questionable assumptions. Among them are the ambiguity or interpretation of such self-report data (discussed above), and the generality of results obtained from a single sample to 42% of the adult U.S. work force. Unfortunately, it is not possible to determine the adequacy of the sample size in the Ylikorkala and Dawood paper cited by Dawood, since Ylikorkala and Dawood (1978) simply assert the "facts" (50%, 10%, 1-3 days of incapacitation) without documentation or original data. Since scientists do not work in a social or political vacuum — and even if they did — investigators have a responsibility to exercise their methods carefully and cautiously when formulating conclusions about matters of empirical fact which bear on social issues (Merton, 1942). Moreover, scientists have in their collective armamentarium the tools of logical and empirical analysis to move toward a clarification of the relationship between PMS and normal menstrual function by means of closer analysis of menstrual beliefs and their significance. To the extent that investigators fail to address this issue rigorously, the research can be seen as serving an ideological function rather than representing the results of a self-corrective, objective search for truth. Thus, scientific research serves an ideological function when it contains conclusions consistent with a negative social image of a vaguely defined group of women and when application of more adequate scientific methods of reasoning that might lead to different or more precise conclusions has not been seriously attempted. The discussion so far has reflected the assumption, embodied in the literature and useful for many purposes, that beliefs about menstruation can be adequately explored using menstrual questionnaires. Given what has been suggested about the conceptual and empirical significance of these beliefs, however, it is relevant to take the next critical step and to ask whether such questionnaires are the only or the best way to investigate them. In particular, is it possible that the methods used in such questionnaire research themselves create or shape the phenomenon they are designed to understand?

When a researcher asks women to indicate on a menstrual questionnaire the degree to which they (or most women or some particular woman) experience certain physical and psychological symptoms at different phases of the cycle, they will do so. These responses can be scored to show that the respondent holds certain beliefs (or perceptions or attitudes) about the intensity of symptom patterns associated with different phases of the menstrual cycle. That is, when a particular method of measurement is used (the menstrual questionnaire), under conditions in which the situation is defined as a research study, where menstruation has been made salient to the respondent and where there is a conventional, hierarchical relationship between the "subject" and "experimenter," the pattern of responses indicates that subjects believe that most women experience premenstrual increases in negative affect and symptomatology. In this situation, however, subjects are constrained by the method to answer only the degree to which they endorse the content of the menstrual beliefs on the experimenter's questionnaire. The method involves a high degree of conceptual control on the part of the experimenter and a low degree of autonomy on the part of the subject in defining the data (Cassell, 1982). Depending on how and with what populations of subjects the questionnaire was developed, the results of this method may or may not accord with the content of the subject's beliefs as they might be expressed in other contexts. Further, such questionnaires have no way of revealing the salience of the menstrual beliefs in the subjects' experience, or how this salience may vary over time or across different groups.

What, then, do women believe about menstrual experience when methods other than questionnaires are used? I recently explored this question using the market research technique known as focus groups. The preliminary results suggest that the content and salience of beliefs about menstruation vary across social groups, and that the media treatment of PMS may play a role in shaping the beliefs and expectations in one particular group.

In focus group research, small groups of women are recruited through random digit telephone dialing (Sudman, 1976) and subsequently screened for particular demographic characteristics. In this study, potential subjects were screened for sex, age, parental status, and total family income. Four groups of eight subjects each were formed. One consisted of teenagers (16-20 years) from families with middle-to-low family income (less than $15,000). Two other groups consisted of women in their 20's with at least one child; one of these groups had a middle-to-low family income, and the other high (greater than $25,000). The fourth group consisted of women in their 20's with high income and no children.

The groups met separately for approximately two hours. During this time, they discussed, in their own terms and with minimal direction from the group leader, their experiences related to menstruation.[1] The role of the "leader" in a focus group is to keep the conversation reasonably well focused on the topic, but not to guide or constrain the conversation by providing particular concepts or terms, or by highlighting some aspects of the topic rather than others. The focus group technique thus enables the researcher to gain information about the way in which the participants spontaneously construe the topic, including their sense of what aspects are salient and what aspects are relatively less important.

In these discussions, only one group spontaneously raised and discussed PMS in their conversation about menstruation. In this group, it was evident that they felt their usual menstrual experience was similar to, although milder than, the clinical syndrome as they

---

[1] The groups were led by Ina Hillebrandt of Hillebrandt Associates, New York, New York.

understood it. The group that did this was the group of unmarried women in their 20's with high income. A comparable group of married women did not bring up PMS, nor did women of similar age with low income, nor did teenagers. As these high-income, single women talked about PMS, it was clear that they had gotten most of their information from the media, primarily print. This is consistent with other data I and my students have collected suggesting that socioeconomic status is an important factor in predicting where people get their information about health-related topics. Upper middle-class women get their information largely from reading; it is scientifically-based and presents knowledge that is abstracted from people and contexts that are personally familiar. Women from lower economic classes, on the other hand, tend to get their information primarily from informal social networks, where the knowledge is more closely linked to direct personal experience of individuals whom they know. Many of these women held negative beliefs and attitudes regarding the menstrual flow itself, but a premenstrual increase in negative moods and symptoms did not emerge as a salient focus in the discussion.

If systematic quantitative analyses of these data support the preliminary indications, the results suggest that the relationships among media treatments of PMS, menstrual research, and individual experience is a highly interactive one. Speculating freely, the relationships might be something like the following:

Media coverage of PMS plays an important role in shaping public discourse (the thinking of opinion leaders and eventually of larger numbers of people) on a socially sensitive topic. In this case, the topic is how female reproductive processes — biological, relatively unchangeable givens — might negatively affect women's performance in the world of paid work and might also cause them to act in ways traditionally associated with the troublesome or "not normal" individuals in society. Acording to the media image, PMS causes women to be unreliable workers and/or to be "mad," "bad," "criminal," or "sick." These latter concepts and the analysis they imply are derived from sociological labeling theory — a perspective on the way social systems respond to undesirable or dysfunctional deviations by an individual from the norms of behavior (Scheff, 1974). Laws (1983) has cogently argued for their applicability to PMS.

At a given point in historical time, the public discourse on PMS has different impacts on different social groups. (Most publicly discussed ideas and activities "trickle down" in the class structure and appear later in the lower than the upper classes.) Upper middle-class women who read and hear about menstruation and PMS in the negative, media-mediated form absorb some of its ideas and connotations; PMS assumes heightened salience in these women's experience of menstruation and plays an active role in the way they formulate (construe, construct) their own experience in a conversational setting (and in other settings that could be identified through research). Since women of all classes within the mainstream, assimilated groups of U.S. society have an opportunity to acquire at least some of the negative views of menstruation from various sources, however, most women can and do endorse a similar set of negative beliefs (perceptions, attitudes) when asked directly to do so on a questionnaire. Because of the way questionnaires exercise implicit conceptual control over the data, such research is not sensitive to — does not and cannot reveal — differences in the salience of a particular belief, or in the way it is organized in the context of other beliefs and values. It is the salience and meaning of the media-mediated image that varies with social class.

If this general view is correct, certain empirical predictions follow. One is that while women of all classes might respond in roughly similar ways on menstrual questionnaires, they might reveal, under a variety of different circumstances, quite different views of menstrual experience (especially differences on the dimension of how much it resembles a mild form of the media-transmitted image of PMS). Furthermore, women of ethnic groups who have been less exposed to mainstream cultural ideas about menstruation might not respond with a negative PMS-based view of normal menstrual experience even when questionnaires are used. Finally, if scientists were able to distinguish PMS more precisely from normal menstrual experience, it would be predicted that the incidence of a clinical, biologically-caused and biologically-treatable syndrome would not vary with social class or ethnic group, even though there might at the same time be group differences in the incidence of women who talk about PMS in conversational settings and who present themselves to the physician as having it.

Scientists, as opinion leaders coming from backgrounds similar to those of journalists, have acquired some of the same "socially-shared" beliefs that are represented by the media coverage. "Socially-shared" now needs to be qualified by saying the beliefs are shared among the upper and upper-middle classes. Like journalists, scientists can perpetuate these beliefs in and through their research — both through failure to distinguish theoretically and empirically between PMS and normal menstrual experience, and through the use of a research method (questionnaires) which allows no information about alternative phenomena or beliefs, or about the salience of particular beliefs, to emerge. The consistency of the image which emerges when scientific knowledge is produced in this way is enhanced when the subjects in the research are socially homogeneous and primarily middle and upper-middle class. It is the scientific views of PMS and of menstruation emerging from this kind of research which is picked up and reported in the media. Scientific research, media coverage, and the experience of individuals (in some social groups more than others) thus represent a system of mutual influences which will be difficult but not impossible to penetrate analytically through research.

CONCLUSIONS

What are the research implications of such speculations about media treatments of PMS and scientific methods and findings? One is that the potential interrelationships suggested here can only be addressed through research on more diverse groups of women. Explicit attention to variations among women on social, psychological, and physiological dimensions continues to be badly needed in menstrual cycle and PMS research (Halbreich et al., 1982; Parlee, 1981b). Secondly, given that some — perhaps many — people will endorse a particular set of beliefs about menstrual experience if asked this directly in an experimental situation, researchers will need to use a variety of methods to determine the nature and range of these beliefs about menstrual experience and their relation to accounts of menstrual experience in different populations of women under different conditions.

Until such data are available, scientists have a responsibility to talk about PMS in and only in the context of what is empirically known about it; that is, some women may experience PMS as a biologically-caused and biologically-treatable entity. They may be a very small proportion of the population. Other women, particularly upper-middle class women, may describe their experiences as similar to a mild form of PMS, but these descriptions are possibly the result of complex constructions of experience, depending in part on their personalities and on the beliefs they have acquired through exposure to cultural institutions, including the media. The nature and range and determinants of normal menstrual experiences — the kinds the vast majority of women have — are not well known or understood. Scientists do not at present know what normal menstrual experiences are (unstructured by methods of measurement) among women in different social groups, how they change with age, how they vary in psychological meaning and significance depending on the personal history and personality of the individual, or how they are related to clinical premenstrual syndromes. These are facts about the context of research on PMS, just as hard and solid as the facts about PMS that are known. Scientists need to be clear about both sets of facts and to do what they can to make the media be clear as well.

REFERENCES

Abraham, S., M. Mira, D. McNeil, J. Vizzard, I. Fraser, and D. Llewellyn-Jones, 1985. Changes in mood and physical symptoms during the menstrual cycle. In: M. Y. Dawood, J. L. McGuire, and L. M. Demers (Eds.), *Premenstrual Syndrome and Dysmenorrhea.* Urban and Schwarzenberg, Baltimore, MD, pp. 41-50.

American Psychological Association, 1981. *Media Guide for Psychologists.* Public Information Office, American Psychological Association, Washington, D.C.

Andersch, B. and I. Milson, 1982. An epidemiological study of young women with dysmenorrhea. *American Journal of Obstetrics and Gynecology 144:* 655-660.

Berger, P. and T. Luckman, 1967. *The Social Construction of Reality.* Doubleday and Co., Garden City, NY.

Brooks-Gunn, J. and D. N. Ruble, 1982. The development of menstrual-related beliefs and behaviors during early adolescence. *Child Development 53:* 1567-1577.

Brooks-Gunn, J. and D. N. Ruble, 1983. The experience of menarche from a developmental perspective. In: J. Brooks-Gunn and A. C. Petersen (Eds.), *Girls at Puberty: Biological and Psychosocial Perspectives.* Plenum Press, New York, NY, pp. 155-177.

Brooks, J., D. N. Ruble, and A. Clarke, 1977. College women's attitudes and expectations concerning menstrual related changes. *Psychosomatic Medicine 39:* 288-298.

Caplow, T. and R. J. McGee, 1965. *The Academic Marketplace.* Doubleday and Co., Garden City, NY.

Cassell, J., 1982. Does risk-benefit analysis apply to moral evaluation of social research? In: T. L. Beauchamp, R. R. Faden, R. J. Wallace, Jr., and L. Walters (Eds.), *Ethical Issues in Social Science Research.* The Johns Hopkins University Press, Baltimore, MD, pp. 144-162.

Clarke, A. and D. N. Ruble, 1978. Young adolescents' beliefs concerning menstruation. *Child Development 49:* 201-234.

Crane, D., 1967. The gatekeepers of science: Some factors affecting the selection of articles for scientific journals. *The American Sociologist 2:* 195-201.

Crane, D., 1972. *Invisible Colleges: Diffusion of Knowledge in Scientific Communities.* The University of Chicago Press, Chicago, IL.

Curran, J., M. Gurevitch, and J. Wollacott (Eds.), 1979. *Mass Communication and Society.* Sage Publications, Beverly Hills, CA.

Curtis, J. E. and J. W. Petras (Eds.), 1970. *The Sociology of Knowledge: A Reader.* Praeger Publishers, New York, NY.

Dalton, K., 1982. Premenstrual tension: An overview. In: R. C. Friedman (Ed.), *Behavior and the Menstrual Cycle.* Marcel Dekker, New York, NY, pp. 217-242.

Dawood, M. Y., 1985. Overall approaches to the management of dysmenorrhea. In: M. Y. Dawood, J. L. McGuire, and L. M. Demers (Eds.), *Premenstrual Syndrome and Dysmenorrhea.* Urban and Schwarzenberg, Baltimore, MD, pp. 177-201.

Dexter, L. A. and D. M. White (Eds.), 1964. *People, Society, and Mass Communication.* The Free Press, New York, NY.

Dick, W. E., 1954. Science and the press. *Impact of Science on Society 5:* 143-173.

Enzensberger, H. M., 1974. *The Consciousness Industry.* Seabury Press, New York, NY.

Gans, H. J., 1979. *Deciding What's News: A Study of CBS Evening News, NBC Nightly News, Newsweek, and Time.* Pantheon, New York, NY.

Gitlin, T., 1983. *Inside Prime Time.* Pantheon, New York, NY.

Halbreich, U., J. Endicott, and J. Nee, 1983. Premenstrual depressive changes: Value of differentiation. *Archives of General Psychiatry 40:* 535-542.

Halbreich, U., J. Endicott, and S. Schacht, 1982. The diversity of premenstrual changes as reflected in the premenstrual assessment form. *Acta Psychiatrica Scandinavica 65:* 46-65.

Halmos, P. (Ed.), 1972. The sociology of science. *The Sociological Review Monograph,* No. 18.

Koeske, R. D. and G. F. Koeske, 1975. An attributional approach to moods and the menstrual cycle. *Journal of Personality and Social Psychology 31:* 473-478.

Laws, S., 1983. The sexual politics of pre-menstrual tension. *Women's Studies International Forum 6:* 19-31.

Mannheim, K., 1936. *Ideology and Utopia.* [Translated from German by L. Wirth and E. Shils.] Harcourt Brace and Co., New York, NY.

Mannheim, K., 1952. *Essays on the Sociology of Knowledge.* Edited by P. Kecskemeti. Routledge and Kegan Paul, London.

Merton, R. K., 1942. Science and technology in a democratic order. *Journal of Legal and Political Sociology 1:* 115-126. [Revised version reprinted in: R. K. Merton, 1968. *Social Theory and Social Structure* (revised and enlarged edition). The Free Press, New York, NY, pp. 604-615.

Merton, R. K., 1972. Insiders and outsiders: A chapter in the sociology of knowledge. *American Journal of Sociology 77:* 9-47.

Merton, R. K., 1973. *The Sociology of Science: Theoretical and Empirical Investigations.* The University of Chicago Press, Chicago, IL.

Paige, K. E., 1973. Women learn to sing the menstrual blues. *Psychology Today 7:* 41-46.

Parlee, M. B., 1973. The premenstrual syndrome. *Psychological Bulletin 80:* 454-465.

Parlee, M. B., 1974. Stereotypic beliefs about menstruation: A methodological note on the Moos Menstrual Distress Questionnaire and some new data. *Psychosomatic Medicine 36:* 229-240.

Parlee, M. B., 1981a. Appropriate control groups in feminist research. *Psychological Women's Quarterly 5:* 637-644.

Parlee, M. B., 1981b. Gaps in behavioral research on the menstrual cycle. In: P. Komnenich, M. McSweeney, J. A. Noack, and S. N. Elder (Eds.), *The Menstrual Cycle, Volume 2: Research and Implications for Women's Health.* Springer Publications, New York, NY, pp. 45-53.

Parlee, M. B., 1982a. New findings: Menstrual cycles and behavior. *Ms.* Magazine, October, pp. 126-128.

Parlee, M. B., 1982b. The psychology of the menstrual cycle: Biological and psychological perspectives. In: R. C. Friedman (Ed.), *Behavior and the Menstrual Cycle.* Marcel Dekker, New York, NY, pp. 77-100.

Parlee, M. B., 1982c. Changes in moods and activation levels during the menstrual cycle in experimentally naive subjects. *Psychological Women's Quarterly 7:* 119-131.

Rodin, J., 1976. Menstruation, reattribution, and competence. *Journal of Perspectives and Social Psychology 33:* 345-353.
Rubinow, D. R. and P. Roy-Byrne, 1984. Premenstrual syndromes: Overview from a methodologic perspective. *American Journal of Psychiatry 141:* 163-172.
Rubinow, D. R., P. Roy-Byrne, and M. C. Hoban, 1985. Menstrually related mood disorders: Methodological and conceptual issues. In: M. Y. Dawood, J. L. McGuire, and L. M. Demers (Eds.), *Premenstrual Syndrome and Dysmenorrhea.* Urban and Schwarzenberg, Baltimore, MD, pp. 27-40.
Ruble, D. N. and J. Brooks-Gunn, 1979. Menstrual symptoms: A social cognitive analysis of perception of symptoms. *Journal of Behavioral Medicine 2:* 171-194.
Scheff, T., 1974. The labeling theory of mental illness. *American Sociological Review 39:* 444-452.
Sigelman, L., 1973. Reporting the news: An organizational analysis. *American Journal of Sociology 79:* 132-151.
Steinem, G., 1978. If men could menstruate: A political fantasy. *Ms.* Magazine, October, p. 110.
Sudman, S., 1976. *Applied Sampling.* Academic Press, New York, NY.
Tuchman, G., 1972. Objectivity as strategic ritual: An examination of newsmen's notions of objectivity. *American Journal of Sociology 77:* 660-670.
Tuchman, G., 1978. *Making News.* The Free Press, New York, NY.
Waite, L. J., 1981. U.S. women at work. *Population Bulletin 37:* 3.
Walkowitz, J., 1980. *Prostitutes and Victorian Society: Women, Class, and the State.* Cambridge University Press, Cambridge, England.
White, D. M., 1950. The "gatekeeper:" A case study in the selection of news. *Journalism Quarterly 27:* 383-390.
Widholm, O., 1985. Epidemiology of premenstrual tension syndrome and primary dysmenorrhea. In: M. Y. Dawood, J. L. McGuire, and L. M. Demers (Eds.), *Premenstrual Syndrome and Dysmenorrhea.* Urban and Schwarzenberg, Baltimore, MD, pp. 3-12.
Ylikorkala, O. and M. Y. Dawood, 1978. New concepts in dysmenorrhea. *American Journal of Obstetrics and Gynecology 130:* 833-847.
Zuckerman, H. A. and R. K. Merton, 1971. Patterns of evaluation in science: Institutionalization, structure and functions of the referee system. *Minerva 9:* 66-100.

A VIEW FROM THE TOP OF A CONSUMER ORGANIZATION

Virginia Cassara, M.S.S.W.

PMS Action, Inc.
P.O. Box 16292
Irvine, California

INTRODUCTION

I spent 19 years seeking help for a complex symptoms I can now identify as "premenstrual syndrome" (PMS). From age 17 to age 36, I sought help from a variety of specialists for a variety of recurring symptoms: fatigue, joint pains, back pains, out-of-control eating binges (resulting in 20-pound weight swings every six weeks), and debilitating depressions, among them.

In spite of being a successful graduate student and teacher, having a special and supportive husband, family, and friends, the sharp division in my life and personality led me to feel not just out of control, but to doubt my sanity.

We are not taught to look at our biochemistry for the answers to our mood swings. (And, as is the case with most women with PMS, the emotional symptoms were the most distressing ones.) So, based on the false assumption that my depressions, in particular, were caused by externals in my life, I changed those "externals" often. Over the course of 19 years, I did a lot of impulsive things, including: dropping out of college, dropping out of graduate school, quitting a college teaching job, running off to Europe "to get my head together," and, perhaps most devastatingly, walking out on a husband who was *la crème de la crème* of husbands. The rationale was: "If I'm unhappy, uncomfortable, or depressed, then I must be doing something wrong." Being a person of action, I often reacted to my symptoms by significantly changing my life's situation. Usually with remarkably positive results — for a few weeks. Feeling better reinforced the "wisdom" of my impulsive behaviors. Now, I realize, I felt better because shortly after whatever change I impulsively made, I started menstruating. The new cycle brought relief, but the relief was always short-lived.

A year after I walked out of my marriage and 15 years after I began experiencing symptoms I never connected with "menstruation," I began keeping a journal. Over the course of two years, I chronicled my symptoms in black and white and coincidentally related them to my menstrual cycle. I then saw the tendency to ascribe them to outside events and, at the same time, the dramatic relief in both the emotional and physical symptoms the day I started menstruating.

It was 1975, I was 32 and still four years from "life on the other side of PMS." With meticulous records in tow, I spent a good part of 1975-1979 seeking help specifically for symptoms related to my menstrual cycle — symptoms which were getting worse with age. For two of the four years, I was a naive medical consumer. I suspected a hormonal disorder and was treated unsuccessfully with a variety of treatments, including tranquilizers, diuretics, and oral contraceptives. Antidepressants were also recommended, but using them didn't make sense to me since I wasn't consistently depressed. (Ironically, for years I had half-jokingly described myself as a "manic-depressive who had been cheated of her mania" and naively yearned for manic episodes to compensate for all the lost time, energy, and productivity resulting from the depressions.)

When, in 1977, one of the leading gynecological-endocrinologists in the country prescribed the oral contraceptive and said, with such certainty, that if it didn't cure me, "You do need a psychiatrist," I thought my help-seeking days were over. When his prescriptiion did not work, I went to the medical library to do my own research. There, I discovered "premenstrual syndrome" and the work of Dr. Katharina Dalton (see chapter by Dalton, this volume). Over the next two years, I went to a dozen physicians — a variety of specialists in several metropolitan areas and at several major university hospitals — specifically seeking progesterone therapy. I was open to other alternatives, but other than the repeated suggestion that I have my ovaries removed, none were proffered.

In 1979, aged 36 — no closer, apparently, to relief than I was 19 years earlier — I went to England to see Dr. Katharina Dalton, who diagnosed my complex of symptoms as premenstrual syndrome. Since 1979, I have been on progesterone therapy and close to asymptomatic. I was spared removal of the ovaries, major surgery which Dr. Dalton maintains is ineffective for PMS anyway.

During my four years of help-seeking for what I considered (but apparently few others saw as) debilitating symptoms, I concluded that there is no such thing as objectivity. We like to think that science is neutral, but the finding of "facts" is dependent upon which questions are asked, how the questions are posed, and what *a priori* expectations the researchers have. Thus, more important than "objectivity" is integrity. If we are honest about our subjective point of view, the reader or listener can evaluate the conclusions we present and, given an awareness of our perspective, decide what to accept or reject.

So I have shared my personal experience and acknowledge a point of view based not just on my struggles with PMS *and* getting help for PMS, but also on my experience as founder and Executive Director of PMS Action, Inc.

PMS ACTION, INC.

Prior to PMS Action, only an esoteric few had heard of premenstrual syndrome. Founded in March, 1980, PMS Action is a nonprofit corporation whose mission is to educate laypersons and professionals about PMS. We were, to my knowledge, the first source of help for women with PMS in the United States and, indeed, are responsible for the fact that PMS is now a household phrase. However, PMS is still not a widely understood concept.

PMS Action's basic premise is that PMS is a biochemical disorder. While we have never adhered to simple theories or answers about the syndrome, we are convinced that progesterone is involved. We thus contend that progesterone therapy ought to be a treatment option for American women — and not just those of us with the financial means to go to England.

Prior to the existence of PMS Action, *progesterone* therapy was not utilized for PMS, although *progestagen* therapy — contraindicated for PMS, according to Dr. Dalton — was used widely. It was not uncommon for women who complained of premenstrual symptoms to be put on the birth control pill (which contains progestagen) or, for that matter, for pure progestagen (such as Provera) to be prescribed. Today, *progesterone* therapy is administered by physicians in all 50 states — in large part thanks to PMS Action and to all the women and physicians who responded to PMS Action's message.

In the form of bibliographies, literature summations, audiotapes, and newsletters, PMS Action has provided information to 100,000 laypersons and 10,000 physicians and other health care professionals. Indirectly, via national television and newspaper coverage, we have reached literally millions.

From 1980-1983, we provided direct service (i.e., counseling) to over 2,000 women, often together with family members. The direct service program was an interim measure necessitated by the lack of recognition of PMS among laypersons and professionals and by the lack of effective treatment within the medical community.

Fortunately, the situation has changed, and today there are medical resources nationwide familiar with PMS and willing to treat it. We have, therefore, discontinued the counseling program and, instead, maintain a national listing of physicians who treat women with PMS. In order to receive referrals from PMS Action, a physician must include progesterone therapy as a treatment option, utilizing dosages corresponding to Dr. Katharina Dalton's protocol. Most physicians to whom we refer prescribe progesterone therapy only after other alternative treatments have proven ineffective.

Since 1982, PMS Action has conducted comprehensive training sessions in major cities across the United States which have been attended by thousands of health care professionals. The expansion of our training program resulted in a major move for the organization from Wisconsin to Irvine, California, in 1984.

THE MYTHS ABOUT PREMENSTRUAL SYNDROME

Given my personal (19 years) and professional (six years) experience with PMS, I would here like to outline and respond to the prevailing myths about PMS and women who experience PMS:

Myth #1: *Premenstrual symptoms result from negative conditioning about menstruation, femininity, and sexuality.* This misconception presupposes that a woman associates her symptoms with her menstrual cycle. In contrast to this presumption, we often find that women experience symptoms for years before they notice that they occur in a pattern related not to menstruation *per se*, but to their menstrual cycles. Working with others suffering from PMS, I discovered that taking 15 years — as I did — to associate recurring symptoms with one's menstrual cycle was not unusual.

The first myth rests on another inaccurate generalization about women: that so little of external importance happens in our lives that we have nothing better to do than pay attention to where we are in our menstrual cycle. Quite the contrary, most of us do not find the time to note, "Today is day 6 of my cycle; today is day 16, etc." Such a menstrual mantra is one upon which most women are *not* meditating.

Myth #2: *PMS is a convenient excuse.* I have never been sure for what it is supposed to be an excuse. The implication is that women with PMS are inherently neurotic hypochondriacs who, furthermore, wish to avoid carrying their share of the load. While granting that there may be some women who are hypochondriacs (just as some men are), my professional experience in working with women with PMS suggests the contrary. The majority of women bend over backwards to take responsibility for their actions. Women do not begin to attribute all the symptoms they experience to PMS. Too, when women actually record their symptoms, they are often surprised to discover that the duration of their symptoms is longer than they had verbalized initially.

Contrary to the notion that women with PMS do not want to "carry their load," women usually seek help only after years of carrying a heavy burden of guilt resulting from repeated out-of-control, impulsive, or acting-out behaviors. Outdated and overused theories about the origins of these symptoms — in which professionals themselves have often been steeped — only add to the guilt. The theories typically "blame the victim:" Women experience these symptoms because they do not accept their sexuality or femininity; because they are immature; or because they lack coping skills (see chapter by Blechman & Clay, this volume), to reiterate a few of the explanations. It is both enlightening and disquieting to note that just 15 years ago, the same theories were offered to explain spasmodic dysmenorrhea.

In sum, the overwhelming majority of women with PMS are not shirking responsibilities. They bend over backwards to assume responsibility for their actions and for their condition. Health care professionals would be more truly helping professionals if they understood that women seeking help for PMS rarely "tell the whole truth and nothing but the truth." PMS sufferers typically understate their symptoms out of guilt and in order to defend themselves against being inappropriately and counterproductively blamed for them.

Myth #3: *Premenstrual syndrome is not a serious disorder because it is self-limiting and because emotional symptoms are not serious symptoms.* True, PMS is "self-limiting" in that the symptoms do go away each month. But they also return, month after month, increasing their impact over time. As for the second point, how easy it is for those who do not experience depression or other mental pain to minimize "emotional" conditions! When evaluating the seriousness of an illness, people — including medical professionals — respond differently when they can see or touch the source of pain. An example of the tendency to dismiss emotional symptoms as inconsequential *vis-à-vis* physical ones is illustrated by a recent *McNeil-Leher Report.* The topic was whether the Food and Drug Administration (FDA) should approve the marketing of a potent injectable progestagen as a birth control product. A physician representing International Planned Parenthood favored its approval stating, "It's been used on millions internationally without serious side effects. In fact, the only side effects we've seen are weight gain and depression." Who says the depression the prestigious physician referred to is not a serious side effect? Probably not the women experiencing it. (Note I say "experiencing" — present tense — since extensive use of progestagens often precipitates PMS which continues after discontinuing the medication, acording to Dr. Dalton.)

Myth #4: *Women seeking help for PMS are looking for simple answers.* This myth is of recent vintage, and appears to have developed in response to the fact that women are no longer willing to suffer silently. On the contrary, our dissatisfaction stems from the purportedly simple answers dispensed to us in the past, answers that really were merely rejections: "If the oral contraceptive doesn't work, then you need a psychiatrist." Or, "If symptoms persist after a hysterectomy, they're 'all in your head.'" In fact, these simple answers are the most frustrating and least effective measures for treating women with PMS. A more honest answer brings a more positive response; e.g., "Much more is not known than is known about PMS." Or, "I don't know how to treat you, but I am willing to work with you." In general, women are not emotionally fragile beings who need protecting. We are capable of dealing with reality (see also chapter by Vergare, this volume).

Myth #5: *Women who report PMS symptoms are setting the women's movement back.* Perhaps, temporarily. There are those who will use the emerging public awareness of PMS to buoy their pre-existing prejudices. But sexism is no more rational than racism. Those who use the "new disease" PMS to judge women incapable of being pilots, paleontologists, or presidents would have said, five years ago, "Women can't hold responsible jobs because of their 'raging hormones.'" Awareness of PMS sheds some light on the stereotypes that are the precursors of prejudice.

Let me quote from *An Essay on Women:*

> She has two different sorts of mood.
> One day she is all smiles and happiness. . .
> There is no better wife. . . nor prettier.
> Then, another day, there'll be no living with her.
> You can't get within sight, or come near her, or
> She flies into a rage and holds you at a distance
> Like a bitch, with pups, cantankerous and cross
> With all the world. . . The sea is like that also.
> Often it will go wild and turbulent. . .
> This woman's disposition is just like the sea's
> Since the sea's temper also changes all the time.

These words were written by Semonides, a Greek poet, in the 6th century B.C. For thousands of years, mankind has been making generalizations about womankind. Like the sea. Hysterical. Irritable. Moody. Unpredictable. Unreliable. Undependable. Inconsistent. Irrational. There are those who, based on observations of some women, some of the time, say that this is the nature of women. It is not. The adjectives do describe, however, the nature of a woman with premenstrual syndrome. That PMS is in the limelight is a positive occurrence not just for the woman with symptoms and those close to her whose lives are directly affected. It is also a ray of hope for society. When PMS is recognized, researched, and treated, the stereotypes will diminish.

Myth #6: Finally, I would like to speak to the *myth of progesterone as placebo.* We do not know why progesterone apparently works for so many. Anecdotal evidence based on Dr. Katharina Dalton's work over the past 30 years in England, as well as anecdotal evidence from over 10,000 women on progesterone in this country, contradicts the placebo theory. Progesterone is not a panacea. It does not work for all women with PMS. But it works for many. For those for whom it is effective, there are factors suggesting its effectiveness is not merely as a placebo. First, most women on progesterone get better results with time. Second, if progesterone is a placebo, why were prior treatments not equally successful? In the United States, by the time progesterone is prescribed for a woman, she has usually tried many of the following treatments: the oral contraceptive, diuretics, anti-prostaglandins, vitamin B6, progestagens, tranquilizers, anti-depressants, and even hysterectomy. This leads to a third factor suggesting progesterone's value is unlikely to be that of a placebo. The placebo effect presupposes faith, a naive acceptance that an omniscient, omnipotent physician has *the* answer. Since progesterone therapy is a therapy of the last resort, by the time women get to progesterone, the prevailing emotion is fear. The thought, "This is my last hope. What if this doesn't work either?" is not very conducive to the placebo effect.

CONCLUSIONS

Just as women do not expect simple answers and just as progesterone is not viewed as a panacea, so we cannot look at PMS as simply a medical problem to the exclusion of a social and political one (see chapters by Bell and by Ericksen, this volume). That this conference was sponsored by the National Science Foundation is the result of a political movement. Five years ago, few lay persons in the United States had heard of PMS. Today, we are discussing whether the emerging public awareness is a positive or a negative occurrence.

Dalton has been consistently publishing on PMS for over 30 years. Until the existence of PMS Action, only a few specialists in this country paid any attention to her work, and most of these are illustrated in this volume. Progesterone was not a treatment option for American women. PMS Action's contribution to the movement has been, first, to encourage women to speak up about the extent and severity of their symptoms; and, second, to emphasize the importance of taking mutual responsibility for our health care. To the extent that we have done — and continue to do — that, women and health care professionals are the beneficiaries. It must be liberating, for instance, for a physician to know that he or she is not expected to have all the answers. On the other hand, as scientist-helping professionals, we do have a responsibility to look for some.

PSYCHOLOGICAL ISSUES

PREMENSTRUAL SYNDROME: IMPLICATIONS FOR PSYCHIATRIC PRACTICE

Michael J. Vergare, M.D.

Department of Psychiatry
Albert Einstein Medical Center
Northern Division
Philadelphia, Pennsylvania

Premenstrual syndrome (PMS) presents a unique challenge to medicine, and to psychiatry in particular. The work reported by the other authors of this volume highlights the diversity of approaches that have been used to understand this syndrome. This chapter will apply these ideas to the current practice of psychiatry.

A full understanding of the nature of this symptom complex must take into account physical, psychological, and sociological influences that have shaped the definition of the syndrome. Failure to do so has led to numerous faulty or incomplete definitions of this "illness," as has been noted by other contributors to the present volume (e.g., Dalton; Halbreich & Endicott; Reid; Rubinow; Sampson; and Steiner & Haskett). This has resulted in needless controversy and confusion for the medical profession and the lay public alike. Furthermore, partial formulations of the cause(s) of the syndrome have led to theories of treatment that frequently have not helped, and on occasion have even harmed, those women suffering from PMS. In many instances, they and their physicians may not be aware of the existence of the condition, or may relate it only to physical symptoms. It therefore becomes a matter of social and medical importance to provide the information necessary to confront this problem in a realistic manner.

Most definitions of PMS emphasize the cyclic occurrence of symptoms prior to the onset of menses, symptoms which are severe enough to interfere with routine functioning. The cessation of symptoms with, or shortly after, the onset of menses is used to differentiate PMS from the broader spectrum of menstrual-related disorders.

Symptoms such as swelling, weight gain, bloating, sleep changes (hypersomnia or insomnia), appetite shifts (appetite loss or food cravings), and pain (e.g., headache, breast tenderness, and musculo-skeletal pain) are often reported. Other symptoms include affective changes such as irritability, restlessness, and sadness, as well as shifts in impulse control, concentration, memory, and social distancing (see also chapters in this volume by O'Brien; and Steiner & Haskett). Some women have reported severe behavioral changes, including suicidal acts, assaultiveness, and substance abuse.

Whether some of these symptoms, particularly the behavioral ones, are primary to this syndrome or are derivative (resulting from discomfort arising from the core symptoms) remains controversial. In some cases, these symptoms may represent an exacerbation during the premenstrual period of other underlying conditions.

HISTORY

The work of Frank (1931) drew attention to the relationship of tension to the premenstrual phase. The focus on this behavioral variable characterized many of the early studies of PMS. More recent efforts have attempted to correlate biological changes with more general mood shifts. Rubinow and Roy-Byrne (1984) reviewed the development of research in this area, and they attribute some of the difficulties in cross-comparison of results to the frequent failure to attend to four important questions:

(1) What are the symptoms that are experienced?
(2) To what degree are the symptoms experienced?
(3) When do they occur in relationship to menstruation? and
(4) What is the symptomatic baseline on which symptoms fluctuate?

I would suggest that these same questions apply not only to research, but are the ones that a clinician must also use to effectively evaluate a woman suspected of having PMS. In order to help these women, it is necessary for the clinician to objectively elicit a description of her symptoms. The questions raised by Rubinow and Roy-Byrne (1984) assume that women are sensitive to fluctuations in day-to-day experience and that clinicians can elicit such a history. Formal efforts at refining this sensitivity have not always been included in the training of clinicians, but would seem to be necessary if these questions are to be addressed.

SOCIAL FACTORS

The emergence of the women's movement has helped to focus interest on the accurate identification of PMS. This reflects the dual concern that it should neither be overstated nor understated. Some feminists have suggested that part of the problem in understanding this syndrome stems from the alleged inability of men to evaluate, treat, or even discuss PMS. I feel that this is an overstatement of a point which nonetheless has merit. While there are limitations that must be confronted when evaluating a syndrome so loaded with myth and folklore that it is likely to color the clinician's approach (as well as that of the patient), these limitations exist for clinicians of either sex. Obviously, men do not have direct experience of PMS, and consequently could overlook the cyclic nature of menstrual changes as they evaluate and treat patients. After all, no similar variation is readily identifiable in men, leaving them somewhat at a loss when they attempt to understand the variation in daily experiences that the cycling of the menses *sometimes* brings. But men are, nevertheless, subject to the same affects and behaviors that characterize this syndrome in women (see also Ginsburg, this volume). Furthermore, it is not necessary to have experienced a condition in order to recognize and treat it. Where evaluation and treatment errors *are* made is in minimizing the effects of cyclical changes, not inquiring into this area, or not appreciating its possible impact on daily behavior. Conversely, overestimating the impact of the cycle can lead to stereotypes of female behavior loaded with negative biases. In the first instance, women who truly suffer with PMS are viewed as merely neurotic; in the second, all women are perceived as intermittently incapacitated or irresponsible.

As is true for the male, the female clinician is not immune from these social influences. Beliefs concerning character weakness, laziness, or female inferiority can also impinge on her evaluation. Men and women alike are mired in the same social milieu encumbered with unsubstantiated and variable beliefs about menstruation (see chapter by Ericksen), and, specifically, about PMS.

The fact that PMS is not an entity listed in standard diagnostic catalogues further complicates the problem of accurate identification. It is not found in the *International Classification of Diseases, 9th Revision* (ICD-9) or the *Diagnostic and Statistics Manual of Mental Disorders, Edition 3* (DSM-III), which are the resources utilized to provide diagnosis in the daily activities of mental health professionals. PMS is given some recognition in medical texts, but frequently it is merged and occasionally confused with the broader spectrum of menstrual-related disorders, such as dysmenorrhea. The same confusion is seen in patients' self-reports of their symptoms.

CURRENT VIEWS OF PREMENSTRUAL SYNDROME IN MEDICAL EDUCATION

Most of formal medical education relies on textbooks. This does not portend well for improved understanding of PMS by those using only medical texts. A review of these texts shows only a superficial presentation of PMS. Some texts even include stereotypes of female behavior and menstruation that have been carried over from Victorian times. The following is a brief review of the treatment this subject in some popular texts.

In the *Comprehensive Textbook of Psychiatry* (1967), Freedman and Kaplan mention the need to differentiate PMS from generalized premenstrual discomfort, using the extent of patient disability as an index. They note that 40% of all women suffer from menstrual disturbances of some kind. The symptoms listed are similar to those described earlier in this chapter and include both physical and psychological changes. The description also emphasizes the relationship to discomfort of anxiety, fear, and fantasies. The authors suggest a spectrum that ranges from those patients whose illness is primarily organic to those who are primarily reacting to the symbolic meaning of menstruation. For most patients, psychotherapy is said to be the treatment of choice, although this has certainly not been supported by research.

By the mid-1970's, we find references to Dalton's work appearing in some textbooks of psychiatry and gynecology. The primary focus is on treatment choice; e.g., progesterone, diuretics, etc. Also cited is the tendency for some women with PMS to be prone to accidents.

The 1980 text by Freedman and Kaplan includes a much broader presentation of what they describe as the premenstrual tension syndrome. They make reference to psychological, social, and biological factors. They also discuss the role of education and expectations in the development of symptoms. Observations of other women and their reaction to menstruation are noted as particularly influential in the development of PMS (see also Ruble & Brooks-Gunn, this volume). Recommendations for treatment are conservative, emphasizing symptomatic approaches.

Other texts (e.g., *New Sex Therapy*, Kaplan, 1974) focus more specifically on the need to externalize rage, and theorize that women suffering from PMS have excessive guilt and fear, which can lead to depression, physical illness, and withdrawal.

A more up-to-date presentation appears in the section on female endocrine disorders in the current edition of the *Comprehensive Textbook of Psychiatry* (Kaplan & Sadock, 1985). It reflects many of the views expressed throughout the present volume, albeit in an abbreviated way. Kaplan and Sadock emphasize that PMS encompasses a variety of physical, psychological, and behavioral symptoms, all of which start after ovulation, peak approximately five days before menstruation, and then rapidly decline. They further describe the period at mid-cycle as a time when there may be an enhanced feeling of well-being, and also suggest that the clinician look for a symptom-free time between menstruation and ovulation. The overview of statistics given in this reference draws attention to the fact that a high percentage (70-90%) of women of childbearing age report some symptoms premenstrually, but they further indicate that less than a third experience any disruption of their routine. Kaplan and Sadock (1985) conclude that the source of the disorder is unknown, but that possibilities range from psychological to hormonal factors, and that PMS may even constitute some variation of normal (see Macklin, this volume, for discussion of the meanings of "normal").

Recent research findings regarding PMS are beginning to find their way into medical textbooks. Nevertheless, for those interested in remaining truly current in their knowledge of this syndrome, critical and continuous review of the rapidly advancing research literature is a must.

ROLE OF THE PSYCHIATRIST

How does one apply current thinking and knowledge about PMS to clinical practice? The psychiatrist interested in helping those suffering from PMS must first recognize the need to achieve an understanding of the range and characteristics of menstrual cycle fluctuations. This is particularly important in relation to PMS, but is also applicable to the evaluation of all women. Although we may be attuned to cyclicity of symptoms associated with diseases such as manic-depressive illness, we are often less sensitive to the variations in affect experienced by a female patient in conjunction with her menstrual cycle. This becomes therapeutically relevant as these fluctuations color our assessment of treatment response. Consider the influence of undiagnosed PMS on the assessment of the efficacy of a tricyclic antidepressant, or any psychotropic medication. Shifts in mood, changes in ability to concentrate, and the presence of physical changes can be reactions to medications, but may also represent symptoms of PMS.

A psychodynamic therapeutic focus is no less influenced by the menstrual cycle. There are numerous writings in the psychiatric literature that deal with the symbolic meaning of menstruation. Negative anticipation and fear are often intensified premenstrually, particularly for those women with PMS. Menstrual concerns can influence self-image and lead to shame and guilt. Although these concerns do not generalize to all women, nor even to all women with PMS, a disservice is done if these concerns are overlooked in psychotherapy.

Since the etiology of PMS has not been established (and there may, in fact, be multiple etiologies), neither laboratory evaluation nor clinical examination will lead to definitive findings. What, then, should the clinician do, beyond the initial development of an empathic stance? Other conditions of metabolic, endocrinologic, and gynecologic origin can be confused with the symptom complex found in PMS, necessitating thorough investigation of these areas. Ideally, the assessment should include both gynecologic and psychiatric evaluation.

Besides physical problems which can obscure or masquerade as PMS, there are psychiatric illnesses that can complicate the evaluation. Research reports contain conflicting results about the association of psychiatric disease with PMS, particularly affective illness (see chapters by Halbreich & Endicott; Steiner & Haskett, this volume). To assist with this differentiation clinically, it is valuable to evaluate the patient both during the premenstruum when she expects to be symptomatic, and at an earlier point in her cycle, when she expects to be asymptomatic. (See chapter by Steiner & Haskett, this volume, for a similar approach in research evaluation.) Self-reports must be reviewed with caution since the evaluation itself may influence the data (see Ruble & Brooks-Gunn, this volume). A daily diary kept over a minimum of two cycles is often informative. Such a diary should include physical and mental symptoms, as well as making note of the events of the day.

It may be helpful to divide patients into three categories: (1) those that have true PMS; (2) those that have psychiatric illness complicated by PMS; and (3) those whose illness masquerades as PMS. One need only think of some of the characteristics of major psychiatric disorders to understand the problem confronting the clinician when establishing a diagnosis. Symptoms such as impulsivity, inappropriate anger, mood instability, and suicidal gestures are part of the diagnostic criteria for Borderline Personality Disorder; they are also symptoms reported by some women with PMS. Sleep disturbance, decreased interest in usual activities, and loss of energy can be associated with Major Depressive Disorder; likewise, these symptoms are found in PMS. Only by a careful review of history combined with direct examination can an appropriate diagnosis be reached.

TREATMENT — A PERSONAL PERSPECTIVE

Currently, no definitive treatments for PMS exist that have as yet withstood strict scientific scrutiny; yet the lay literature and advertising industry regularly report "cures." Symptomatic treatment is helpful for some women. Supportive interventions such as increasing awareness of how to "cope" with transient changes in personality and physical function are helpful for some, but are mistrusted by others who contend that this approach can be used to reinforce impressions of female inferiority. Other interventions include monitoring dietary excesses to avoid carbohydrate imbalance (i.e., sugar binges).

When a diagnosable psychiatric disorder is present, the appropriate pharmacologic treatment of this disorder sometimes alleviates some of the PMS symptoms as well. Such treatments must take into account that a worsening of symptoms during the premenstrual period does not signal failure of treatment for the psychiatric illness, but that symptoms may be intensified by the coexistence of PMS (see especially Steiner & Haskett, this volume). Some patients benefit from a temporary increase in medication five or six days prior to the expected onset of menstruation. Psychotherapy has also been found useful for some women, particularly if it takes into account cultural issues relevant to the patient's current milieu as well as psychodynamic issues that have a bearing on the individual's perception of self. Psychotherapy may also be effectively combined with medication.

When spouse, family, and friends reinforce negative expectations about menstruation, there is diminished opportunity for a symptom-free cycle. Interpersonally-derived negative expectations may reinforce a view of self already distorted intrapsychically by feelings of inferiority and a sense of being untouchable.

My own experience has confirmed the view that a supportive and educative treatment works best for the patient with classic PMS. The clinician must be "cycle sensitive" in order to remain relevant to the patient's experience from week to week. Even for those women who have a psychiatric disorder and who may not have classic PMS, an awareness of variations of behavior over the course of a menstrual cycle can be highly useful in therapy.

Those with severe PMS can learn to anticipate the premenstrual shifts of mood and behavior that can lead to maladaptive acts. It may be advisable for some to avoid highly stressful situations at this time of the cycle. Most women benefit from careful attention to diet and to health maintenance. Of course, this same advice has general merit for all of us. Surprisingly, a portion of those women reporting PMS overlook the benefits of this approach while experimenting with untested treatments.

The knowledge that a shift in emotional reactivity is more likely during the premenstrual phase can also prove effective in resolving interpersonal conflicts. It may be useful to engage other family members, particularly the spouse, in the treatment process in order to broaden this awareness. The danger here is that a multitude of behaviors might be wrongly ascribed to "that time of the month," thus bypassing the identification and resolution of problems that are independent of PMS. Psychotherapy can help in untangling this web by bringing into clearer focus those issues that are rooted in generalized intrapsychic or interpersonal conflict. In contrast, when the premenstrual period is the only time a couple experiences significant interpersonal friction, a preventive education approach might be the primary intervention.

Although attention has been focused on how disruptive, and even dangerous, premenstrual behavioral shifts can be for some PMS patients, it is very important to recognize that the opposite is sometimes true (see also Halbreich & Endicott, this volume). I have found that, for some women in psychotherapy, premenstrual mood changes actually liberate feelings that are so deeply suppressed at other points in their cycle as to be virtually inaccessible. Affective changes that initially might cause distress for the patient can be used to foster insight, if appropriately handled. For the woman who is highly restricted in her ability to be in touch with her impulses, the premenstrual period can be a period of heightened accessibility. What at first might be deprecated as labile affect can, for some, be a true expression of underlying suppressed emotion.

THE CHALLENGE OF PREMENSTRUAL SYNDROME

The implications that PMS holds for psychiatry are multifaceted. It challenges our ability to bring together a diverse group of social, physical, and psychological variables. Our approach must be individualized, and we must incorporate the assistance of other professionals to ensure accomplishment of a broad-based evaluation. Although some would argue that the clustering of symptoms described throughout this book does not constitute a diagnosis, it is clear that a subgroup of women experience personally significant suffering from this ailment. Even though no single treatment has been identified with proven consistent effectiveness, there are persuasive reports of some women benefiting from some of the current symptomatic approaches (detailed by others in this volume; e.g., Dalton; O'Brien; Reid; Steiner & Haskett).

In addition to the problems that PMS poses for the clinician, there are also the problems that the educator faces in training physicians. Teaching a multidisciplinary, bio-psycho-social approach is no easier than practicing this model. Educating medical students and residents about female development and health has typically been overshadowed by a focus on illness (see Bell, this volume, for further discussion of the biomedical model and its implications). Yet, to effectively evaluate for PMS, one must first develop a sense of the normal menstrual cycle shifts in both the physical and psychological realms. Hopefully, continued research in this area will help us with the twin problems of diagnosis and treatment.

REFERENCES

Frank, R. T., 1931. The hormonal causes of premenstrual tension. *Archives of Neurology and Psychiatry 26:* 1053-1057.

Freedman, A. M. and H. Kaplan, 1967. *Comprehensive Textbook of Psychiatry.* Williams and Wilkins, Baltimore, MD.

Freedman, A. M. and H. Kaplan, 1980. *Comprehensive Textbook of Psychiatry.* Williams and Wilkins, Baltimore, MD.

Kaplan, H., 1974. *New Sex Therapy.* Brunner-Mazel, Inc., New York, NY.

Kaplan, H. and B. Sadock, 1985. *Comprehensive Textbook of Psychiatry.* Williams and Wilkins, Baltimore, MD.

Rubinow, D. R. and P. Roy-Byrne, 1984. Premenstrual syndrome: Overview from a methodologic perspective. *American Journal of Psychiatry 141:* 163-172.

THE SCIENTIFIC METHOD AND ETHICAL TREATMENT OF PREMENSTRUAL COMPLAINTS

Elaine A. Blechman, Ph.D. and Connie J. Clay, M.S.

Albert Einstein College of Medicine/Montefiore Medical Center
Bronx, New York

INTRODUCTION

> "Dozens of clinics specializing in PMS have appeared throughout the country, some hospital-based but others independently operated. . . Many clinics 'are being merchandised like many of the fast-food chains' and 'frequently provide unproved or ineffective forms of therapy' for women who are desperate enough to try anything. Although a score of remedies for PMS have been tested with varying degrees of success, no one method has thus far emerged as the 'treatment of choice.' Nor have the underlying causes of the syndrome been clearly explained. There is even disagreement among physicians and psychologists as to how PMS should be defined. Indeed, judging from the highly variable symptoms and treatment successes and failures, it appears that PMS may be a multifaceted problem, with different causes in different women, each therefore requiring an individualized therapy."
>
> — J. E. Brody (1986, p. C-10)

Many women seek help for premenstrual complaints and many practitioners are eager to sell them services. The quality of the medical and psychiatric services they receive is questionable, reflecting inadequate scientific knowledge about premenstrual complaints and unjustified acceptance by practitioners of unverified assumptions about etiology and treatment. In the legal arena as well, decisions are made regarding women with premenstrual complaints that are simply not supported by credible, empirical evidence. Here again, the problem is twofold: Premenstrual complaints have only recently become the target of methodologically rigorous scientific inquiry (see chapters by Halbreich & Endicott, O'Brien, Reid, Rubinow, Sampson, and Steiner & Haskett, this volume); as a result, relevant knowledge is limited. In addition, the courts have accepted assumptions about premenstrual complaints, some of which are unverified and some of which are inconsistent with available, albeit scarce, empirical evidence.

Ethical and just treatment of women with premenstrual complaints requires, therefore, that this problem increasingly becomes the target of scientific inquiry and that the medical and legal professions adopt higher standards in their scrutiny of key assumptions.

This chapter begins with a description of what in our view are the properties of ethical and just treatment of premenstrual complaints. On the assumption that such treatment is hindered by a paucity of rigorous scientific inquiry into premenstrual complaints, the next sections of the chapter provide operational definitions of relevant terms and a theoretical guide for future inquiry. The closing sections of the chapter consider the implications of this model for assessment, treatment, and future research on premenstrual complaints.

PROPERTIES OF ETHICAL TREATMENT FOR PREMENSTRUAL COMPLAINTS

In our view, ethical treatment (medical, psychiatric, or psychological) of women with premenstrual complaints has the following properties:

1. A particular treatment modality (e.g., drug treatment) and components of that modality (e.g., prostaglandin inhibitors) are only offered when there is compelling evidence supporting the effectiveness of such treatment. Compelling evidence is substantial enough to have been published in a peer-reviewed journal of unimpeachable scientific repute.

2. Assessment of the individual patient's behavioral and biological excesses and deficits is always the first step in treatment, followed by design of an individualized course of treatment tailored to the patient's needs.

3. Baseline (pretreatment) assessment continues during and after treatment assessing short- and long-term effects on target problems (e.g., premenstrual irritability), adjunctive problems (e.g., arguments with family members), and competence. When assessment reveals deficits in the treatment's effects (e.g., an increase in arguments accompanying a decrease in self-reported irritability), treatment is altered to overcome these deficits (e.g., reducing arguments and irritability).

PROPERTIES OF JUST LEGAL DETERMINATIONS REGARDING PREMENSTRUAL COMPLAINTS

Just legal decisions reflect awareness of the following aspects of premenstrual complaints:

1. A substantial body of evidence contradicts the common belief that most women's behavior deteriorates during the premenstrual phase (Bäckström, Sanders, Leask, Davidson, Warner, & Bancroft, 1983; Englander-Golden & Barton, 1983; Parlee, 1982; Scambler & Scambler, 1985).

2. Evidence supporting the belief that the physiology of the premenstrual phase causes otherwise well-functioning women to become psychiatrically disabled or engage in antisocial behavior is extremely weak and derived from methodologically unsound research. Careful inspection of these studies suggests that the women in question evidence psychiatric disturbance or antisocial behavior throughout the month. The belief that deviant behavior can be attributed to the premenstrual phase is a product of studies relying on biased clinical samples and subjective and biased self-report and observer data.

3. There is limited and anecdotal evidence of premenstrual exacerbations in the behavior of women suffering from psychiatric or physical illness (Endicott, Halbreich, Schacht, & Nee, 1981; Halbreich

& Endicott, 1982; Halbreich, Endicott, & Nee, 1983). Although many people attribute such exacerbations to the physiology of the premenstrual phase, supporting evidence is sparse. In contrast, some evidence suggests that cultural expectations might account for these exacerbations (Bäckström et al., 1983; Clark & Ruble, 1978; Widholm, 1979).

4. Evidence supporting the existence of a distinctive, diagnostically useful premenstrual symptom cluster or syndrome is weak and flawed by an absence of operational definitions and objective measurement standards. Credible, albeit limited, evidence points to enormous variability in premenstrual complaints both between and among women. In contrast, existence of a syndrome would be supported by evidence of: common and consistently occurring symptoms, a common etiological pathway, or a common response to intervention. As we have already mentioned, none of these commonalities are supported by credible evidence.

Many writers in this volume feel that common usage of the term "syndrome," in combination with self-reported, cyclic irritability, warrants scientific adoption of the term "syndrome." We respectfully disagree, since evidence that cyclic irritability is confined to the premenstrual phase is not persuasive, and we believe that scientific practice should lead, not follow, popular beliefs. Therefore, in the remainder of this chapter we use the terms "premenstrual complaints" and "premenstrual distress" to refer to what others in this volume call "premenstrual syndrome."

5. Biological causes for premenstrual complaints have not been established. If a biological cause could be isolated, a rational treatment, based on remediation of such pathophysiology, could be instituted. To date, numerous biological explanations have been advanced, although not one has been consistently supported either by data descriptive of preexisting differences between groups of women with and without premenstrual complaints, or by data resulting from attempts to treat premenstrual complaints through alteration of a relevant biological process.

6. Psychological causes for premenstrual complaints have not been established. Speculation about an intrapsychic psychological mechanism responsible for premenstrual complaints has centered on women's conflicts about their sexuality and their rejection of socially prescribed feminine role obligations. These hypotheses have often been formulated in a manner defying empirical test and rarely have they been subjected to rigorous inquiry. Even so, evidence supporting a psychodynamic process underlying premenstrual complaints has not emerged. Later, we describe a conditioning hypothesis pertaining to the development of premenstrual complaints which requires substantial empirical verification.

7. Premenstrual complaints are a "political football" in feuds among medical, psychiatric, and behavioral science professionals and between professionals and feminists. As a result, statements of presumed experts are more often based on political considerations than on unassailable and objective evidence.

OPERATIONAL DEFINITIONS OF RELEVANT TERMS

Poorly defined terms have been the rule rather than the exception where premenstrual complaints are concerned. Before premenstrual complaints can be subjected to rigorous scientific inquiry, relevant terms require operational definitions. We use the following terms and definitions, in accord with the recommendations of The Society for Menstrual Cycle Research (SMCR, 1986).

The menstrual phases are: menses, ovulatory, postovulatory, premenstrual, postmenses, and perimenstrual. The key reference point, menses, is synonymous with bleeding; it includes all days when blood flow occurs and is of variable length. Bleeding is a continuous flow of visible blood, as opposed to spotting, intermittent times when blood is visible. The ovulatory phase estimates the time of ovulation by including the 14th day prior to onset of menses, plus and minus 2 days. The postovulatory phase includes the days from the end of the ovulatory phase to the beginning of the premenstrual phase. The premenstrual phase includes the seven days before menses. The postmenses phase includes the time from the end of menses to the beginning of the ovulatory phase. Perimenstrual refers to a combination of premenstrual and menstrual phases. The term midcycle is rejected as too vague. The terms follicular and luteal are reserved for phase designations based on direct biological measures of follicular and corpus luteal function.

Perimenstrual complaints can be defined as descriptions of unpleasant physical and behavioral experiences in the premenstrual phase and during menses.

Menstrual complaints, usually of abdominal cramps, are traditionally called dysmenorrhea. Cramps may be accompanied by nausea, vomiting, diarrhea, headache, fatigue, nervousness, or dizziness. Physical exam, age, and menstrual history are used to distinguish between primary dysmenorrhea (no known organic cause) and secondary dysmenorrhea (a known organic cause such as endometriosis) (Coppen & Kessel, 1963).

The unpleasant behavioral and physical experiences a woman describes in the premenstrual phase can be defined as premenstrual complaints (PMCo). The nature, number, and severity of PMCo may vary greatly from one woman to the next, perhaps as much as the length of their menstrual cycles. These complaints include physical and behavioral changes which interfere with daily activities and disrupt interpersonal relationships (Reid, 1985). Frequently reported physical complaints include headache, backache, bloating, edema, abdominal discomfort and pain, breast tenderness, acne, intestinal distress such as constipation and diarrhea, and exacerbation of chronic illness such as asthma and epilepsy. The behavioral complaints may be excesses or deficits relative to typical performance and include: increased tension, irritability, aggressiveness, overuse of analgesic or sedative medication and alcohol, decreased energy, and disrupted patterns of eating, sleeping, sex, interpersonal relationships, and work. Tension or irritability appears to be the only universal premenstrual complaint (Hoes, 1980; Reid & Yen, 1981; Widholm, 1979; Wood, Larsen, & Williams, 1979).

When, for three months in a row a woman reports severe, uniform PMCo that abate during the postmenstruum, she suffers from premenstrual distress.

Two popular terms are unnecessary: premenstrual symptom and premenstrual syndrome. The term premenstrual symptom implies existence of covert pathophysiology. To date, however, evidence does not support an underlying cause of PMCo. The term premenstrual syndrome connotes a group of signs and symptoms that occur together and characterize a particular abnormality, such as an illness or disease. Yet, PMCo is extraordinarily heterogeneous, making use of the term syndrome quite inappropriate. Premenstrual distress is a better label for consistently recurring PMCo.

The term premenstrual dysphoric disorder is also unnecessary, even though it is likely to be included in the main section or as an appendix of DSM-IIIR (*The Diagnostic Statistical Manual*, American Psychiatric Association, in press) (The Society for Menstrual Cycle Research, 1986). Many clinicians feel the need for such a diagnostic category so that patients who seek treatment for PMCo can receive reimbursement. In the absence of evidence that some women suffer from premenstrual dysphoria unaccompanied by mood disorder during the rest of the month or by other psychiatric symptomatology, we recommend that when a diagnosis is required, clinicians rely upon available diagnostic categories for this purpose.

EPIDEMIOLOGY OF COMPLAINTS

Most women report physical and behavioral changes over the course of the menstrual cycle. Epidemiological surveys have varied in their definition of terms and their measurement methods. As a result, it is hard to determine how many women in the general population are truly disabled by PMCo. Judging by frequently cited studies, the prevalence of all levels of severity of PMCo varies from 70% to 90% of adult women (Hoes, 1980; Reid & Yen, 1981; Widholm, 1979; Wood et al., 1979). Perhaps 50% of women present mild complaints, 30 to 40% present moderate complaints, and 5 to 10% present severe, disabling complaints (Coppen & Kessel, 1963; Janiger, Riffenburgh, & Kersh, 1972; Wood, Most, & Dery, 1982). We can only guess that the latter group of women suffer from premenstrual distress as we defined it earlier. Dysmenorrhea is diagnosed in 30 to 50% of postpubescent females, approximately 10% of whom are disabled for one to three days a month (Bergsjo, Jenssen, & Vellar, 1975; Kistner, 1971; Svennerund, 1959).

RELATIONSHIP BETWEEN MENSTRUAL AND PREMENSTRUAL COMPLAINTS

The relationship between premenstrual and menstrual complaints is not firmly established. Some clinicians and researchers maintain that premenstrual and menstrual complaints are unrelated (Dalton, 1969; Chesney & Tasto, 1975a, 1975b). Yet, a growing body of evidence suggests the contrary. Although there are great differences in their perimenstrual complaints, women seem to report similar complaints in their premenstrual and menstrual phases, with the exception of uterine cramps which are restricted to the menstrual phase (Coppen & Kessel, 1963; Cox, 1977; Halbreich & Endicott, 1985; Moos, 1968; Most, Woods, Dery, & Most, 1981; Taylor, 1979).

A THEORETICAL GUIDE FOR INQUIRY

Haphazard and unproductive research on premenstrual complaints has been the rule rather than the exception. One way to escape this state of affairs and to elevate relevant scientific inquiry is by relying on a fundamental, testable theoretical model, which can be either proved or disproved, to guide inquiry. Elsewhere, Blechman and colleagues (Blechman, Clay, Kipke, & Bickel, in press) have proposed such a model and called it the danger-signal hypothesis of premenstrual complaints.

The Danger-Signal Hypothesis

Perhaps premenstrual complaints are the product of avoidance conditioning. Avoidance conditioning could begin with a woman who, at about the time bleeding should begin, searches for any physical or behavioral precursor to bleeding. Because of her hypervigilance, such a woman's premenstrual mood might seem very irritable. Premenstrual irritability is, of course, the only premenstrual complaint common to all women who request help with such complaints.

All women are aware of normal bodily and behavioral changes right before menstruation begins. These changes are slight and neutral. For a hypervigilant woman, however, these changes would function as early warning signals of the onset of bleeding. Constant attention to these changes could amplify them in frequency and intensity until they become premenstrual complaints. Which premenstrual complaints capture her attention would be determined by her physiology, culture, and individual history of reinforcement. This would account for the great differences in premenstrual complaints among women requesting help for such complaints (see chapter by Cassara, this volume, for a different view).

The hypervigilant woman's search for information about the onset of bleeding allows her to begin engaging in avoidant routines before bleeding and even before premenstrual complaints begin (e.g., staying home from work). When these avoidant routines lead to massive negative reinforcement unrelated to menses (e.g., relief from responsibilities at work), generalization of hypervigilance, premenstrual complaints, and avoidant routines to the entire month is likely. It may be for this reason that women with "pure" premenstrual complaints which occur only during the premenstrual phase are very hard to find.

Two groups of women are likely to be hypervigilant prior to menses. The organic PMCo group includes women with excessive uterine prostaglandins and menstrual cramps. For these women, hypervigilance allows them to prevent menstrual cramps from causing too much disruption in their lives. The behavioral PMCo group includes women with exceptionally adverse attitudes toward menstruation; these women, who may or may not suffer from menstrual cramps, find bleeding and other natural bodily functions distasteful. For these women, hypervigilance allows them to prevent bleeding from causing too much disruption in their lives. Cultures in which menstruating women are segregated would be likely to promote behavioral PMCo.

Origin of the Danger-Signal Hypothesis

Seligman's safety-signal hypothesis (1968), which applies to escape and avoidance learning, proposes that an aversive event such as electric shock accompanied by a signal will be preferred over an unsignalled aversive event. According to Seligman, the signalled aversive event provides useful information by reducing uncertainty about the onset of punishment. Once a signal is associated with reward or punishment, it can promote vigilance — a constant search for the beginning of the signal. Humans describe the state of vigilance as anxious anticipation, tension, or stress. When vigilance was defined as choosing to listen for a cue signalling shock over listening to recorded music (Averill & Rosen, 1972; Miller, 1979), vigilance increased along with shock intensity, particularly when the shock could be avoided. Even when shock could not be avoided, subjects preferred to listen for the signal over listening to music (Miller, 1979).

The safety-signal hypothesis is a parsimonious explanation for the irrational anxiety and maladaptive coping behavior common to many forms of psychopathology. Signalled punishment promotes the emergence of vigilance and avoidant, coping behavior. Occasional moderation of the signal or of the punishment strengthens vigilance and avoidance via reinforcement and promotes generalization of these habits to other signals and other punishments. As a result, these habits persist even when circumstances change. The original signal may disappear or provide less useful information, the original punishment may disappear or moderate, yet vigilance and avoidance endure.

For those women with organic PMCo who experience painful uterine cramps on the first two days of menstruation, their cramps function, like shock, as a punishment. For those women with behavioral PMCo (with or without cramps) who have adverse attitudes toward menstruation, their bleeding functions, like shock, as a punishment. For both groups, the beginning of menstrual discomfort and bleeding signals the end of safety and the proximity of punishment or negative events.

Both groups of women are inclined to premenstrual vigilance, a constant search during the premenstrual days for any indication that bleeding and cramps are about to begin. Premenstrual vigilance, the primary premenstrual complaint, focuses the woman's attention on minor, benign physical and behavioral changes. Over time, due to vigilance, these changes become pronounced and aversive, resulting in various secondary, premenstrual complaints (e.g., headaches, backaches, and intestinal disturbance) and avoidant habits, such as inactivity, sleep, excessive and inappropriate eating, drinking, and drug-taking.

Empirical support for the danger-signal hypothesis would require convincing evidence that PMCo never develop in the absence of painful menstrual cramps or adverse attitudes toward menstruation, that PMCo always develop after the emergence of cramps or adverse attitudes toward menstrual function, and that premenstrual vigilance or irritability is always the first premenstrual complaint to emerge.

Thus far, two groups of women with premenstrual complaints have been described, one with an organic basis to their complaints, and the second with a behavioral basis to their complaints. The danger-signal hypothesis implies the presence of two additional groups. One "healthy" group experiences no menstrual pain and has no adverse attitudes toward menstruation; as a result, they evidence no premenstrual hypervigilance and acquire no premenstrual complaints. A second "stoic" group experiences menstrual pain unaccompanied by adverse attitudes toward menstruation; these women ignore or minimize their pain and as a result, they evidence little or no premenstrual hypervigilance and acquire few premenstrual complaints. Investigation of the danger-signal hypothesis must include inquiry into the distribution in the normal population of the four groups of women we have described. The skill repertoires of the stoic group are a particularly important target for future investigators, since the aim of intervention with women who suffer from premenstrual complaints might well be to help these women behave like their more stoic peers.

IMPLICATIONS OF THE DANGER-SIGNAL HYPOTHESIS FOR CLINICAL RESEARCH

Ethical treatment of women with premenstrual complaints and just legal determinations are most likely to result when guiding assumptions derive from scientific inquiry of the highest quality. The danger-signal hypothesis has implications both for future scientific inquiry and for clinical practice. In fact, science and clinical practice must be combined where premenstrual complaints are concerned. This is because so little is known about premenstrual complaints, that ethical treatment of women with these complaints should, in our opinion, be conducted as clinical research. Implications of the danger-signal hypothesis for clinical research follow.

The Measurement of Premenstrual Complaints

The danger-signal hypothesis suggests the following measurement procedures. These apply to basic and applied research and to clinical practice.

(1) There is likely to be a discrepancy between women's self-reported complaints and objective measures of these complaints (Parlee, 1974; Ruble, 1977), particularly among women with adverse attitudes toward menstruation. As a result, multiple subjective and objective measures of PMCo are necessary (Abplanalp, Donnelly, & Rose, 1979; McCance, Luff, & Widdowson, 1937; Parlee, 1982; Silbergeld, Brost, & Nobel, 1971; Vila & Beech, 1980).

(2) Premenstrual physical and behavioral complaints may have important precursors (e.g., vigilance) and important consequences (e.g., avoidant habits). Therefore, measurement should target multiple parameters, including: menstrual cramps, attitudes toward menstruation, bleeding, premenstrual vigilance, secondary premenstrual complaints, and avoidant habits.

(3) Menstrual cramps may be a critical parameter in the acquisition of premenstrual complaints. Nevertheless, women's self-reports of cramps may be biased; some women may minimize their severity, while others may exaggerate their severity. Therefore, measurement should involve objective quantification of cramps. The presence of prostaglandins (PGs) of the E and F series in the menstrual blood is a reliable indicator of uterine cramps in primary dysmenorrhea. The level of these PGs in menstrual blood can be estimated from tampons (Chan & Dawood, 1980; Chan & Hill, 1978; Janbu, Lokken, & Nesheim, 1979; Michael, Bonsall, & Kutner, 1975).

(4) There are likely to be many individual differences in the etiology of premenstrual complaints, even within the four groups we have described. These individual differences might manifest themselves in phase-dependent patterns of premenstrual complaints and avoidant habits. Therefore, measures of PMCo should be collected repeatedly from individual women throughout the month. Individual patterns over time should be inspected before summing an individual's scores or grouping the scores of several individuals.

(5) When data are gathered only from women with PMCo, important information is likely to be overlooked. For example, there may well be a group of stoic women who experience severe menstrual pain but nonetheless do not acquire premenstrual complaints. The aim of treatment for women who suffer from premenstrual complaints should be, in our view, to help them function like stoic women. To promote such socially valid treatment, it is important to collect information on all measures, not only from women who seek treatment for PMCo, but also from a representative sample of menstruating women in the general population.

(6) Premenstrual complaints are most severe when they interfere with a woman's competence; that is, her relative success compared to peers at interpersonal and academic/occupational tasks (Blechman, 1984). The acquisition of avoidant habits and their generalization to month-long functioning would appear to jeopardize women's competence. It remains to be established, of course, how many women in the general population

are debilitated by premenstrual complaints, and how much conditioning contributes to the emergence of premenstrual complaints. In the meantime, routine and repeated measurement of competence seems important. Such measurement would, at the very least, encourage clinicians to make improved competence a goal of intervention with women who suffer from premenstrual complaints.

The Treatment of Premenstrual Complaints

The danger-signal hypothesis suggests the following treatment procedures:

(1) *Involvement of the patient in treatment monitoring, planning, and implementation.* Too little is known about the origin of premenstrual complaints and their effective treatment for any clinician to occupy the expert role with women who suffer from these complaints. In our view, at this stage, only clinical researchers should be involved in treatment of premenstrual complaints. Women who suffer from these complaints should be treated as partners in the treatment enterprise. All available information about the problem should be shared with them prior to treatment so that they can make an informed decision about participation. They should be relied upon to gather data; and their self-reported data, even though they may vary from objective data, should be taken seriously. After all, premenstrual complaints are only known about through self-report. No treatment which fails to alter this self-report, even though it alters a woman's status on objective measures, is of much use. As data are collected, they should be shared with the woman, and she should be involved in the planning of subsequent treatment.

Some women, it is true, will take a passive role in this process, finding it both alien and uncomfortable. Some women may even prefer a more authoritarian approach to treatment. We see selective participation in clinical research on premenstrual complaints as good for women and good for treatment development. When a treatment has been found to be highly effective for a self-selected group of premenstrual sufferers, it will be appropriate to encourage widespread adoption of this treatment.

(2) *Continuous measurement of treatment results.* Since effective treatments for premenstrual complaints have not been established, continuous evaluation following the guidelines for measurement presented above seems a mandatory treatment component. Data should be used to estimate the impact of treatment components (e.g., relaxation training) on component targets (e.g., anxiety) and on adjunctive behaviors (e.g., arguments with spouse). When treatment components fail to bring about the desired impact on targets or bring mixed results (less anxiety, more arguments), a revised treatment component should be introduced. When a treatment component is demonstrably effective, a component with a new target can be introduced. Data should also be used to estimate when treatment has achieved its desired short-term effects and when follow-up has achieved its desired goals for long-term maintenance and generalization. Demonstration that a woman has reached criterion in response to a particular treatment component is as important in research employing group comparisons as it is in research employing single-case experimental designs (Barlow, Hayes, & Nelson, 1984).

(3) *Individualized treatment.* There are two routes through which PMCo may be acquired (behavioral, organic). Although premenstrual vigilance (irritability) is common to most women with PMCo, there are enormous differences among women with respect to the types of secondary premenstrual complaints and avoidant habits they acquire. As a result,

effective treatment must begin with an assessment of the individual woman's behavioral deficit and excess, followed by design of a relevant, tailor-made treatment plan.

(4) *Multiple treatment goals.* Premenstrual complaints and avoidant habits, once established, are likely to quickly proliferate, interfering with numerous skill repertoires. As a result, most women with premenstrual complaints will benefit from a treatment that has multiple goals. Pretreatment assessment data should be used to determine deficiencies on the following parameters and to plan treatment accordingly: attitudes toward menstruation, premenstrual vigilance, premenstrual complaints, avoidant behavior, and competence (Fordyce, Roberts, & Sternback, 1985). Elsewhere (Blechman et al., in press), we have reviewed behavioral treatment components relevant to premenstrual complaints.

(5) *Improved functioning throughout the month.* Premenstrual complaints and avoidant habits, once established, are likely to generalize until they occur throughout the month. As a result, most women with premenstrual complaints will benefit from a treatment that aims for improved functioning throughout the month (for an alternate view, see chapter by Dalton, this volume).

(6) *Engineering the social environment.* Premenstrual complaints are likely to impede interpersonal competence by setting in motion a pernicious, coercive (Patterson & Reid, 1984) spiral of discomfort, depression, anger, and demands for help, met by withdrawal and anger by family and friends. The product of the spiral may be chronic depression (Biglan, Hops, Sherman, Friedman, Arthur, & Osteen, 1985). Pretreatment assessment should be designed to detect environmental influences on premenstrual complaints. The treatment plan should be designed either to directly alter these influences (e.g., by instructing family members to ignore premenstrual temper tantrums) or to teach skills that will alter the environment (e.g., teaching the woman to reduce her premenstrual requests for help and sympathy). When skill training is adopted, it is important to assess whether the woman acquires the skills she has been taught and whether the skills have the desired impact on the environment. Simply teaching a woman to reduce her premenstrual requests for help is not enough. A demonstration that reduced requests for help leads to reduced attention to premenstrual complaints is also necessary.

(7) *Combination of behavioral and biological treatment components.* Women with organic PMCo may acquire their premenstrual complaints in response to painful menstrual cramps. Once these complaints have been established, elimination of the cramps via drug treatment would be insufficient. However, combination of a drug treatment component targeting cramps and a behavioral treatment component targeting premenstrual vigilance, secondary premenstrual complaints, and avoidant behavior might constitute an effective treatment for some women. Antiprostaglandin drugs which have been demonstrated to be an effective method of reducing menstrual cramps (Chan, 1983; Chan, Dawood, & Fuchs, 1979, 1981; Chan, Fuchs, & Powell, 1983; Chan & Hill, 1978; Csapo, 1980; Dawood, 1981; Halbert & Demers, 1978; Halbert, Demers, & Jones, 1976; Shangold, Aksel, Schomberg, & Hammond, 1976; Ylikorkala & Dawood, 1978) would seem to be an ideal candidate for the biological component of such a biobehavioral treatment and should be considered when pretreatment assessment data indicate persisting, severe menstrual cramps.

PREMENSTRUAL COMPLAINTS: A WINDOW ON BEHAVIORAL MEDICINE FOR WOMEN

We began this chapter with a description of the many women who seek help for premenstrual complaints and the numerous clinicians willing to provide help. Unfortunately, the treatments so willingly provided have, in some cases, already been found to be ineffective or harmful, and in other cases have never been evaluated. We consider this approach to treatment to be highly unethical. With respect to premenstrual complaints, we contend that unethical treatment of women by medical and mental health professionals and unjust legal determinations continue because premenstrual complaints have not been sufficiently subjected to rigorous scientific inquiry. As a result, important decisions are often based on implausible, untested, untestable, and false assumptions.

In our opinion, application of the scientific method to premenstrual complaints is the best way to achieve ethical and fair treatment of women who suffer from these complaints. Toward this end, we presented relevant operational definitions and a conditioning hypothesis which we believe is a useful guide to scientific inquiry. Since so little data exist about the etiology or treatment of premenstrual complaints, we believe that all treatment of women with this problem should be conducted as clinical research. Accordingly, we considered the implications of the danger-signal hypothesis for assessment and treatment conducted in the spirit of clinical research.

In sum, our recommendations about inquiry into premenstrual complaints are integral to our view of the broader fields of behavior therapy and behavioral medicine for women (Blechman, 1984; Blechman & Brownell, in press-a). Premenstrual complaints provide a window on the development of behavioral and physical vulnerability in women (Blechman & Brownell, in press-b). The danger-signal hypothesis is a primitive, albeit testable, theory about how physiology, behavior, and the environment conspire to trap formerly competent, hardy girls into incompetence and physical vulnerability during adolescence (see also chapter by Ruble & Brooks-Gunn, this volume).

How do young women overcome biological changes and cultural constraints, remaining physically hardy despite problems which would otherwise promote ill health and interfere with achievement and interpersonal competence? We believe that through problem-solving, women find ways to remain relatively free from physical illness, to recover relatively quickly from physical injury and stress, and to cope relatively well with chronic illness compared to their peers (Blechman & Brownell, in press-b).

We strongly suspect that the young women who are most vulnerable to the conditioning of premenstrual complaints are those who lack accurate information about their bodies, who are relatively incompetent in interpersonal and academic domains, and whose surroundings (family, school, health care system, peer group) obstruct risk-taking and refinement of problem-solving skills. Prevention and intervention efforts aimed at improving the physical hardiness of these high-risk young women are most likely to succeed if they convey a rich mixture of information, skills, and environmental engineering.

REFERENCES

Abplanalp, J. M., A. F. Donnelly, and L. M. Rose, 1979. Psychoendocrinology of the menstrual cycle: I. Enjoyment of daily activities and moods. *Psychosomatic Medicine 41:* 587-604.

American Psychiatric Association, in press. *Diagnostic and Statistical Manual of Mental Disorders* (revised edition). Washington, D.C.

Averill, J. and M. Rosen, 1972. Vigilant and nonvigilant coping strategies and psychophysiological stress reactions during the anticipation of electric shock. *Journal of Personality and Social Psychology 23:* 128-141.

Bäckström, T., D. Sanders, R. Leask, D. Davidson, P. Warner, and J. Bancroft, 1983. Mood, sexuality, hormones, and the menstrual cycle. II. Hormone levels and their relationship to the premenstrual syndrome. *Psychosomatic Medicine 45:* 503-507.

Barlow, D. H., S. C. Hayes, and R. O. Nelson, 1984. *The Scientist Practitioner: Research and Accountability in Clinical and Educational Settings.* Pergamon Press, New York, NY.

Bergsjo, P., H. Jenssen, and O. D. Vellar, 1975. Dysmenorrhea in industrial workers. *Acta Obstetrica et Gynecologica Scandinavica 54:* 255-259.

Biglan, A., H. Hops, L. Sherman, L. F. Friedman, J. Arthur, and V. Osteen, 1985. Problem solving interactions of depressed women and their husbands. *Behavior Therapy 16:* 431-451.

Blechman, E. A., 1984. Women's behavior in a man's world: Sex differences in competence. In: E. A. Blechman (Ed.), *Behavior Modification with Women.* Guilford Press, New York, NY.

Blechman, E. A. and K. B. Brownell (Eds.), in press-a. *Behavior Medicine with Women.* Pergamon Press, New York, NY.

Blechman, E. A. and K. B. Brownell, in press-b. Competence and physical hardiness. In: E. A. Blechman and K. B. Brownell (Eds.), *Behavior Medicine with Women.* Pergamon Press, New York, NY.

Blechman, E. A., C. J. Clay, M. D. Kipke, and W. B. Bickel, in press. Premenstrual complaints. In: E. A. Blechman and K. B. Brownell (Eds.), *Behavior Medicine with Women.* Pergamon Press, New York.

Brody, J. E., 1986. Treatment techniques vary for premenstrual syndrome. *The New York Times*, April 16, p. C-10.

Chan, W. Y., 1983. Prostaglandins and nonsteroidal antiinflammatory drugs in dysmenorrhea. *Annual Review of Pharmacological Toxicology 23:* 131-149.

Chan, W. Y. and M. Y. Dawood, 1980. Prostaglandin levels in menstrual fluid of nondysmenorrheic and of dysmenorrheic subjects with and without oral contraceptive or ibuprofen therapy. In: B. Samuelsson, P. W. Ramwell, and R. Paoletti (Eds.), *Advances in Prostaglandin and Thromboxane Research, Vol. 8.* Raven Press, New York, NY.

Chan, W. Y., M. Y. Dawood, and F. Fuchs, 1979. Relief of dysmenorrhea with the prostaglandin synthetase inhibitor ibuprofen: Effect on prostaglandin levels in menstrual fluid. *American Journal of Obstetrics and Gynecology 135:* 102-108.

Chan, W. Y., M. Y. Dawood, and F. Fuchs, 1981. Prostaglandins in primary dysmenorrhea. *American Journal of Medicine 70:* 535–540.

Chan, W. Y., F. Fuchs, and A. M. Powell, 1983. Effects of naproxen sodium on menstrual prostaglandins and primary dysmenorrhea. *Journal of Obstetrics and Gynecology 61:* 285-291.

Chan, W. Y. and J. C. Hill, 1978. Determination of menstrual prostaglandin levels in nondysmenorrheic and dysmenorrheic subjects. *Prostaglandins 15:* 365-375.

Chesney, M. A. and D. L. Tasto, 1975a. The development of the menstrual symptom questionnaire. *Behavior Research and Therapy 13:* 237-244.

Chesney, M. A. and D. L. Tasto, 1975b. The effectiveness of behavior modification with spasmodic and congestive dysmenorrhea. *Behavior Research and Therapy 13:* 245-253.
Clark, A. and D. N. Ruble, 1978. Young adolescents' beliefs concerning menstruation. *Child Development 49:* 231-234.
Coppen, W. R. and N. Kessel, 1963. Menstruation and personality. *British Journal of Psychiatry 109:* 711-721.
Cox, D. J., 1977. Menstrual symptom questionnaire: Further psychometric evaluation. *Behavior Research and Therapy 15:* 506-508.
Cox, D. J. and R. G. Meyer, 1978. Behavioral treatment parameters with primary dysmenorrhea. *Journal of Behavioral Medicine 1:* 297-309.
Csapo, A. I., 1980. A rationale for the treatment of dysmenorrhea. *Journal of Reproductive Medicine 25:* 213-221.
Dalton, K., 1969. *The Menstrual Cycle.* Pantheon Books, New York, NY.
Dawood, M. Y., 1981. Dysmenorrhea and prostaglandins: Pharmacological and therapeutic considerations. *Drugs 22:* 42-56.
Endicott, J., U. Halbreich, S. Schacht, and J. Nee, 1981. Premenstrual changes and affective disorders. *Psychosomatic Medicine 43:* 519-529.
Englander-Golden, P. and G. Barton, 1983. Sex differences in absence from work: A reinterpretation. *Psychology of Women Quarterly 8:* 185-188.
Fordyce, W. E., A. H. Roberts, and R. A. Sternback, 1985. The behavioral management of chronic pain: A response to critics. *Pain 22:* 113-125.
Halbert, D. R. and L. M. Demers, 1978. A clinical trial of indomethacin and ibuprofen in dysmenorrhea. *The Journal of Reproductive Medicine 21:* 219-222.
Halbert, D. R., L. M. Demers, and D.E.D. Jones, 1976. Dysmenorrhea and prostaglandins. *Obstetrical and Gynecological Survey 31:* 77-81.
Halbreich, U. and J. Endicott, 1982. Classification of premenstrual syndromes. In: R. C. Friedman (Ed.), *Behavior and the Menstrual Cycle.* Marcel Dekker, New York, NY.
Halbreich, U. and J. Endicott, 1985. Methodological issues in studies of premenstrual changes. *Psychoneuroendocrinology 10:* 10-32.
Halbreich, U., J. Endicott, and J. Nee, 1983. Premenstrual depressive changes. *Archives of General Psychiatry 40:* 535-542.
Hoes, M. J., 1980. The chronopathology of premenstrual psychopathology. *Medical Hypotheses 6:* 1063-1075.
Janbu, T., P. Lokken, and B. I. Nesheim, 1979. Effect of acetylsalicyclic acid, paracetamol and placebo on pain and blood loss in dysmenorrheic women. *Acta Obstetrica et Gynecologica Scandinavica 87:* 81-85.
Janiger, O., R. Riffenburgh, and R. Kersh, 1972. Cross cultural study of premenstrual symptoms. *Psychosomatics 13:* 226.
Kistner, R. W., 1971. *Gynecology, Principles, and Practices.* Year Book Medical Publishers, Chicago, IL, pp. 584-587.
McCance, R. A., M. C. Luff, and E. E. Widdowson, 1937. Physical and emotional peridocity in women. *Journal of Hygiene 37:* 571-605.
Michael, R. P., R. W. Bonsall, and M. Kutner, 1975. Volatile fatty acids, "copulins," in human vaginal secretions. *Psychoneuroendocrinology 1:* 153-163.
Miller, S. M., 1979. Coping with impending stress: Psychophysiological and cognitive correlates of choice. *Psychophysiology 16:* 572-581.
Moos, R. H., 1968. The development of a Menstrual Distress Questionnaire. *Psychosomatic Medicine 30:* 853-867.
Most, A. F., N. F. Woods, G. K. Dery, and B. M. Most, 1981. Distress associated with menstruation among Israeli women. *International Journal of Nursing Studies 18:* 61-71.
Parlee, M. B., 1974. Stereotypic beliefs about menstruation: A methodological note on the Moos Menstrual Stress Questionnaire and some new data. *Psychosomatic Medicine 36:* 229-240.

Parlee, M. B., 1982. Changes in moods and activation levels during the menstrual cycle in experimentally naive subjects. *Psychology of Women Quarterly 7:* 119-131.

Patterson, G. R. and J. B. Reid, 1984. Social interactional processes within the family: The study of moment-by-moment family transactions in which human social development is imbedded. *Journal of Applied Developmental Psychology 5:* 237-262.

Reid, R. L., 1985. Premenstrual Syndrome. In: J. M. Leventhal (Ed.), *Current Problems in Obstetrics, Gynecology and Fertility, Vol. 8.* Year Book Medical Publishers, Chicago, IL, pp. 2-57.

Reid, R. L. and S. C. Yen, 1981. Premenstrual syndrome. *American Journal of Obstetrics and Gynecology 139:* 85-104.

Ruble, D. N., 1977. Premenstrual symptoms: A reinterpretation. *Science 197:* 291.

Scambler, A. and G. Scambler, 1985. Menstrual symptoms, attitudes, and consulting behavior. *Social Science Medicine 20:* 1065-1068.

Seligman, M.E.P., 1968. Chronic fear produced by unpredictable (unsignalled) electric shock. *Journal of Comparative and Physiological Psychology 66:* 402-411.

Shangold, M. M., S. Aksel, D. W. Schomberg, and C. B. Hammond, 1976. Plasma prostaglandin F2a levels in dysmenorrheic women. *Fertility and Sterility 27:* 1171-1175.

Sibergeld, S., N. Brost, and E. P. Nobel, 1971. The menstrual cycle: A double-blind study of symptoms, mood, and behavior, and biochemical variables using Enovid and placebo. *Psychosomatic Medicine 33:* 411-428.

Society for Menstrual Cycle Research, 1986 (Winter). Task Force report on guidelines for menstrual cycle research. *Newsletter 2:* 1-2.

Svennerund, S., 1959. Dysmenorrhea and absenteeism: Some gynaecological and medicosocial aspects. *Acta Obstetrica Gynecologica Scandinavica 38 (Suppl. 2):* 5-16.

Taylor, J. W., 1979. The timing of menstruation-related symptoms assessed by a daily symptom rating scale. *Acta Psychiatrica Scandinavica 60:* 87-105.

Vila, J. and H. R. Beech, 1980. Premenstrual symptomatology: An interaction hypothesis. *British Journal of Social and Clinical Psychology 19:* 73-80.

Widholm, O., 1979. Dysmenorrhea during adolescence. *Acta Obstetrica Gynecologica Scandinavica 87:* 61-66.

Wood, C., L. E. Larsen, and R. Williams, 1979. Menstrual characteristics of 2,343 women attending the Shepard Foundation. *Australia and New Zealand Journal of Obstetrics and Gynecology 19:* 107-110.

Wood, N. F., A. Most, and G. K. Dery, 1982. Prevalence of perimenstrual symptoms. *American Journal of Public Health 72:* 1257.

Ylikorkala, O. and M. Dawood, 1978. New concepts in dysmenorrhea. *American Journal of Obstetrics and Gynecology 130:* 833-847.

PERCEPTIONS OF MENSTRUAL AND PREMENSTRUAL SYMPTOMS: SELF-DEFINITIONAL PROCESSES AT MENARCHE

Diane N. Ruble, Ph.D.* and Jeanne Brooks-Gunn, Ph.D.**

*Department of Psychology
New York University
New York, New York

**Educational Testing Service
Princeton, New Jersey

INTRODUCTION

Two lines of inquiry appear to characterize research related to premenstrual syndrome (PMS) (for example, see descriptions in Debrovner, 1982, and Friedman, 1982). Those two lines overlap and do not seem to be clearly delineated. The first concerns symptom reports associated with premenstrual and menstrual bases of the cycle and represents most of the literature. This line of research concerns the study of a wide range of symptoms — anything that might constitute menstrual or premenstrual distress in even its mildest form. Thus, terms such as premenstrual blues, negative affect, premenstrual tension, etc., apply to this line of research. But regardless of the term, the symptoms studied are not viewed as constituting a syndrome. The other line of research refers to a PMS syndrome characterized by a very specific cluster or clusters of symptoms. It is characterized as well by a greater level of severity, such that it may be disruptive to a woman's functioning, and by precise timing in relation to menstruation. The latter is what is usually referred to as PMS, and what we will use as the definition of PMS for the purposes of this chapter.

INCIDENCE OF PREMENSTRUAL SYNDROME

The distinction noted above is important for a number of reasons. Obviously, for etiological reasons, it is very important to know which kind of phenomenon it is. It is also important for interpreting reports of incidence of PMS. The popular press and other forms of popular media seem to be leading us to the conclusion that PMS is a very prevalent phenomenon. Certainly, magazines and some movies lead us to think that. PMS is presented as a significant malady of the 1980's and, more importantly, it is perceived as something that applies to almost every woman. This conclusion is not, in fact, supported by the scientific literature, but the lack of clarity between the two lines of research described above may lead to confusion about the incidence of PMS. Indeed, we would conclude from the scientific literature that the incidence of PMS, in the more strictly defined sense as a syndrome ("severe and characterized by precise timing") is really very small. Most relevant studies recruit subjects who identify themselves as having PMS; even of those, the numbers who actually meet the specific criteria for PMS are very small.

In one study, for example, of the 130 individuals responding to an advertisement for women with severe PMS, only 24 met the interview criteria: Suffering from moderate-to-severe premenstrual symptoms that remitted shortly after the onset of menses, and currently free of other significant physical or psychiatric disorders (Haskett & Abplanalp, 1983). Only eight of these met the more specific diagnostic criteria for PMS developed by Steiner, Haskett, and Carroll (1980). As the authors conclude, these findings imply that "only relatively few women reporting these difficulties are in fact suffering from a strictly defined disorder which is suitable for systematic investigation."

A second point in terms of incidence is that even the other line of research leads to an over-estimation. Our earlier review of prospective studies using a variety of measures of premenstrual negative affect found that about half such studies failed to show even marginally significant mean differences across cycle phase, although significant effects of pain and water retention were consistently reported (Ruble & Brooks-Gunn, 1979). In contrast, when studies involved retrospective reports, mean cycle phase differences were large and significant. Moreover, when retrospective studies are compared with general knowledge or stereotyping studies, the pattern of means is almost indistinguishable. Furthermore, studies with adolescent subjects have found that ratings for self and ratings for others are highly correlated and that adolescent boys and premenarcheal girls have similar symptom beliefs to postmenarcheal girls (Brooks-Gunn & Ruble, 1980; Clarke & Ruble, 1978). These similarities support the suggestion by Parlee (1974) that there is a set of cultural beliefs regarding cyclic changes and that direct knowledge of menstrual and premenstrual symptoms cannot fully account for reports of cyclic fluctuations. Of course, problems in the data base *per se* do not indicate necessarily the existence of biased beliefs, only that assumptions regarding cyclic changes are not yet justified by the data. However, the comparisons across different types of self-report studies and recent experimental data suggest that a set of beliefs exists that require explanation beyond knowledge based on direct physical experience with symptoms. For example, the results of studies which experimentally manipulated women's perceptions of their cycle phase (Ruble, 1977) and women's awareness of the purpose of the study as menstrual-related (Aubuchon & Calhoun, 1985; Englander-Golden, Whitmore, & Dienstbier, 1978) both suggest that women's self-reported experience of symptoms is distorted by labeling them as menstrual-related.

It could be argued, of course, that these conclusions are no longer valid because they were based on the Moos Menstrual Distress Questionnaire (MDQ) (see Moos, 1985, and Appendix) and other older instruments that did not take advantage of more precise definitions of symptom clusters or because they did not use objective measures to identify the phase of the cycle. Also, these studies were not measuring PMS *per se* but rather cycle-related symptoms. More recent studies employing multiple psychological and physiological measures, however, also fail to show significant negative changes during the premenstrual phase of the cycle in prospective daily reports (e.g., Abplanalp, Rose, Donnelly, & Livingston-Vaughn, 1979; Lahmeger, Miller, & Deleon-Jones, 1982; Parlee, 1983). Thus, it appears that most menstruating women (those without significant psychopathology) show, at most, minor affective changes premenstrually. These data should not be interpreted to mean that no women experience severe symptoms, but rather that the number of these women is probably small, and assumptions concerning ubiquitous effects are unfounded.

In summary, findings from retrospective and stereotyping studies suggest that it is widely believed that women experience symptoms premenstrually and menstrually. Findings from prospective reports, however, which presumably are closer to actual experiences, present a different picture. These discrepancies between prospective and retrospective reports are troubling, in part, because it is apparently generally believed that women are debilitated during certain times of the month. In the past, this has led to statements that result in prejudice and discrimination against women. In fact, that is the reason we initially began this program of research. People believe that women experience debilitating symptoms. Women, themselves, believe that they experience such symptoms. Yet, a closer examination of the data does not reveal the extent, the incidence, and the severity of symptoms suggested by the beliefs.

INTERPRETING THE DATA

How can we explain this apparent discrepancy across measures? What does it say about etiology? We contend the data suggest that something other than direct experience of symptoms may account, in part, for symptom reports. The utility of this hypothesis is reinforced by the consistent conclusions of reviews on the etiology and treatment of PMS that definitive evidence for the physiological basis of PMS has yet to be reported, in spite of the large number of theories advanced (Green, 1982; Rausch & Janowsky, 1982). Indeed, the predominant findings of placebo effects led one recent reviewer to conclude, "At present, positive attitude appears to be the most potent item in the premenstrual treatment armamentarium" (Green, 1982, p. 388). Thus, symptom reports may be influenced by a set of biased or erroneous beliefs.

In an earlier paper, we examined the question of what processes could account for the development and persistence of such beliefs (Ruble & Brooks-Gunn, 1979). Based on findings concerning biases and errors in the way people process information when making judgments (e.g., Ross, 1977; Tversky & Kahneman, 1974), we suggested how perceptions of cyclicity may be acquired and maintained by such information-processing errors. For example, once a set of symptoms is labeled as menstrual-related, individuals may continue to perceive an association between these symptoms and the phases of the cycle, even in the absence of a true relationship. This "illusory correlation" (e.g., Chapman & Chapman, 1967; Hamilton, 1976) continues because, for example, the evidence can be distorted to be consistent with pre-existing beliefs (e.g., the same somatic sensation may be labeled and perceived differently — cramps vs. indigestion — depending on the time of the month it occurs).

Moreover, distinctive events — distinctive in terms of being unusual, statistically improbable, or highly salient for some reason — tend to become associated with each other, even if in reality, they have no association at all (Chapman, 1967; Hamilton & Gifford, 1976). What that would mean for the menstrual cycle is that distinctive events like bleeding and outbursts of irritability could become associated, even if, in fact, irritability were equally distributed throughout the menstrual cycle. Another example is distortion. Once a belief exists or a conclusion is formed, information becomes distorted to fit with the pre-existing belief (Ross, 1977). For example, occurrence of a symptom at other times of the month may not be noticed. In fact, there is fairly clear evidence that what people notice is a positive, positive co-association; that is, irritability coinciding with menstruation or changes associated with the premenstrual phase will be noticed and will be labeled as a positive association. In contrast, irritability at some other time of the month is not perceived as evidence relevant to the hypothesis, and it does not become part of the data on which the hypothesis is evaluated.

Such processes seem important to keep in mind in evaluating the literature. Most importantly, we need to be concerned about possible chance associations in current PMS formulations. For example, although recent research identifying subtypes (e.g., Halbreich & Endicott, 1982) represents an important advance, it also leads to a proliferation of possible symptoms to be associated with PMS, making chance associations more likely. This problem is compounded when, as some suggest, PMS is no longer limited to a few premenstrual days, but rather is said to occur at almost any time of the month (Rausch & Janowsky, 1982; Stone, 1982) or to occur for 3 or 4 weeks (Dalton, 1982).

SOCIOCULTURAL FACTORS AND THE MENSTRUAL EXPERIENCE

The preceding analysis suggests how beliefs about menstrual changes may be acquired and maintained independent of their association with physiological state, but it cannot in itself account for individual variation in the types of associations reported or their magnitude. Thus, a more complete understanding of such beliefs seems dependent on an analysis at a more individualized level. Variations in physiological factors such as hormone levels and sensitivity to hormones are an obvious possible source of such individual differences. Physiological variables may also have indirect effects on some symptom reports, as, for example, the association of pain with menstruation may itself result in emotional changes such as irritability (Moos & Leiderman, 1978; Paige, 1973a). However, recent research suggests that there should be increasing attention to the role of sociocultural factors in producing variations in reports of symptoms (Matthews & Carra, 1982; Paige, 1971, 1973b; Parlee, 1978). Findings that reports of menstrual distress and its correlates vary cross-culturally (e.g., Janiger, Riffenburgh, & Kersh, 1972; Snowden & Christian, 1983) and subculturally by religion (Paige, 1973c) emphasize the need to examine the socialization context in which an individual learns about or experiences menstruation.

Consider the hypothetical example of how premenstrual symptomatology may come about that is displayed in Figure 1. A cultural taboo against discussing menstruation leads to, in some cases, little information being passed on to a girl about to experience menstruation because it is considered an uncomfortable topic for discussion. That means that the girl is unprepared for menarche. This, in turn, leads to a distressing initial experience of menarche, which, as discussed subsequently, could lead to a continued expectation for negative experiences, and to anxiety surrounding the event. The anxiety surrounding the event, given all these social influences, could affect hormones (e.g., Michael, 1968), could lead to psychologically increased awareness of symptoms, could lead to labeling of the states as psychologically related, and/or could lead to an exaggeration of the experience.

This is one hypothetical example of how these complicated sets of social, psychological, and physiological factors may interact in influencing perceptions of symptoms. Most of our recent research has been

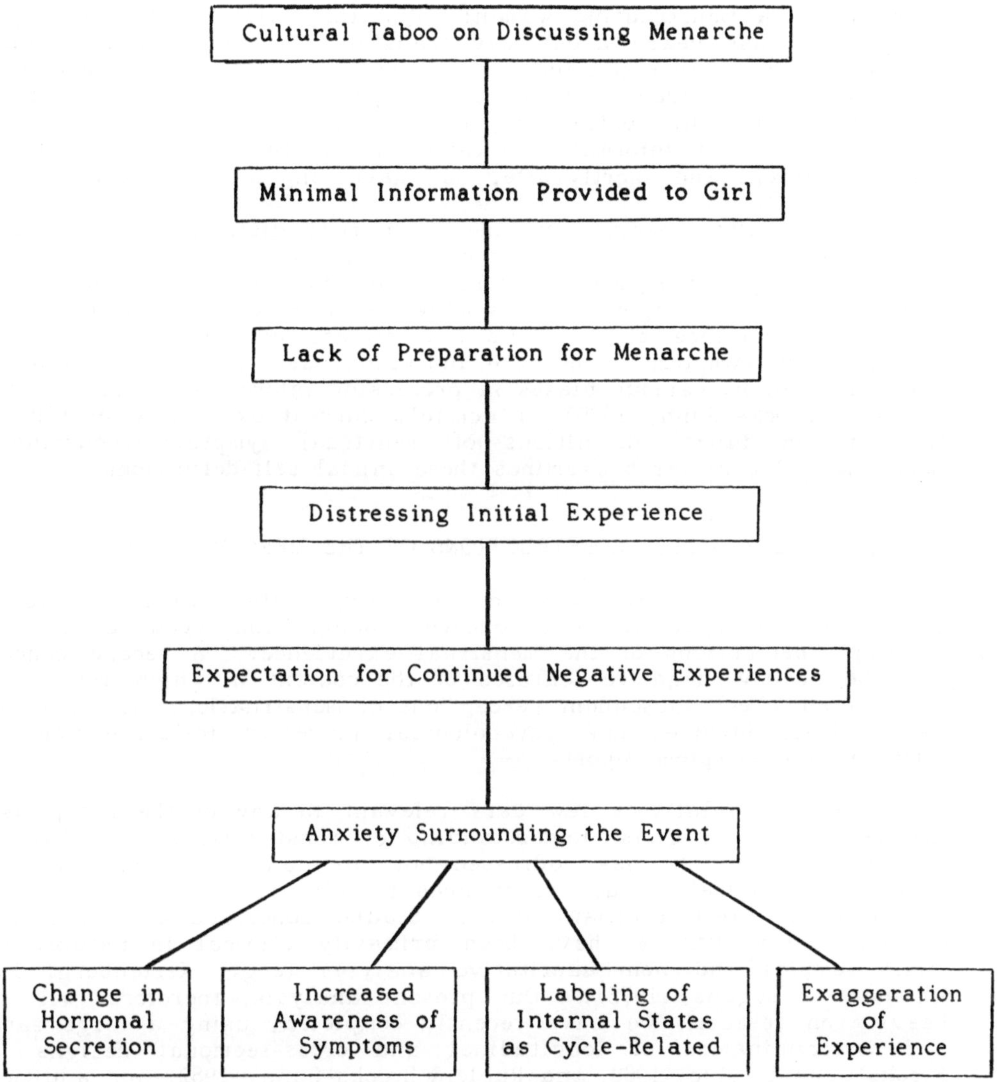

Fig. 1. Possible interactions between factors contributing to perceptions of symptoms.

concerned with the social context in which learning about menstruation occurs during adolescence. It is important to note that we, as well as most researchers in this field, use as our main dependent variables measures that are very much influenced by such social expectation effects; namely, self reports of symptoms. It therefore seems important to understand how social factors influence perceptions of symptoms.

THE IMPACT OF MENARCHE

The study of these socialization processes has been the goal of our research during the last several years. We have focused on menarche because, as the biological symbol of a shift from child to woman, it may represent a time of change in self-identity or self-definition. At a minimum, this event signals a need for the girl to determine what it means to be a menstruating woman: How the somatic and psychological changes she has heard about may translate into personal experiences. The definition of the experience established at this time may be difficult to change: Subsequent experiences are perceived in terms of and may be distorted by this definition (Ruble & Brooks-Gunn, 1979). Thus, perceptions of and information received about the menstrual experience during menarche and shortly after may have long-lasting impact.

Although our research examines menstrual distress more generally, rather than PMS *per se*, both terms involve a perception of symptoms influenced by psychological processes. We would argue that the specific constellation(s) of symptom reports known as PMS represent a combination of direct experience of symptoms and sociocultural factors influencing beliefs about symptoms. Because individual associations feed into and are reinforced by various biases in processing information about cyclicity (Ruble & Brooks-Gunn, 1979), a woman's current experience of PMS may originate in initial definitions of menstrual symptoms occurring at menarche. Our research examines these initial self-definitions.

ADOLESCENT GIRLS' CONSTRUCTIONS OF THE MENSTRUAL EXPERIENCE

We will discuss two ways of examining self-definitional processes related to menstruation. One concerns changes that occur at menarche in girls' perceptions of the menstrual experience. A second concerns how the positive/negative features of the context in which menarche is experienced affect subsequent perceptions of menstruation. In each case, the analysis involves how psychological processes influence menstrual attitudes and symptom reports.

There are relatively few data relevant to any of these aspects of the development of girls' understanding of menstruation. Most previous research on menarche has addressed how pre- and postmenarcheal girls differ psychologically, such as changes in self-image or sexual differentiation (c.f., Greif & Ulman, 1982). Studies concerned with perceptions of menstruation *per se* have been primarily clinical in nature, with small samples and non-quantitative analyses (e.g., Kestenberg, 1965; Whisnant & Zegans, 1975). Our present analysis, therefore, will rely heavily on research we have recently completed, using a large sample and a combination of longitudinal and cross-sectional designs (see Brooks-Gunn & Ruble, 1982, and Ruble & Brooks-Gunn, 1982, for additional details of the investigation).

The cross-sectional sample consisted of 639 public school girls in 5th to 8th and 11th to 12th grades. The longitudinal sample consisted of an initial group of 120 5th and 6th graders who were premenarcheal at the time of first testing. The longitudinal design employed a matching procedure to control for repeated testing: A premenarcheal girl, matched on age and school, was paired with each girl who reached menarche. Using this procedure, 46 pairs of girls completed both the pre- and postmenarcheal phases of testing. At each testing, the girls completed a lengthy questionnaire that included sections on incidence and severity of menstrual and premenstrual symptoms, attitudes about menstruation, and sources of menstrual-related information (for questionnaires, see Appendix). In addition, girls from the longitudinal sample were interviewed at the second testing.

PERCEPTION OF THE MENSTRUAL EXPERIENCE: PRE-/POSTMENARCHEAL DIFFERENCES

What are girls' beliefs and attitudes as they approach their first experience with menstruation? Our data show that even the youngest premenarcheal girls we studied expected to experience the symptom cluster commonly associated with the menstrual cycle. Thus, when girls enter menarche, they expect to experience premenstrual and menstrual distress. Responses to attitude measures are quite mixed, although when averaged, they appear to be largely neutral in terms of general negative evaluation, comfort, embarrassment, and so on. Interestingly, the strongest agreement is with items suggesting that menstruation is normal and natural. Thus, young girls are aware of the positive as well as the negative aspects of menstruation. These findings are generally consistent with previous research (e.g., Clarke & Ruble, 1978; Petersen, 1983; Williams, 1983).

Do girls' expectations become a self-fulfilling prophecy? Findings of few pre- vs. postmenarcheal differences appear to provide an initial affirmative answer. In the cross-sectional sample, the only difference in symptom reports is that postmenarcheal girls reported experiencing *less* pain than premenarcheal girls expected. Similarly, in the longitudinal sample, girls' reports of symptoms were either the same or less severe after menarche than what they had expected premenarcheally and what their premenarcheal counterparts expected at the second testing. Similar results were obtained for the attitude and feeling measures. Menarcheal status affected responses on only two of nine scales, and these effects were shown only in the longitudinal analysis. Consistent with differences in symptom reports, postmenarcheal girls viewed menstruation as *less* debilitating than premenarcheal girls.

In general, then, girls' perceptions of menstruation appear to show little change as a function of initial direct experience. Moreover, in contrast to what might be expected, direct experience, if anything, seems to result in perceptions of fewer symptoms and less debilitation. Perhaps the premenarcheal girls receive or attend to more negative information about menstrual symptoms than postmenarcheal girls. Alternatively, premenarcheal girls may adhere to the same information more strongly because they do not have any contrary evidence.

These findings appear to conflict with previous reports that postmenarcheal girls are more negative than premenarcheal girls (Clarke & Ruble, 1978; Koff, Rierdan, & Jacobson, 1981). This apparent discrepancy, however, may indicate little more than the complexity of defining the experience. Girls' responses seem to be quite sensitive to the timing of the interview in relation to age and menarcheal status. In cross-sectional studies, age or grade and menarcheal status are almost inevitably confounded. Thus, the greater negativity of postmenarcheal girls in previous research may be due to age-related factors rather than the direct experience of menstruation. Indeed, there is a considerable amount of research suggesting increasingly negative reactions to menstruation with age among postmenarcheal girls and women (Golub & Harrington, 1981; Ruble & Brooks-Gunn, 1982; Widholm & Kantero, 1971). Moreover, in our longitudinal study in which age effects could be examined separately from menarcheal status, we found that overall negative evaluations (e.g., "Menstruation is something I would prefer not to have") and perceptions that it is bothersome (e.g., "Menstruation is something I just have to put up with") increased as a function of age only, not menarcheal status. Finally, girls appear to be particularly sensitive or secretive about menstruation immediately after menarche, the time that we interviewed girls in our longitudinal study. This sensitivity is indicated, in part, by our findings of decreased comfort in talking to others about menstruation reported by post- compared to premenarcheal girls. It is also indicated by responses during a telephone interview within two months after each girl's first period. Although most girls reported telling someone soon after the event, almost all of these initial discussions were with their mothers. Only 18 percent said they specifically told a friend. By the time girls had had two to three periods, however, most were no longer extremely secretive. Indeed, about half of the girls appear to discuss menstruation regularly with a friend. It is noteworthy, in the contrast of reports of increasing symptoms during the first few years after menarche (Ruble & Brooks-Gunn, 1982), that the most frequent topic of discussion was symptomatology. To the extent that discussing symptoms represents a social comparison process, a form of "one upmanship" or "undirectional drive upward" (Festinger, 1954) may exacerbate the frequency or severity of psychosomatic complaints (Mechanic, 1972; Ruble & Brooks-Gunn, 1979). Age-related increases could also indicate physiological changes, such as increased frequency of ovulation occurring within the first few years after menarche (Vollman, 1977), although cross-cultural differences in symptom reports during these years suggest that socialization processes are involved as well (Ruble & Brooks-Gunn, 1982).

In summary, the literature suggests that by the time girls reach menarche they have negative expectations regarding somatic and emotional effects of menstruation and mixed feelings and attitudes. The actual experience of menstruation changes little except that girls appear to find the event less debilitating than they expected. Thus, a girl enters menarche with a clear set of expectations, many of which are quite negative, and most of her peers, male as well as female (Clarke & Ruble, 1978), hold similar expectations. Her experience of menstruation is, therefore, primed to be a self-fulfilling prophecy. Indeed, additional analyses of our longitudinal data suggest that the prophecy is fulfilled, at least to some extent. Symptom reports of postmenarcheal girls at the second testing were significantly correlated with their premenarcheal expectations at the first testing. The fact that no significant relationships were found between expectations at Time 1 and at Time 2 for the girls who remained premenarcheal seems to rule out response-bias explanations of this relationship. Instead, it is as if expectations present at the time a girl begins to menstruate provide the definition of that experience, while expectations of premenarcheal girls continually change, presumably in response to age-related changes in the information available.

THE CONTEXT IN WHICH MENARCHE IS EXPERIENCED

If, as we are suggesting, self-definitions with long-lasting significance occur at menarche, then it is important to examine factors that influence how positive or negative the experience is. Negative menarcheal experiences may have deleterious consequences for a girl's subsequent experience of the menstrual cycle; and, because of the intimate link between menstruation, womanhood, and sexuality, menarcheal experiences may affect more general aspects of a girl's self-concept as well. In our research, we have examined this issue by relating girls' reports or recollections of context factors affecting the experience of menarche to subsequent self-perceptions and symptoms.

One such factor, adequacy of preparation, has often been referred to as necessary for later menstrual adjustment (e.g., Deutsch, 1944; Rees, 1953). Relevant studies, however, have relied on retrospective reports and are inconsistent and difficult to interpret (May, 1976; Paige,

Table 1. Means of Symptoms and Medication Reported as a Function of Preparedness for the Cross-Sectional Sample.

Variable	Preparedness	
	Not Prepared	Prepared
Incidence of any symptoms at first menstruation (0-2)	0.47	0.57
Incidence of taking medication at first menstruation (0-1)	0.70	0.53*
Current incidence of particular symptoms (0-6)	3.89	3.31*
Number of other current menstrual symptoms	0.45	0.24*
Number of other current premenstrual symptoms	0.55	0.24*
Current incidence of taking medication (0-2)	0.76	0.62

Note: Higher numbers represent higher scores. Incidence variables represent combinations of "Yes/No" responses on scales ranging from 1-6 questions (Ruble & Brooks-Gunn, 1982).

* $p < .05$

1973c; Shainess, 1961). Recently, for example, Woods, Dery, and Most (1983) found little relation between recollections of menarche and the current attitudes and symptoms of college women. If anything, the relationship was in the reverse direction: Positive recollections were associated with more current symptoms. The one finding consistent with the general hypothesis is that being "surprised" at menarche was related to more current reports of pain. Rierdan (1983), however, found that college women who recalled being poorly prepared at menarche reported less positive experience.

A second related context factor is timing of menarche. An important source of information during a period of self-definitional change is social comparison, and the values and norms that peers provide may be particularly significant because of heightened conformity pressures at that time (Costanzo & Shaw, 1966). Reaching menarche at about the same age as her peers can provide a girl with a sense of sharing and closeness. Reaching menarche earlier than most peers, however, may generate insecurity about being different from the group and make the experience more negative than it is for average-maturing girls. Previous data on age of maturation are consistent with the present analysis (e.g., Brooks-Gunn, Petersen, & Eichorn, in press; Faust, 1983; Jones & Mussen, 1958; Petersen, in press), although these studies do not focus on the effects of timing of menarche on symptoms *per se*.

Our analysis of the effects of timing and preparation differed from previous studies in several ways: (a) the girls were younger and thus recollections were based on more recent experience; (b) the sample was very large and thus we could look at more extreme variations; and (c) a longitudinal sample reporting on immediate experiences was included. The results of analyses of differences in reported symptoms and medication are shown in Tables 1 and 2. Although many of the differences failed to reach statistical significance, effects which did emerge were generally in the predicted direction (see "Methods of

Table 2. Means of Symptoms and Medication Reported as a Function of Timing of Menarche for the Cross-Sectional Sample.

Variable	Grade That Menarche Occurred		
	$\leq$ 6th	7th	$\geq$ 8th
Incidence of any symptoms at first menstruation (0-2)	0.71	0.58	0.39*
Incidence of taking medication at first menstruation (0-1)	0.71	0.48	0.49*
Current incidence of particular symptoms (0-6)	3.64	3.20	3.39
Number of other current menstrual symptoms	0.32	0.17	0.33
Number of other current premenstrual symptoms	0.35	0.14	0.38*
Current incidence of taking medication (0-2)	0.86	0.54	0.55**

Note: Higher numbers represent higher scores. Incidence variables represent combinations of "Yes/No" responses on scales ranging from 1-6 questions (Ruble & Brooks-Gunn, 1982).

* $p < .01$

** $p < .001$

Evaluation" in Appendix). Girls who were unprepared or menstruated early reported more negative reactions, more symptoms, and (in the 7th grade) their self-image ratings were more negative. In addition, the data are, at least indirectly, supportive of the idea of long-lasting effects of these aspects of the menarcheal experiences. Some effects on current experiences were evident for girls as old as 11th and 12th graders, in that there was no interaction with grade level.

It is possible, of course, that the effects of feeling prepared represent a response bias; that is, if girls feel negatively about the experience generally, they may respond negatively to all relevant items, including reports of preparation. It is noteworthy, therefore, that not all relevant variables showed similar effects. The lack of symptoms experienced at menarche is particularly important because it rules out the alternative explanation that girls felt totally unprepared *because* they had severe symptoms.

A third factor likely to affect positive/negative experiences at menarche is girls' perceptions of the reactions of significant others. We examined this issue in two ways in our longitudinal sample. The first concerned the relationship between the amount of information received from different sources and menstrual attitudes of postmenarcheal girls. Since overall, female and health sources are viewed as having positive attitudes and male sources as having negative attitudes, we would expect positive attitudes to be related to more learning from female and health sources. The correlations were generally consistent with these predictions. Perceiving menstruation as a natural event and comfort in talking about it were positively correlated with amount learned from female sources and parents and doctor.

Table 3. Correlations Between Amount Learned from Male Sources and Degrees of Menstrual Distress for the Menarcheal Subsample of the Longitudinal Study.

	Menstrual	Premenstrual
Negative affect	0.42	NS
Water retention	0.53	0.57
Pain	NS	0.52

Note: All p's $<$ .01

A second type of analysis concerned the relationship between girls' perceptions of sources premenarcheally (Time 1) and their subsequent experience of symptoms (Time 2). Interestingly, girls who reported learning more from male sources premenarcheally reported greater menstrual and premenstrual distress postmenarcheally (see Table 3). Similar significant correlations were found for perceptions of symptoms at Time 2 and perceptions of male sources as having negative feelings about menstruation at Time 1. Thus, receiving information premenarcheally from sources perceived to be negative appears to be associated with more negative perceptions of symptoms after menarche.

In summary, several context variables have been identified that affect how positively or negatively menarche is experienced. Consistent with a self-definitional perspective, these factors influence menstrual attitudes and symptoms at menarche or shortly after, and even appear to influence symptom reports as late as senior high scnool.

IMPLICATIONS OF A SELF-DEFINITIONAL ANALYSIS FOR THE STUDY OF PREMENSTRUAL SYNDROME

We have argued that around the time of menarche, girls construct a definition of the menstrual experience from various sources of information, of which direct knowledge of symptoms is only one. Our data suggest that adolescent girls' symptom reports are correlated with their own premenarcheal expectations, suggesting that the direct experience of menstruation is interpreted in terms of expectations previously formed. Moreover, individual differences in symptom reports can be predicted from the context in which self-definitions are initially formed. Current negative reports of symptoms in postmenarcheal girls from 7th to 12th grades are related to being unprepared for menarche, being early to mature, or receiving information from sources perceived as negative.

Findings that psychological factors (expectations and context) influence individual differences in girls' perceptions of menstruation have several implications for understanding PMS. First, adolescent experiences may create a foundation for an association between the premenstrual phase and negative affect, particularly if premenarcheal expectations are based on informational sources that emphasize this association. Thus, menarcheal experiences may prime some women to be ready to attribute new problems to the menstrual cycle. As PMS receives increasing attention and publicity, therefore, the likelihood increases that PMS will be part of girls' premenarcheal expectations and, presumably, subsequent reported experiences. This account of the impact of menarche differs from previous suggestions that menstrual-related symptoms reflect maladjustment to the trauma of the first menstruation and the effect of that trauma on the unconscious (Dalton, 1982). In contrast, we would argue that mechanisms linking menarcheal experience to symptoms could be quite direct: Specifically, girls interpret their experience in light of the prior expectations they construct, some of which are quite negative. In addition, other aspects of the experience, such as timing, may make it more or less positive or negative. Once the definition is formed, it can be maintained by fairly straightforward biases inherent in processing information about cyclicity (Ruble & Brooks-Gunn, 1979). In short, if girls' initial definitions involve PMS symptom clusters, this perception is likely to remain. It seems important, then, that the uncertain status and questions about the incidence of PMS become more widely recognized by the scientist and general public alike.

A second implication of this analysis concerns the suggestion by some PMS researchers that finding variations in PMS symptom clusters across subgroups of women rules out explanations based on social factors or stereotypes (e.g., Halbreich & Endicott, 1982). In contrast, we would argue that multiple differences (e.g., across individual families and significant others, cultures and subcultures with regard to specific menstrual beliefs and practices including medication, and more general values) affect the kinds of symptom associations found. Processes other than socialization may also create individual differences in expectations. Problems not initially associated with menstruation, such as depression or anxiety neurosis, may become labeled a premenstrual response as a woman seeks to explain what is happening to her. Thus, one would expect to find the incidence of different PMS symptom clusters to differ across subgroups of women with different forms of psychological distress; and available evidence does seem to support this hypothesis (Endicott, Halbreich, Schacht, & Nee, 1981; Hurt, Friedman, Clarkin, Corn, & Aronoff, 1982; Schuckit, Daly, Hernman, & Hineman, 1975). Although this relationship is usually assumed to reflect the physiological changes associated with the menstrual cycle, it is not intuitively obvious why the same hormonal changes should result, for example, in premenstrual depression in depressed women and premenstrual anxiety in women with anxiety neurosis. It is reasonably easy to explain, however, why depressed versus anxious women might differ in which symptoms they emphasize and thus report PMS symptoms that are consistent with their form of psychological distress.

CONCLUSIONS

Severe PMS is a serious health problem regardless of its etiology. Even if some women are mistaken in attributing physical or emotional difficulties to the menstrual cycle, they may suffer loss of self-esteem, lack of proper treatment, or side effects of needless medication. Our research suggests the need to further examine the influence of socialization and social expectation processes at the same time that important advances continue in carefully defining and examining physiological concomitants of the syndrome.

ACKNOWLEDGMENTS

Preparation of this chapter and some of the research was supported, in part, by grants SOC-76 02137 and SOC-76 02179 from the National Science Foundation; in part, by RSDA grant MH00484 from the National Institute of Mental Health to Ruble; and, in part, by a grant from The Grant Foundation to Brooks-Gunn.

REFERENCES

Abplanalp, J. M., R. M. Rose, A. F. Donnelly, and L. Livingston-Vaughn, 1979. Psychoendocrinology of the menstrual cycle: The relationship between enjoyment of activities, moods, and reproductive hormones. *Psychosomatic Medicine 41:* 605-615.

Aubuchon, P. G. and K. S. Calhoun, 1985. Menstrual cycle symptomatology: The role of social expectancy and experimental demand characteristics. *Psychosomatic Medicine 47:* 35-45.

Brooks-Gunn, J., A. C. Petersen, and D. Eichorn (Eds.), in press. Timing of maturation and psychosocial functioning in adolescence. *Journal of Youth and Adolescence* (special issue).

Brooks-Gunn, J. and D. N. Ruble, 1980. Menarche: The interaction of physiological, cultural, and social factors. In: A. J. Dan, E. A. Graham, and C. P. Beecher (Eds.), *The Menstrual Cycle: A Synthesis of Interdisciplinary Research.* Springer, New York, NY.

Brooks-Gunn, J. and D. N. Ruble, 1982. The development of menstrual-related beliefs and behaviors during early adolescence. *Child Development 53:* 1567-1577.

Chapman, L. J., 1967. Illusory correlation in observational report. *Journal of Verbal Learning and Verbal Behavior 6:* 151-155.

Chapman, L. J. and J. P. Chapman, 1967. Genesis of popular but erroneous psychodiagnostic observations. *Journal of Abnormal Psychology 72:* 193-204.

Clarke, A. E. and D. N. Ruble, 1978. Young adolescents' beliefs concerning menstruation. *Child Development 49:* 231-234.

Costanzo, P. R. and M. E. Shaw, 1966. Conformity as a function of age level. *Child Development 35:* 1217-1231.

Dalton, K., 1982. Premenstrual Tension: An overview. In: R. C. Friedman (Ed.), *Behavior and the Menstrual Cycle.* Marcel Dekker, New York, NY, pp. 217-242.

Debrovner, C. H. (Ed.), 1982. *Premenstrual Tension: A Multidisciplinary Approach.* Human Sciences Press, Inc., New York, NY.

Deutsch, H., 1944. *The Psychology of Woman.* Grune & Stratton, New York, NY.

Endicott, J., U. Halbreich, S. Schacht, and J. Nee, 1981. Premenstrual changes and affective disorders. *Psychosomatic Medicine 43:* 519-529.

Englander-Golden, P., M. R. Whitmore, and R. A. Dienstbier, 1978. Menstrual cycle as a focus of study and self reports of moods and behaviors. *Motivation and Emotion 2:* 75-86.

Faust, M. A., 1983. Alternative constructions of adolescent growth. In: J. Brooks-Gunn and A. C. Petersen (Eds.), *Girls at Puberty.* Plenum, New York, NY, pp. 105-125.

Festinger, L., 1954. A theory of social comparison. *Human Relations 7:* 117-140.

Friedman, R. C. (Ed.), 1982. *Behavior and the Menstrual Cycle.* Marcel Dekker, New York, NY.

Golub, S. and D. M. Harrington, 1981. Premenstrual and menstrual mood changes in adolescent women. *Journal of Personality and Social Psychology 4:* 961-965.

Green, J., 1982. Recent trends in the treatment of premenstrual syndrome: A critical review. In: R. C. Friedman (Ed.), *Behavior and the Menstrual Cycle.* Marcel Dekker, New York, NY, pp. 367-369.

Greif, E. B. and K. J. Ulman, 1982. The psychological impact of menarche on early adolescent females: A review of the literature. *Child Development 53:* 1413-1430.

Halbreich, U. and J. Endicott, 1982. Classification of premenstrual syndromes. In: R. C. Friedman (Ed.), *Behavior and the Menstrual Cycle.* Marcel Dekker, New York, NY, pp. 243-266.

Hamilton, D. L., 1976. Cognitive biases in the perception of social groups. In: J. S. Carroll and J. W. Payne (Eds.), *Cognition and Social Behavior*. Lawrence Erlbaum Associates, Hillsdale, N.J., pp. 81-93.

Hamilton, D. L. and R. K. Gifford, 1976. Illusory correlation in interpersonal perception: A cognitive basis of stereotypic judgements. *Journal of Experimental and Social Psychology 12:* 392-407.

Haskett, R. F. and J. M. Abplanalp, 1983. Premenstrual tension syndrome: Diagnostic criteria and the selection of research subjects. *Psychiatric Research 9:* 125-138.

Hurt, S. W., R. C. Friedman, J. Clarkin, R. Corn, and M. S. Aronoff, 1982. Psychopathology and the menstrual cycle. In: R. C. Friedman (Ed.), *Behavior and the Menstrual Cycle*. Marcel Dekker, New York, NY, pp. 299-316.

Janiger, O., R. Riffenburgh, and R. Kersh, 1972. Cross-cultural study of premenstrual symptoms. *Psychosomatics 13:* 226-235.

Jones, M. C. and P. H. Mussen, 1958. Self-conceptions, motivations, and interpersonal attitudes of early- and late-maturing girls. *Child Development 29:* 491-501.

Kestenberg, J. S., 1965. Menarche. In: S. Lorand and H. Schneer (Eds.), *Adolescents*. Dell, New York, NY, pp. 19-50.

Koff, E., J. Rierdan, and S. Jacobson, 1981. The personal and interpersonal significance of menarche. *Journal of the American Academy of Child Psychiatry 20:* 148-158.

Lahmeger, H. W., M. Miller, and F. Deleon-Jones, 1982. Anxiety and mood fluctuations during the normal menstrual cycle. *Psychosomatic Medicine 44:* 183-194.

Matthews, K. A. and J. Carra, 1982. Suppression of menstrual distress symptoms: A study of Type A behavior. *Personality and Social Psychology Bulletin 8:* 146-151.

May, R. R., 1976. Mood shifts and the menstrual cycle. *Journal of Psychosomatic Research 20:* 125-130.

Mechanic, D., 1972. Social psychological factors affecting the presentation of bodily complaints. *New England Journal of Medicine 286:* 1132-1139.

Michael, R. P., 1968. *Endocrinology and Human Behavior*. Oxford University Press, London.

Moos, R. H., 1985. *Premenstrual Symptoms: A Manual and Overview of Research*. Department of Psychiatry, Stanford University and Veterans Administration, Palo Alto, CA.

Moos, R. H. and D. B. Leiderman, 1978. Toward a menstrual cycle symptom typology. *Journal of Psychosomatic Research 22:* 31-40.

Paige, K. E., 1971. The effects of oral contraceptives on affective fluctuations associated with the menstrual cycle. *Psychosomatic Medicine 33:* 515-537.

Paige, K. E., 1973a. "The curse:" Possible antecedents of menstrual distress. In: A. A. Harrison (Ed.), *Explorations in Psychology*. Brooks-Cole, Monterey, CA, pp. 36-51.

Paige, K. E., 1973b. Women learn to sing the menstrual blues. *Psychology Today 7:* 41-46.

Paige, K. E., 1973c. Determinants of menstrual distress: Stress, feminity, and religion. Paper presented at the meeting of the American Sociological Association, September.

Parlee, M. B., 1974. Stereotypic beliefs about menstruation: A methodological note on the Moos Menstrual Distress Questionnaire and some new data. *Psychosomatic Medicine 36:* 229-240.

Parlee, M. B., 1978. Psychological aspects of menstruation, childbirth, and menopause. In: J. A. Sherman and F. L. Denmark (Eds.), *Psychology of Women: Future Directions of Research*. Psychological Dimensions, New York, NY, pp. 179-238.

Parlee, M. B., 1983. Future directions for research. In: S. Golub (Ed.), *Menarche*. Lexington Books, Lexington, MA, pp. 309-314.

Petersen, A. C., 1983. Menarche: Meaning of measures and measuring meaning. In: S. Golub (Ed.), *Menarche*. Lexington Books, Lexington, MA, pp. 63-76.

Petersen, A. C., in press. Pubertal development as a cause of disburbance: Myths, realities, and unanswered questions. *Journal of Genetic Psychology*.

Rausch, J. C. and D. S. Janowsky, 1982. Premenstrual tension: Etiology. In: R. C. Friedman (Ed.), *Behavior and the Menstrual Cycle*. Marcel Dekker, New York, NY, pp. 397-427.

Rees, L., 1953. The premenstrual tension syndrome and its treatment. *British Medical Journal 1:* 1014-1016.

Rierdan, J., 1983. Variations in the experience of menarche as a function of preparedness. In: S. Golub (Ed.), *Menarche*. Lexington Books, Lexington, MA, pp. 119-126.

Ross, L. D., 1977. The intuitive psychologist and his shortcomings: Distortions in the attribution process. In: L. Berkowitz (Ed.), *Advances in Experimental Social Psychology*. Academic Press, New York, NY, pp. 173-220.

Ruble, D. N., 1977. Premenstrual symptoms: A reinterpretation. *Science 197:* 291-292.

Ruble, D. N. and J. Brooks-Gunn, 1979. Menstrual symptoms: A social cognition analysis. *Journal of Behavioral Medicine 2:* 171-194.

Ruble, D. N. and J. Brooks-Gunn, 1982. The experience of menarche. *Child Development 53:* 1557-1566.

Schuckit, M. A., V. Daly, G. Hernman, and S. Hineman, 1975. Premenstrual symptoms and depression in a university population. *Diseases of the Nervous System 36:* 516-517.

Shainess, N., 1961. A re-evaluation of some aspects of femininity through a study of menstruation: A preliminary report. *Comparative Psychiatry 2:* 20-26.

Snowden, R. and B. Christian (Eds.), 1983. *Patterns and Perceptions of Menstruation*. St. Martin's Press, New York, NY.

Steiner, M., R. F. Haskett, and B. J. Carroll, 1980. Premenstrual tension syndrome: The development of research diagnostic criteria and new rating scales. *Acta Psychiatrica Scandinavica 62:* 177-190.

Stone, M. H., 1982. Premenstrual tension in borderline and related disorders. In: R. C. Friedman (Ed.), *Behavior and the Menstrual Cycle*. Marcel Dekker, New York, NY, pp. 317-344.

Tversky, A. and D. Kahneman, 1974. Judgment under uncertainty: Heuristics and biases. *Science 185:* 1124-1131.

Vollman, R. F., 1977. *The Menstrual Cycle*. Saunders, Toronto, Canada.

Whisnant, L. and L. A. Zegans, 1975. A study of attitudes toward menarche in white middle-class American girls. *American Journal of Psychiatry 132:* 809-814.

Widholm, O. and R. C. Kantero III, 1971. Menstrual pattern of adolescent girls according to chronological and gynecological ages. *Acta Obstetrica et Gynecologica Scandinavica 1* (Suppl. 14): 19-29.

Williams, L. R., 1983. Beliefs and attitudes of young girls regarding menstruation. In: S. Golub (Ed.), *Menarche*. Lexington Books, Lexington, MA, pp. 139-148.

Woods, N. F., G. K. Dery, and A. Most, 1983. Recollections of menarche, current menstrual attitudes, and premenstrual symptoms. In: S. Golub (Ed.), *Menarche*. Lexington Books, Lexington, MA, pp. 87-97.

APPENDIX

The Menstrual Attitude Questionnaire
Form for Adolescent Females

Jeanne Brooks-Gunn
Associate Director and Research Scientist
Institute for the Study of Exceptional Children
Educational Testing Service

Assistant Professor of Pediatric Psychology
College of Physicians and Surgeons
Columbia University

and

Diane Ruble
Associate Professor of Psychology
University of Toronto

This form of the MAQ was developed from research supported by the National Science Foundation (SOC-02179) and the Educational Testing Service. It was developed as a clinical research instrument, and any data should be interpreted with this in mind. If you use the MAQ, we would appreciate a summary or reprint/preprint of your results. For more information, please write Dr. Jeanne Brooks-Gunn, Educational Testing Service, Princeton, N.J. 08541.

Brooks-Gunn, J. & Ruble, D. N. The menstrual attitude questionnaire. *Psychosomatic Medicine*, 1980, *42*, 503-512.

Brooks, J., Ruble, D. N., & Clarke, A. College women's attitudes and expectations concerning menstrual-related changes. *Psychosomatic Medicine*, 1977, *29*, 288-298.

Menstrual Attitude Questionnaire

Jeanne Brooks-Gunn and Diane N. Ruble
Educational Testing Service
Princeton, N.J. 08541

We would like you to read the following sentences and tell us how much you agree or disagree with each one. We will be asking you what <u>your</u> attitudes are and what you think <u>other people's</u> attitudes are.

Your Attitudes

Please read the sentences below and tell us how much you agree or disagree with each one. If you disagree a lot, circle "1". If you just disagree, circle "2". If you disagree a little bit, circle a "3". If you agree a little bit, circle "4". If you agree with it, circle "5". If you agree a lot, circle a "6".

1	2	3	4	5	6	X
disagree a lot	disagree	disagree a little bit	agree a little bit	agree	agree a lot	don't know

FACTOR										
	1.*	I don't mind talking about menstruation with a good female friend.	1	2	3	4	5	6	X
VI	2.	When I have (or will have) my menstrual period, I am (or I think I will be) worried that someone will know.	1	2	3	4	5	6	X
VI	3.	When I have (or will have) my menstrual period, I am (or I think I will be) worried that I'll have an accident (like spots on a skirt).	1	2	3	4	5	6	X
II	4.	I envy boys because they don't have menstruation.	1	2	3	4	5	6	X
	5.*	I don't mind talking about menstruation with my mother.	1	2	3	4	5	6	X
	6.*	I don't mind talking about menstruation with my father.	1	2	3	4	5	6	X
II	7.	Menstruation is something to be happy about.	1	2	3	4	5	6	X

1	2	3	4	5	6	X
disagree a lot	disagree	disagree a little bit	agree a little bit	agree	agree a lot	don't know

FACTOR										
II	8.	Menstruation is something I would prefer not to have.	1	2	3	4	5	6	X
	9.*	I don't mind talking about menstruation with a male friend (a friend who is a boy).	1	2	3	4	5	6	X
I	10.	I make (or will make) an extra effort not to be crabby during my period.	1	2	3	4	5	6	X
II	11.	You shouldn't talk to just anyone about menstruation.	1	2	3	4	5	6	X
II	12.	Menstruation gives women a way to keep in touch with their bodies.	1	2	3	4	5	6	X
I	13.	Women are more tired than usual when they are menstruating.	1	2	3	4	5	6	X
I	14.	I hope it will be possible someday to get a menstrual period over within a few minutes.	1	2	3	4	5	6	X
	15.	I feel as fit (or think I will feel as fit) during menstruation as I do during any other time of the month.	1	2	3	4	5	6	X
II	16.	Menstruation is a sign of womanhood.	1	2	3	4	5	6	X
IV	17.	I can tell (or think I will be able to tell) my period is coming because of breast soreness, backache, cramps, or other physical signs.	1	2	3	4	5	6	X
	18.	Most women make too much of the minor (little) physical effects of menstruation.	1	2	3	4	5	6	X

1	2	3	4	5	6	X
disagree a lot	disagree	disagree a little bit	agree a little bit	agree	agree a lot	don't know

FACTOR

III	19.	Menstruating every month is a sign of a woman's general good health.	1 2 3 4 5 6 X
IV	20.	I am (or think that I will be) more easily upset just before or during my menstrual period than at other times of the month.	1 2 3 4 5 6 X
V	21.	Cramps bother you only if you pay attention to them.	1 2 3 4 5 6 X
V	22.	Others should not be critical of a woman who is easily upset before or during her menstrual period.	1 2 3 4 5 6 X

* These four items are <u>not</u> part of the MAQ paper and should be scored separately.

Factors:

I Menstruation as a debilitating event
II Menstruation as a bothersome event
III Menstruation as a natural event
IV Anticipation of the onset of menstruation
V Denial of any effect of menstruation
IV Embarrassment about menstruation

Adolescent Menstrual Distress Questionnaire

Part II

An Explanation of What is Coming

In the following three pages you will be answering questions about how you feel or think you will feel at three different times of the month. The drawing below shows how we are dividing the month.

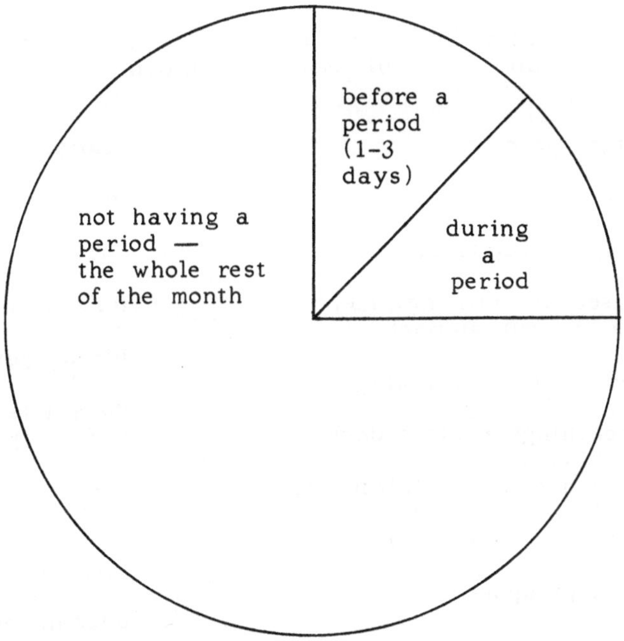

On the next three pages we will ask how you feel just before a period (1-3 days before), during a period (during the menstrual flow itself), and during the rest of the month. The next three pages will look the same but each page will ask about a different time of the month. Read the underlined words carefully.

Part II

Now we would like to ask you what you, yourself, feel or think you will feel <u>when you have your menstrual period</u> (that is, during the time of the menstrual flow). Mark each item using the scale below. A "1" means you don't feel that way at all, a "2" or a "3" means you feel that way a little bit, a "4" or "5" means you feel that way pretty much, and a "6" means you feel that way a lot. Use only one number for each item. Try to answer each item the best you can. If you have not yet begun to menstruate, and have absolutely no idea how you will feel, mark an "X" for that item.

1	2	3	4	5	6
not at all	a little bit	a little bit more	a fair amount	pretty much	a lot

_____ weight gain

_____ crying

_____ fatigue, feel tired

_____ nausea or vomiting; feel sick to your stomach

_____ have trouble breathing

_____ keep things neat; orderly

_____ avoid meeting or talking to people; don't want to see or talk to your friends

_____ anxiety; upset

_____ backache

_____ don't do so well in school

_____ get mixed up; confused

_____ take naps; stay in bed longer than usual

_____ headaches

_____ pimples

_____ stay away from school

_____ cramps

_____ feel dizzy or faint

_____ change in how you eat

_____ feel clumsy

_____ blind spots or fuzzy vision

_____ have lots of energy; bursts of activity

_____ don't pay attention well; difficulty in concentrating

_____ sore breasts

_____ buzzing or ringing in the ears

_____ swelling; feel heavier; swollen

_____ crabby or irritable

_____ mood swings; how you feel changes rapidly

_____ heart poundings

_____ depressed; feeling blue or sad

_____ have feelings of well-being; feel good

Part II

Now we would like to ask what your, yourself, feel or think you will feel just before you have your menstrual period (that is, one to three days before the period). Mark each item using the scale below. A "1" means you don't feel that way at all, a "2" or "3" means you feel that way a little bit, a "4" or a "5" means you feel that way pretty much, and a "6" means you feel that way a lot. Try to answer each item the best you can. If you have not yet begun to menstruate and have absolutely no idea how you will feel, mark an "X" for that item.

1	2	3	4	5	6
not at all	a little bit	a little bit more	a fair amount	pretty much	a lot

______ weight gain

______ crying

______ feeling tired, fatigue

______ nausea or vomiting; feel sick to your stomach

______ have trouble breathing

______ keep things neat; orderly

______ avoid meeting or talking to people; don't want to see or talk to your friends

______ upset, anxiety

______ backache

______ don't do so well in school

______ get mixed up; confused

______ take naps; stay in bed longer than usual

______ headache

______ pimples

______ stay away from school

______ cramps

______ feel dizzy or faint

______ change in how you eat

______ feel clumsy

______ blind spots or fuzzy vision

______ have lots of energy; bursts of activity

______ don't pay attention well; difficulty concentrating

______ sore breasts

______ buzzing or ringing in the ears

______ swelling, feel heavier; swollen

______ crabby or irritable

______ mood swings; how you feel changes rapidly

______ heart poundings

______ depressed; feeling blue or sad

______ feel good; have feelings well-being

Part II

Now we would like to ask what you, yourself, feel or think you will feel when you are not having your menstrual period (that is, the rest of the month). Mark each item using the scale below. A "1" means you don't feel that way at all, a "2" or "3" means you feel that way a little bit, a "4" or "5" means you feel that way pretty much, and a "6" means you feel that way a lot. Use only one number for each item. Try to answer each item the best you can. If you have not yet begun to menstruate and have absolutely no idea how you will feel, mark an "X" by that item.

1	2	3	4	5	6
not at all	a little bit	a little bit more	a fair amount	pretty much	a lot

_____ weight gain

_____ crying

_____ fatigue, feel tired

_____ nausea or vomiting; feel sick to your stomach

_____ have trouble breathing

_____ keep things neat; orderly

_____ avoid meeting or talking to people; don't want to see or talk to your friends

_____ anxiety; upset

_____ backache

_____ don't do so well in school

_____ get mixed up; confused

_____ take naps; stay in bed longer than usual

_____ headache

_____ pimples

_____ stay away from school

_____ cramps

_____ feel dizzy or faint

_____ change in how you eat

_____ feel clumsy

_____ blind spots or fuzzy vision

_____ have lots of energy; bursts of activity

_____ don't pay attention well; difficulty in concentrating

_____ sore breasts

_____ buzzing or ringing in the ears

_____ swelling; feel heavier; swollen

_____ crabby or irritable

_____ mood swings; how you feel changes rapidly

_____ depressed; feeling blue or sad

_____ heart poundings

_____ have feelings of well-being; feel good

MOOS MENSTRUAL DISTRESS QUESTIONNAIRE

Menstrual Symptom Questionnaire

Write the approximate dates of your most recent menstrual period (flow) in the space marked "A" below. Then write the dates of the menstrual period which preceded the most recent one in the space marked "D".

from_______ to_______	other times during most recent cycle	week before most recent flow	most recent flow from_______ to_______
D	C	B	A

On the next three pages is a list of symptoms women and girls sometimes experience. Please describe your experience of each of these symptoms during the three different time periods listed below:

Column 1 during your most recent menstrual flow (the dates indicated by area A on the diagram above).

Column 2 during the one week before your most recent menstrual flow (area B on the diagram above).

Column 3 during the remainder of your most recent menstrual cycle (area C on the diagram above).

Note: The answers you put in Columns 1, 2, and 3 should describe your experience specifically during your most recent menstrual cycle. Please do not simply report your general experience. Also, please report any experience of these symptoms whether or not they seem to you to be related to your menstrual cycle.

For each answer choose the category listed which best describes your experience of that symptom during that time. Write the number of that category in the space provided. Even if none of the categories are exactly correct, choose the one that best describes your experience. Do not leave any blank spaces.

Categories:

1 = no experience of symptom
2 = barely noticeable
3 = present, mild
4 = present, moderate
5 = present, strong
6 = acute or partially disabling

		1. most recent flow (A)	2. the week before (B)	3. the rest of the month (C)
(WR)	1. Weight gain	____	____	____
(CO)	2. Insomnia.	____	____	____
(NA)	3. Crying	____	____	____
(BC)	4. Lowered school or work performance. .	____	____	____
(P)	5. Muscle stiffness	____	____	____
(CO)	6. Forgetfulness.	____	____	____
(CO)	7. Confusion	____	____	____
(BC)	8. Take naps or stay in bed.	____	____	____
(P)	9. Headache	____	____	____
(WR)	10. Skin disorders	____	____	____
(NA)	11. Loneliness	____	____	____
(C)	12. Feelings of suffocation	____	____	____
(A)	13. Affectionate	____	____	____
(A)	14. Orderliness	____	____	____
(BC)	15. Stay home from work or school	____	____	____
(P)	16. Cramps (uterine or pelvic)	____	____	____
(AR)	17. Dizziness or faintness	____	____	____
(A)	18. Excitement	____	____	____
(C)	19. Chest pains	____	____	____

Categories:

1 = no experience of symptom
2 = barely noticeable
3 = present, mild
4 = present, moderate
5 = present, strong
6 = acute or partially disabling

			1. most recent flow (A)	2. the week before (B)	3. the rest of the month (C)
(BC)	20.	Avoid social activities	_____	_____	_____
(NA)	21.	Anxiety	_____	_____	_____
(P)	22.	Backache.	_____	_____	_____
(AR)	23.	Cold sweats	_____	_____	_____
(CO)	24.	Lowered judgment	_____	_____	_____
(P)	25.	Fatigue	_____	_____	_____
(AP)	26.	Nausea or vomiting	_____	_____	_____
(NA)	27.	Restlessness	_____	_____	_____
(AR)	28.	Hot flashes	_____	_____	_____
(CO)	29.	Difficulty in concentration	_____	_____	_____
(WR)	30.	Painful or tender breasts	_____	_____	_____
(A)	31.	Feelings of well-being.	_____	_____	_____
(C)	32.	Buzzing or ringing in ears	_____	_____	_____
(CO)	33.	Distractable	_____	_____	_____
(WR)	34.	Swelling (e.g., abdomen, breasts, ankles)	_____	_____	_____
(CO)	35.	Accidents (e.g., cut fingers, break dish).	_____	_____	_____
(NA)	36.	Irritability	_____	_____	_____
(P)	37.	General aches and pains	_____	_____	_____
(NA)	38.	Mood swings	_____	_____	_____
(C)	39.	Heart pounding	_____	_____	_____
(NA)	40.	Depression (feeling sad or blue) . . .	_____	_____	_____
(BC)	41.	Decreased efficiency	_____	_____	_____

Categories:

1 = no experience of symptom
2 = barely noticeable
3 = present, mild
4 = present, moderate
5 = present, strong
6 = acute or partially disabling

		1. most recent flow (A)	2. the week before (B)	3. the rest of the month (C)
(CO)	42. Lowered motor coordination	____	____	____
(C)	43. Numbness or tingling in hands and feet	____	____	____
	44. Change in eating habits	____	____	____
(NA)	45. Tension	____	____	____
(C)	46. Blind spots or fuzzy vision	____	____	____
(A)	47. Bursts of energy or activity	____	____	____

In what ways, if any, was your most recent menstrual cycle unusual?

MOOS SUBSCALES

WR =	water retention	(4 items)
CO =	concentration	(9 items)
NA =	negative affect	(8 items)
BC =	behavior change	(5 items)
P =	pain	(6 items)
AR =	autonomic reactions	(3 items)
A =	arousal	(5 items)
C =	control	(6 items)

44 = change in eating habits

Menstrual Distress

Each girl rated the severity of 30 symptoms taken from the Moos Menstrual Distress Questionnaire (MDQ; Moos, 1968) but modified by including more familiar adjectives for the younger girls (i.e., "crabby" as well as "irritable"). Each symptom was rated for severity on a six-point scale (experience the symptom "not at all" to "a lot") for the menstrual, the premenstrual, and the intermenstrual phases of the cycle. A definition of each of the cycle phases was given prior to filling out the MDQ. For example, girls were told that "the premenstrual phase is those 1 to 3 days just before the period starts. Please fill out the questionnaire items for what you typically feel or think you will feel premenstrually or *just before your menstrual period.*" Postmenarcheal subjects filled out the MDQ for their own experience, premenarcheal subjects for their expected experience. The eight factors by Moos (1968) are pain (cramps), water retention (swelling), negative affect (crying), arousal (bursts of energy), autonomic reactions (feel dizzy), behavioral change (school performance), concentration (confused), and control (symptoms not believed to vary with cycle phase). Psychometric information is provided by Moos. To control for response bias in overall symptom reporting, menstrual-intermenstrual and premenstrual-intermenstrual mean difference scores were used. Since the girls filled out the MDQ three times (for each of the cycle phases), the order of presentation was counterbalanced across subjects. No significant effects were found for the order in which the cycle-phase symptom data were collected.

Menstrual-Related Attitudes

The Adolescent Menstrual Feeling Scale (AMFS) is composed of 13 menstrual-related attitude items which are rated on a six-point scale ("disagree a lot" to "agree a lot"). The factor analysis using a varimax rotation generated four factors with Eigen values more than one (accounting for 53% of the variance). The factor loading for each item was $\leq .40$. The four factors were labeled: (1) negative evaluation ("menstruation is something I would prefer not to have"); (2) comfort talking to other persons about menstruation (male friends, female friends, mother, and father); (3) embarrassment ("when I have or will have my menstrual period, I am worried or will be worried that I will have an accident like spots on a skirt"); and (4) concern about acting normal ("I make an extra effort not to be crabby during my period" or "I will make an extra effort not to be crabby during my period").

The Menstrual Attitude Questionnaire (adolescent form) (MAQ) also was filled out by one-half of the longitudinal samples. The MAQ is comprised of 12 items which subjects rate on a seven-point scale (from "strongly disagree" to "strongly agree"). The MAQ was developed for college women; it was extended to college men and adolescent girls; and its alpha coefficients are high (Brooks-Gunn & Ruble, 1980). The five factors are: (1) menstruation is a natural event ("menstruation gives women a way to keep in touch with their bodies"), (2) menstruation is a debilitating event ("I am more easily upset just before and during my menstrual period than at other times of the month"), (3) menstruation is a predictable event ("I can tell my period is coming because of breast soreness, backache, cramps or other physical signs"), (4) menstruation is a bothersome event ("I hope it will be possible someday to get a period over in a few minutes"), and (5) denial of any effects of menstruation ("Most women make too much of minor [little] physical effects of menstruation"). Subjects were asked to fill out the MAQ in terms of their own attitudes, their perception of maternal attitudes, and their perceptions of girlfriends' attitudes.

Sources of Information

Subjects were asked to rate the amount they had learned about menstruation from each of 15 potential sources on a four-point scale ("learned nothing" to "learned a lot"). These responses were factor analyzed using a varimax rotation, and five factors had an Eigen value of more than one (accounting for 51% of the variance). All items had factor loadings of .40 or higher. The five sources were: (1) females (girlfriends, female adults, sisters, and overheard conversations), (2) males (male friends, male adults, and brothers), (3) media (television, magazines, and books), (4) health (nurses and health education classes), and (5) parents and doctor (mother, father, and doctor).

In addition, the subjects were asked how each of the 15 potential informational sources felt about menstruation, rating each source on a four-point scale ("feels very negative" to "feels very positive"). Using a varimax rotation, four factors had Eigen values of more than one (accounting for 69% of the variance). All items had factor loadings of .40 or higher. The four factors for perceptions of sources' feelings were: (1) females (mothers, older sisters, female friends, and female adults), (2) males (father, brothers, male friends, and male adults), (3) health (health education classes, nurses, and doctors), (4) media (television, magazines, and books). The source "overheard conversations" did not load on any of the factors.

From: J. Brooks-Gunn and D. N. Ruble, 1982. The development of menstrual-related beliefs and behaviors during early adolescence. *Child Development 53:* 1570-1571.

BIOMEDICAL ISSUES

HISTORICAL DEVELOPMENT OF PROGESTERONE THERAPY

Ronald V. Norris, M.D.

Corporate Medical Director
Healthcare Services of America, Inc.
Birmingham, Alabama

INTRODUCTION

The crash of the stockmarket was not the only momentous event of 1929. It was also an exciting year in our knowledge of female reproductive endocrinology. The use of the experimental method as a means of elucidating the origin and functional significance of the ovarian luteal body stems only from the beginning of this century. Prior to the turn of the century, there were approximately 2,000 years of curiosity, erroneous observation, and unfounded speculations embodied in the dialectical approach (Greep, 1977). One must keep in mind that the ovary had no known functional significance other than the production of ova until the works of Beard (1897), Prenant (1898), and Fraenkel (1903) were published. This is quite remarkable considering that the endocrine function of the testes had been established 50 years earlier (Berthold, 1849).

An explosion of meaningful research in reproductive endocrinology began in 1923 when Edgar Allen and Edward Doisy (1923) discovered the estrone-inducing hormone in the ovarian follicular fluid of the pig. In parallel work in the chemistry laboratories of Europe, the structure and nature of steroids were being elucidated, resulting in Nobel prizes being awarded to H. Wieland in 1927 and A. Windaus in 1928. Doisy, Veler, and Thayer (1929) isolated crystalline estrone from the urine of pregnant women on July 13, 1929 to culminate the first step in the long quest to identify the female sex hormones. There was great excitement in the budding world of female reproductive endocrinology, but back to that in a moment.

FIRST DESCRIPTIONS OF PREMENSTRUAL TENSION

At about this same time, R. T. Frank (1929) published a book entitled *The Female Sex Hormone*, based upon lectures he had given at the University of Illinois School of Medicine in December 1928. In this book, he first described the symptom complex of "premenstrual tension" and coined the term. Premenstrual disturbances of manifold nature had been described for centuries in women and had appeared in the world medical literature beginning early in the 19th century (Bullough & Voght, 1973; DeWees, 1847; Macht, 1943). In the later 1800's and early 1900's, reports appeared in American medical literature describing certain disorders which occurred in certain women only premenstrually. A popular gynecological textbook (Novak, 1924) described such phenomena without viewing them as part of a symptom-complex or syndrome. Although Frank was among the researchers publishing extensively on the quest for an understanding of female sex hormones during the previous 25 years, he is now remembered only for his published description of premenstrual tension in 1929 [and erroneously had his first publication concerning the subject cited as 1931 (Frank, 1931)]. It is interesting that this journal article was published outside of Frank's discipline of gynecology and was based upon a lecture he had delivered to the Section of Neurology and Psychiatry of the New York Academy of Medicine. The article received little comment at the time as the phenomenon of premenstrual tension was well known, if not well understood, and was recognized by many physicians, although not by all (Norris & Sullivan, 1983). With the isolation and identification of the female sex hormones, many disorders, including premenstrual tension, were being attributed to reproductive endocrine changes.

ISOLATION AND PURIFICATION OF PROGESTERONE

With the first isolation of an estrogen in 1929, attention rapidly shifted to the second important step in the quest for the female sex hormones — the isolation of the progestin. George Corner (1928), at the University of Rochester, mated rabbits and soon thereafter removed the corpora lutea from the females. When these rabbits were killed a few days later, the embryos were found to be degenerating, their fate tied to the progestational change in the endometrium of the uterus, which had been arrested as a result of the corpus luteum ablation. In an effort to identify the active agent in the corpus luteum, Corner invited Willard Allen, a student in the medical school with a background in organic chemistry, to join him (Allen, 1974; Corner, 1974). Within a year, they obtained crude extracts from pig ovaries which were successful in inducing full progestational changes and maintaining pregnancy in castrated female rabbits (Allen & Corner, 1929; Corner & Allen, 1929). Within two years, Allen had purified the material extracted from the corpus luteum and obtained a product in crystalline form. In 1934, with Wintersteiner of Columbia University, he confirmed, in the laboratory, the empirical formula of the hormone (Wintersteiner & Allen, 1934), subsequently named progesterone (Allen, Butenandt, Corner, & Slotta, 1935). Slotta, Raschig, and Fels (1934) had also proposed this formula, but on a purely speculative basis. In record time, the synthesis of progesterone from stigmasterol and pregnanediol (Allen, 1939) was achieved by the combined chemical ingenuity of Butenandt (see Butenandt & Westphal, 1934) and Fernholz (1934). Both progesterone and related synthetic steroid compounds with similar biologic action were given the generic name "progestins" (Fernholz, 1934).

CLINICAL USE OF PROGESTERONE FOR PREMENSTRUAL TENSION

Shortly after Allen had isolated and purified progesterone in the laboratory in 1934, he used some of it to successfully relieve one of his patients of premenstrual tension (W. M. Allen, personal communication, 1982). At the time, the most popular lay treatment for premenstrual tension and other female disorders was Lydia E. Pinkham's Vegetable Compound, which had attained sales of over $3 million annually by 1925. Although it was not known to contain progesterone or any other female sex hormones, Miss Pinkham's vegetable compound did contain botanicals consisting of Unicorn root *(Aletris farinosa)*, Life root

(Senecio aureus), Black Cohosh *(Cimicifuga racemosa)*, Pleurisy root *(Asclepias tuberosa)*, and Fenugreek seed *(Foenum graceum)* suspended in 18% alcohol (Stage, 1979). Some have thought the alcohol was the explanation for the relief it brought. However, these botanicals are among those known to contain plant steroid estrogens and glycosides, and more importantly, sapogenins from which progesterone was subsequently converted by the remarkable Russell Marker (1947), as we shall see a little later in our story.

RESEARCH ON THE ROLE OF PROGESTERONE IN PREMENSTRUAL SYNDROME

Israel (1938) was the first to suggest a rationale for the use of progesterone in the treatment of premenstrual syndrome (PMS). He demonstrated proliferative endometrial changes as a result of estrogen stimulation in four severely affected women during the premenstruum, when one would expect to see secretory endometrial changes as a result of progesterone stimulation. He postulated that an unopposed estrogen effect due to a deficiency of progesterone production was the cause of the symptoms. Later reports (Morton, 1950; Widholm, Frisk, & Tenhunen, 1967) of other indirect measurements of progesterone effects obtained from endometrial biopsies and vaginal smears supported this view. Studies of luteal (premenstrual) phase steroid levels in women suffering from PMS have documented a relative progesterone deficiency in relation to a possible estrogen excess (Backstrom & Mattsson, 1975; Backstrom, Wide, & Sodergard, 1976; Munday, Brush, & Taylor, 1977, 1981). Other conflicting data have been reported from measurement of basal body temperature and endometrial biopsies, and from assessments of urinary and serum ovarian steroid levels (Anderson & Larsen, 1979; Bickers & Wood, 1951; Greenblatt, 1940). A problem in assessing these discrepant reports (and a continuing recurrent problem in assessing all studies related to PMS) is that selection criteria for patients and the definition of PMS varied between studies, and the study populations were not homogeneous.

Following Allen's use in 1934 and Israel's use in 1938 of progesterone to successfully treat PMS, three similar reports were published in the 1940's (Albaux-Fernet & Loublie, 1946; Gray, 1941; Puech, 1942). This leads us back to the extraordinary and eccentric Russell Marker.

PRACTICAL ISSUES IN THE SYNTHESIS OF PROGESTERONE

Initially, science left to nature the task of producing the minute quantity of hormone needed for testing purposes, and progesterone was painstakingly extracted from the ovaries of sows. It required the ovaries of 50,000 sows to recover 20 milligrams of progesterone! Laboratory methods (degradation of higher substances down to the hormone, conversion of similar steroids, and/or assembly from suitable precursors) were subsequently perfected for synthesizing steroid hormones, chiefly from bile acids and cholesterol, and large scale production for therapeutic applications resulted. The manufacture and sale of synthetic sex hormones during the period prior to World War II was controlled by Schering in Germany, Ciba in Switzerland, Organon in Holland, and Parke-Davis in the United States. This monopoly, plus the use of raw materials which were in limited supply, resulted in a price of $100 per gram of progesterone produced via cholesterol or pregnenolone recovered from urine. It became imperative to locate raw materials which would be available in abundance even if war broke out and which were suitable for economical conversion using newly designed processes. The first search was limited to steroids closely related to the hormones occurring naturally in large amounts, such as cholesterol from lambs' wool, stigmasterol from soybeans, and bile acids from ox bile. These sources proved to be neither inexhaustible nor suitable for high yield conversion.

As Witzman (1981) tells it, in 1928, while Corner was ablating the corpora lutea of rabbit ovaries, as we have previously discussed, Russell Marker accepted a position at the Rockefeller Institute to take charge of the production of various materials they had not been able to synthesize. Subsequently, he was to publish 32 scientific papers in six years on molecular structure and optical rotation, an unusual feat at any time. During the two years prior to joining the Institute while working for the Ethyl Gasoline Corporation, he developed a method still valid today for determining the antiknock quality of gasoline according to "octane rating." (He accomplished all of this after being refused a Ph.D. by the University of Maryland despite a brilliant doctoral dissertation. He was late in filling out the proper paper work in order to receive the degree!) To pursue his new interest in steroid synthesis, he left the Institute and accepted a junior position at Pennsylvania State University and a grant from Parke-Davis.

It was clear to Marker that the raw materials for steroid synthesis had to come from plants whose steroids could be easily converted. It was his conviction that the sapogenins (the steroid portion of the saponins which produce foam in water and were used by primitive peoples as soap) found in the sarsaparilla plant were the desired source. By a simple and still common process (called "Marker degradation"), he converted the sapogenin of the sarsaparilla plant into progesterone in 1939. However, available amounts of sarsaparilla plant were not sufficient to support an industry. Reviewing botany textbooks, he learned that sarsaparilla is one of the Liliaceae, the lily family, which includes additional species containing sapogenin such as the roots in Lydia E. Pinkham's famous vegetable compound and the Dioscorea plant from Japan. Marker obtained a sapogenin from Dioscorea called diosgenin and successfully converted it to progesterone. But how could one ensure a continuous supply of Dioscorea from Japan in 1940? The resourceful Marker discovered a variety of Dioscorea root, called *cabeza de negro*, which protruded from the ground like a bushy head of hair, and grew in the Tehuantepec Jungle in the province of Veracruz in Mexico. A few days prior to the attack on Pearl Harbor, he went to Mexico and called upon the President of the Republic for assistance in finding this root. Needless to say, he was gently escorted to the American embassy and out of the country. True to his character, he returned to Mexico in January 1942 and found the *cabeza de negro* roots, and took them with him back to Pennsylvania State. There he confirmed that the root was full of diosgenin which could be converted to progesterone. When Parke-Davis refused to set up the necessary laboratory, he discontinued his relationship with them and returned to Mexico virtually penniless. In 1943, working in a potter's shed with makeshift equipment, he converted several tons of *cabeza de negro* root into about three kilograms of progesterone worth $160,000 at the going market price. With the two chemist-owners of the nearby small Laboratorios Hormona, he formed what was to become one of the largest steroid manufacturers of the world today — Syntex. Large scale manufacturing of progesterone began, but Marker did not patent the process. He soon tired of the manufacturing business and in 1947 sold his share of Syntex to the other owners for a small amount of money and returned to the jungle. In his travels, he found yet another variety of Dioscorea, called barbasco root. It was used by the Indians for fishing by whipping the water with the roots until the amount of sapogenin leached-out was sufficient to reduce the water's surface tension to the point where the fish actually drowned without being poisoned. The barbasco root contained ten times the diosgenin found in the *cabeza de negro* root and took only three years to mature as opposed to twenty. As one might expect, Marker worked at converting diosgenin from the barbasco root into progesterone for only a short time and then also grew tired of the endeavor. In 1949, at the age of 47, he tore up all his work, flushed thousands of dollars of progesterone down the drain, and returned to Pennsylvania State University never to work with steroids again!

Dr. George Rosenkranz, a former student of the 1939 Nobel prize winner L. Ruzicka, came to Mexico by way of Cuba and replaced Marker at Syntex. The company became a major producer of synthetic progesterone for the American and international markets. The price of progesterone dropped from $80 per gram in 1941 when first produced by Marker to $18 per gram when Syntex first mass-produced it, to 48¢ per gram in 1952 when Syntex sold tons of it.

It was also discovered at about this time that a mold, *Rhizopus arrhizus*, would cause an oxygen atom to attach to the C-11 position of the progesterone molecule creating the corticosteroids (Peterson, 1952). Further, it was discovered that a bacterium would create a double bond in ring A of the progesterone molecule, leading to the creation of estrogens. Thus, Marker's economical progesterone synthesis and his discovery of the diosgenin-abundant barbasco root attained their true significance in modern medicine. Progesterone rapidly became the most important substance in the steroid-producing industry. The free enterprise system soon sought a way out of the Mexican raw materials monopoly, and improved chemical techniques permitted utilization of steroids that had been unsuitable previously. Stigmasterol, which is recovered in large quantities as a by-product of soybean oil production, was used once again. Roussel, a French company, developed a process of total synthesis of progesterone. Now progesterone is abundantly available in a highly micronized form to improve absorption.

DALTON'S ROLE IN THE USE OF PROGESTERONE THERAPY FOR PREMENSTRUAL SYNDROME

Having progressed to the 1950's in our history of the development of progesterone therapy, we must now discuss another remarkable individual, Katharina Dalton. Dalton, a general practitioner, and Raymond Greene, an endocrinologist who had successfully treated Dalton's premenstrual migraine headaches with progesterone, published a paper in May 1953 in which they coined the term "premenstrual syndrome" (Greene & Dalton, 1953). [To place ourselves in the proper historical perspective from a reproductive endocrinology standpoint, this was about the same time that Gregory Pincus and M. C. Chang (1953) were publishing their classical paper on the effects of progesterone and related compounds on ovulation and early development in the rabbit.] Greene and Dalton analyzed 84 cases of PMS and described the successful treatment of 72 of 78 cases with ethisterone or progesterone. Rees (1953) and Mukherjee (1954) also reported successful treatment of PMS with progesterone. Dalton (1959) then published a report in which she compared several progestins in the treatment of PMS and concluded that progesterone was the superior hormone. Dalton has relentlessly pursued the description and treatment of PMS since that time, and has evaluated more women with PMS than any physician or group of physicians in the world (Dalton, 1977, 1984). Further, she has treated thousands of women with progesterone during the past 30 years — undoubtedly encompassing the largest uncontrolled trial in history of a single medication by one physician for one disorder! Unfortunately, Dalton has never completed any randomized double-blind placebo-controlled trials of progesterone in the treatment of PMS. Nor has she conducted long-term, epidemiologically sound, follow-up studies as to possible deleterious side effects. She has described the follow-up monitoring of 120 women on continuous progesterone for five years, and of 19 women on progesterone therapy for over 15 years (Dalton, 1984), none of whom experienced adverse effects. Our own follow-up study of 50 women who have been on various cyclical doses of progesterone for over three years has shown no significant change in prolactin, estradiol, follicle-stimulating hormone (FSH), luteinizing hormone (LH), cortisol, aldosterone, cholesterol, high density lipoprotein, triglycerides, serum glutamic pyruvic transaminase, bilirubin, alkaline phosphatase, urinalysis, blood pressure, or in results of physical examination.

THE PREMENSTRUAL SYNDROME-PROGESTERONE CONTROVERSY

In the 1960's, two reports appeared concerning successful use of progesterone in PMS, but both were uncontrolled studies (Parker, 1960; Waxman, 1968). During this time, progesterone was available in injectable, suppository, and oral lozenge forms as it was in the 1950's (Norris, 1985). Clinical and research interest in progesterone was diminishing throughout this time and continued until the present, as the focus moved to the other synthetic progestins and "the pill" (McLaughlin, 1982).

Unfortunately, all of the studies reporting success with progesterone in PMS cited to this point have not used a controlled, double-blind research design as is now required for scientific acceptance (Spodick, 1982). Numerous scientific writers (for example, Glick, 1985) cite a paper by Smith (1976) as being a controlled study and state he "found no significant difference between results with progesterone and those with placebo." Those actually reading this paper of Smith's will discover that it is an exceedingly brief review article on mood and the menstrual cycle, and presents no data whatsoever! Smith's previous book chapter (Smith, 1975) does little better, although it also is often cited similarly. In fact, Smith, Cleghorn, Streiner, and Younglai (1975) did publish a paper on the negative results of a "double-blind controlled study of intramuscular progesterone as therapy for premenstrual depression." Unfortunately, they did not indicate in the paper how the PMS subjects were selected, how they defined the disorder, nor any confirmation on the diagnosis. The authors did state that intramuscular injections were given "every two days starting about ten days prior to the expected onset of menses," but they fail to state the dose of progesterone used. Further, their table (indicating the mean plasma progesterone levels measured) fails to demonstrate a significant difference between progesterone-treated cycles and placebo-treated cycles. This leads one to wonder if the progesterone was actually given or if it was only poorly absorbed.

The other study often cited (Sampson, 1979) is superior in design to the Smith et al. study and does represent a double-blind controlled trial of progesterone given by suppository or pessary and compared with placebo. Sampson worked with Dalton, so one would assume that the study design, diagnostic selection criteria, and use of progesterone essentially conform to Dalton's. One of the major flaws of this study is that it uses the Moos Menstrual Distress Questionnaire (MDQ; Moos, 1977) to make the diagnosis of PMS. This assessment tool is a poor instrument for this purpose, as it cannot differentiate between PMS and a premenstrual exacerbation of an affective or other disorder which may be present throughout the menstrual cycle but worsen premenstrually. Review of how the Moos MDQ was derived makes this obvious (Moos, 1968). The study population consisted of wives of university graduate students with an average age of 25.2 $\pm$ 3.9 years and varying degrees of parity, hardly a population representative of women who would be most likely to have PMS. Women who might have been pregnant or on oral steroidal contraceptives were not excluded from the study. The variety of changes assessed during the various phases of the menstrual cycle in these women used *retrospective* methods which have been shown to be invalid because of the tendency of women with randomly occurring or chronic changes or symptoms to selectively remember these changes as occurring during the premenstrual phase of the cycle (Abplanalp, Donnelly, & Rose, 1979; Rubinow, Roy-Byrne, & Hoban, 1984; Ruble & Brooks-Gunn, 1979). Sampson's (1981) case descriptions suggest that some women were suffering from an affective disorder and possibly PMS as well. Another flaw of this study is that only two doses of progesterone were used, the levels being 200 milligrams twice a day and 400 milligrams twice a day. Dalton's (1984) work indicates, and our report confirms (Norris, 1983), that 62% or less of a population of PMS sufferers would respond positively to these doses of that particular progesterone suppository. Other studies indicate there is wide variation in absorption of progesterone from suppositories from one woman to another (Nillius & Johansson, 1971), and absorption is dependent upon the suppository base used (Price, Ismail, Gorwill, & Sarda, 1983). Suffice it to say that an adequate randomized, double-blind, placebo-controlled, cross-over study has yet to be completed. An adequate study would at least include: (1) an acceptable operational definition of premenstrual syndrome; (2) a homogeneous study population; (3) prospective daily assessment through several menstrual cycles of mood, behavior, and physical symptoms using either a 6-point daily rating form (Endicott & Halbreich, 1982) or a visual analogue scale (DeJong, Rubinow, Roy-Byrne, Hoban, Grover, & Post, 1985) to quantify changes; (4) use of the same daily assessment instrument during the progesterone-placebo phase of the trial; and (5) regardless of route of administration, measurement of serum progesterone concentrations to confirm absorption.

CURRENT STATUS OF PROGESTERONE THERAPY AND RESEARCH RELATING TO PREMENSTRUAL SYNDROME

Renewed interest in PMS and progesterone developed in this country in 1981 when we opened the first diagnostic and treatment center specializing in PMS, and Dalton began to gain public recognition in the United States (Clark & Shapiro, 1981; Toufexis, Simpson, & Wymelenberg, 1981). We applied to the Food and Drug Administration (FDA) to conduct a double-blind, placebo-controlled trial of progesterone suppositories in the treatment of PMS. The study was to be financed by L.D. Collins, Ltd., the British manufacturer of the progesterone suppositories (Cyclogest) to be used. We proposed to use the progesterone in the study in the manner described by Dalton (1977). It was our contention that Dalton's near 30-year claims for the efficacy of progesterone in PMS needed to be put to a test. It was our concern, and our prediction, that with the rapidly developing physician and public awareness of PMS, and with progesterone being an approved prescription drug available through pharmacists, that the demand for treatment with progesterone would quickly increase. If our proposed controlled trials, and those of others, demonstrated progesterone to be efficacious, then other side-effect and safety studies could be begun forthwith. However, if it were to be demonstrated that progesterone was not an effective treatment, physicians and the public could be so advised, and its growing use could be discouraged and diminished. The FDA was not persuaded. At a hearing of the FDA Fertility and Maternal Health Drugs Advisory Committee (1981) in November, the question of "What is the maximum safe dose of progesterone that may be administered for the treatment of premenstrual syndrome?" was briefly addressed at the very end of a long day. Without presentations of data or opinion on the question, the Committee agreed on 200 milligrams a day! The Committee Chairman admitted that the Committee had not reviewed our study proposal prior to making their decision (Today Show, 1981). Based upon our experience and that of Dalton (1977) and Sampson (1979), we could confidently predict that a 200 milligram Cyclogest suppository a day would be ineffective. It seemed hardly fair to the women suffering from PMS who would be the study subjects, or to those who would be committing considerable time, energy, and money to the study, to proceed. In our opinion, the only study worth doing was one which used dose ranges like those used in clinical practice in England during the previous 15 years and now used in the United States. The study was therefore abandoned. The FDA Committee did subsequently hold a hearing on progesterone and PMS in February 1983 (see chapter by Rubinow, this volume). Essentially, they confirmed their prior position and urged pharmacokinetic studies of progesterone. To date, no credible double-blind controlled study of progesterone in the treatment of PMS has been published.

In June 1983, we formulated detailed plans for an epidemiologic study into the long-term effects of progesterone treatment. We proposed to use the PMS patients at University College Hospital in London who had been treated with progesterone as an index group, and to use patients from other PMS centers in England who had been treated with vitamins and other medications as the comparison group. We intended to follow-up patients who had been treated in the previous 10-20 years, specifically assessing them for cancer, liver disease, cardiovascular, and cerebrovascular disease. The proposal was met with enthusiasm, but died in its infancy as we failed to gain cooperation from a key physician (K. Dalton, personal communication, July 8, 1983).

CONCLUSIONS

Progesterone is increasingly being prescribed in this country for premenstrual syndrome, luteal phase defect, and *in vitro* fertilization. It is the responsibility of any physician prescribing progesterone for any disorder to inform the patient that an approved drug is being administered for an unlabeled or nonapproved use (FDA, 1982; Kapp, 1981). Review of the endocrinologic and metabolic literature might reveal other instances where progesterone might prove beneficial, as in the treatment of hypertension (De Soldati, De Forteza, Pellegatta, & Cammarota, 1966) or respiratory control disorders (Goldman, Morrison, & Foster, 1981). Such a circumstance requires that the efficacy of progesterone be well established by randomized controlled clinical trials for each disorder. Further investigations into safety are also required.

The studies published during the past five years concerning the non-contraceptive health benefits of steroidal contraceptives are reassuring (Mishell, 1982). So, too, are the studies which support the concept that C-21 steroids, such as progesterone, do not cause major anomalies when given to pregnant women (McDonough, 1985). Numerous reports support the view that progesterone does not cause gross adverse metabolic effects (Bardin, Milgrom, & Mauvais-Jarvis, 1983; Kalkhoff, 1982; Ottosson, Johansson, & von Schoultz, 1985). In evaluating these studies and others, one must keep in mind that there has been far too much "lumping" (Chez, 1978) when it comes to discussing the progestins, and that the 19-nortestosterone derivatives and C-21-substituted progestins have different properties from 17-alpha-hydroxyprogesterone and progesterone (Rozenbaum, 1982). Therefore, each progestin must be studied individually.

With the expected increased availability and use in clinical practice of progesterone in the oral micronized form (Lane, Siddle, Ryder, Pryse-Davies, King, & Whitehead, 1983; Maxson & Hargrove, 1985; Whitehead, Townsend, Gill, Collins, & Campbell, 1980) or intranasal spray (Anand, David, & Puri, 1977), the studies of efficacy and safety become even more imperative. No one possesses a patent for progesterone, and only a unique delivery vehicle is likely to be patentable. Therefore, the ethical drug industry has little financial incentive to support this research. This is additionally true, as positive proof of the efficacy and subsequent increased use of progesterone would likely reduce the use of other of their medications. Therefore, it is incumbent upon governmental agencies and foundations to vigorously support this research.

The history of the development of progesterone therapy has been fascinatingly full of human interest and controversy. One might surmise that its future will continue to be the same for some time to come.

REFERENCES

Abplanalp, J. M., A. F. Donnelly, and R. M. Rose, 1979. Psychoendocrinology of menstrual cycle, I: Enjoyment of daily activities and moods. *Psychosomatic Medicine 41:* 587-604.

Albaux-Fernet, M. and G. Loublie, 1946. *Seminar Hospital Paris 22:* 1487-1490.

Allen, E. and E. A. Doisy, 1923. An ovarian hormone. A preliminary report on its localization, extraction, and partial purification and action in test animals. *Journal of the American Medical Association 81:* 819-824.

Allen, W. M., 1939. Biochemistry of the corpus luteum hormone, progesterone. In: E. Allen, C. H. Danforth, and E. A. Doisy (Eds.), *Sex and Internal Secretions*. Williams & Wilkins, Baltimore, MD, pp. 901-928.

Allen, W. M., 1974. Recollections of my life with progesterone. *Gynecological Investigations 5:* 142-182.

Allen, W. M. and G. W. Corner, 1929. Physiology of the corpus luteum: IV. *Proceedings of the Society for Experimental Biology and Medicine 27:* 403-405.

Allen, W. M., A. Butenandt, G. W. Corner, and K. H. Slotta, 1935. Nomenclature of corpus luteum hormone. *Science 82:* 153.

Anand, Kumar T. C., G.F.X. David, and V. Puri, 1977. Ovulation in rhesus monkeys suppressed by intranasal administration of progesterone and norethisterone. *Nature 270:* 532-535.

Anderson, A. W. and J. F. Larsen, 1979. Bromocriptine in the treatment of premenstrual syndrome. *Drugs 17:* 383-385.

Backstrom, T. and B. Mattsson, 1975. Correlation of symptoms in premenstrual tension to oestrogen and progesterone concentrations in blood plasma. *Neuropsychobiology 1:* 80-86.

Backstrom, A. W., L. Wide, and R. Sodergard, 1976. FSH, LH, TeBG-capacity, estrogen and progesterone in women with premenstrual tension during the luteal phase. *Journal of Steroid Biochemistry 7:* 473-476.

Bardin, C. W., E. Milgrom, and P. Mauvais-Jarvis (Eds.), 1983. *Progesterone and Progestins*. Raven Press, New York, NY.

Beard, J., 1897. *The Span of Gestation and the Cause of Birth. A Study of the Critical Period and Its Effects in Mammalia.* Gustav Fischer, Jena, German Democratic Republic.

Berthold, A. A., 1849. Transplantation der hoden. *Archive Anatomie Physiologie und Wizzenschaft Medicine 16:* 42-46.

Bickers, N. and M. Wood, 1951. Premenstrual tension: Rational treatment. *Texas Report on Biology and Medicine 9:* 406-419.

Bullough, V. and M. Voght, 1973. Women, menstruation and nineteenth-century medicine. *Bulletin of the History of Medicine 47:* 66-82.

Butenandt, A. and U. Westphal, 1934. Uber die Darstellung des Corpus-luteum-Hormons aus Stigmastrin: Die Konstition des Corpus-luteum-Hormons. *Berichte Deutschen Chemische Gesellschaft 67:* 2085-2087.

Chez, R. A., 1978. Proceedings of the symposium "Progesterone, Progestins, and Fetal Development." *Fertility and Sterility 30:* 16-26.

Clark, M. and D. Shapiro, 1981. The monthly syndrome. *Newsweek,* May 4, p. 74.

Corner, G. W., 1928. The effect of very early ablation of the corpus luteum on embryos and uterus. *American Journal of Physiology 86:* 74-81.

Corner, G. W., 1974. The early history of progesterone. *Gynecological Investigations 5:* 106.

Corner, G. W. and W. M. Allen, 1929. Physiology of the corpus luteum: II. *American Journal of Physiology 88:* 326-346.

Dalton, K., 1959. Comparative trials of new oral progestagenic compounds in the treatment of the premenstrual syndrome. *British Medical Journal 2:* 1307-1309.

Dalton, K., 1977. *Premenstrual Syndrome and Progesterone Therapy.* William Heinemann Medical Books, Ltd., London.

Dalton, K., 1984. *Premenstrual Syndrome and Progesterone Therapy* (second edition). William Heinemann Medical Books, Ltd., London.

Dejong, R., D. R. Rubinow, P. Roy-Byrne, M. C. Hoban, G. N. Grover, and R. M. Post, 1985. Premenstrual mood disorder and psychiatric illness. *American Journal of Psychiatry 142:* 1359-1361.

De Soldati, L., I. E. De Forteza, C. R. Pellegatta, and H. Cammarota, 1966. The antihypertensive action of progesterone. *Cardiologia 48:* 489-503.

DeWees, W. P., 1847. *A Treatise on the Disease of Females.* Lea and Blanchard, Philadelphia, PA.

Doisy, E. A., C. D. Veler, and S. Thayer, 1929. Folliculin from urine of pregnant women. *American Journal of Physiology 90:* 392.

Endicott, J. and U. Halbreich, 1982. Psychobiology of premenstrual change. *Psychopharmacology Bulletin 18:* 109-112.

Fernholz, E., 1934. Zur synthese des corpus-luteum-hormons. *Berichte Deutschen Chemische Gesellschaft 67:* 1855-1862.

Food and Drug Administration, 1981. *Safety and Efficacy of Progesterone and 17-Hydroxyprogesterone for Treatment of Reproductive Disorders.* Fertility and Maternal Health Drugs Advisory Committee. FDA, Rockville, MD, November.

Food and Drug Administration Bulletin, 1982. *Use of Approved Drugs for Unlabeled Indications.* FDA, Rockville, MD, April 4-5.

Fraenkel, L., 1903. Die function des corpus-luteum. *Archive Gynakologischen 68:* 438-445.

Frank, R. T., 1929. *The Female Sex Hormone.* Charles C. Thomas, Baltimore, MD, p. 236.

Frank, R. T., 1931. The hormonal causes of premenstrual tension. *Archives of Neurology and Psychiatry 26:* 1053-1057.

Glick, I. D., 1985. Treatment of premenstrual syndrome in psychiatric practice. In: H. J. Osofsky and S. J. Blumenthal (Eds.), *Premenstrual Syndrome: Current Findings and Future Directions.* American Psychiatric Press, Washington, D.C., pp. 57-65.

Goldman, A. L., D. Morrison, and L. J. Foster, 1981. Oral progesterone therapy: Oxygen in a pill. *Archives of International Medicine 141:* 574-575.
Gray, L. A., 1941. The use of progesterone in nervous tension states. *Southern Medical Journal 34:* 1004-1006.
Greenblatt, R. B., 1940. Syndrome of major menstrual molimina with hypermenorrhea alleviated by testosterone propionate. *Journal of the American Medical Association 115:* 120-124.
Greene, R. and K. Dalton, 1953. The premenstrual syndrome. *British Medical Journal 1:* 1007-1014.
Greep, R., 1977. The genesis of research on the progestins. *Annals of the New York Academy of Sciences 286:* 1-8.
Israel, S. L., 1938. Premenstrual tension. *Journal of the American Medical Association 110:* 1721-1723.
Kalkhoff, R. K., 1982. Metabolic effects of progesterone. *American Journal of Obstetrics and Gynecology 142:* 735-738.
Kapp, M. B., 1981. Prescribing approved drugs for nonapproved uses. Physicians' disclosure obligations to their patients. *Law, Medicine and Health Care,* October, pp. 20-23.
Lane, G., N. C. Siddle, T. A. Ryder, J. Pryse-Davies, R.J.B. King, and M. I. Whitehead, 1983. Dose-dependent effects of oral progesterone on the oestrogenized postmenopausal endometrium. *British Medical Journal 287:* 1241-1245.
Macht, D. I., 1943. Further historical and experimental studies on menstrual toxin. *American Journal of Medicine & Science,* September, pp. 281-305.
Marker, R., 1947. New sources of sapogenins. *Journal of the American Chemical Society 69:* 2242.
Maxson, W. S. and J. T. Hargrove, 1985. Bioavailability of oral micronized progesterone. *Fertility and Sterility 44:* 622-626.
McDonough, P. G., 1985. Progesterone therapy: Benefit versus risk. *Fertility and Sterility 44:* 13-16.
McLaughlin, L., 1982. *The Pill, John Rock, and the Church.* Little, Brown and Co., Boston, MA.
Mishell, D. R., 1982. Noncontraceptive health benefits of oral steroidal contraceptives. *American Journal of Obstetrics and Gynecology 142:* 809.
Moos, R. H., 1968. The development of a menstrual distress questionnaire. *Psychosomatic Medicine 30:* 853-867.
Moos, R. H., 1977. *Menstrual Distress Questionnaire Manual.* Social Ecology Laboratory, Department of Psychiatry and Behavioral Sciences, Stanford University, Stanford, CA.
Morton, J. H., 1950. Premenstrual tension. *American Journal of Obstetrics and Gynecology 60:* 343.
Mukherjee, C., 1954. Premenstrual tension: A critical study of the syndrome. *Journal of the Indiana Medical Association 24:* 81-97.
Munday, M. R., M. G. Brush, and R. W. Taylor, 1977. Progesterone and aldosterone levels in premenstrual tension syndrome. *Journal of Endocrinology 73:* 21.
Munday, M. R., M. G. Brush, and R. W. Taylor, 1981. Correlation between progesterone, oestradiol and aldosterone levels in the premenstrual syndrome. *Clinical Endocrinology 14:* 1-9.
Nillius, S. J. and E.D.B. Johansson, 1971. Plasma levels of progesterone after vaginal, rectal, or intramuscular administration of progesterone. *American Journal of Obstetrics and Gynecology 110:* 470-477.
Norris, R. V., 1983. Progesterone for premenstrual tension. *Journal of Reproductive Medicine 28:* 509-516.
Norris, R. V., 1985. Clinical management of the premenstrual tension syndrome. In: M. Y. Dawood, J. L. McGuire, and L. M. Demers (Eds.), *Premenstrual Syndrome and Dysmenorrhea.* Urban and Schwarzenberg, Baltimore, MD, pp. 67-76.

Norris, R. V. and C. Sullivan, 1983. *PMS: Premenstrual Syndrome.* Rawson Associates, New York, NY.

Novak, E., 1924. *Menstruation and Its Disorders.* Appleton, New York, NY.

Ottosson, U. B., B. G. Johansson, and B. von Schoultz, 1985. Subfractions of high-density lipoprotein cholesterol during estrogen therapy: A comparison between progestogens and natural progesterone. *American Journal of Obstetrics and Gynecology 151:* 746-750.

Parker, A. S., 1960. The premenstrual tension syndrome. *Medical Clinics of North America 44:* 339-348.

Peterson, D. H., 1952. Microbiological transformation of steroids. *Journal of the American Chemical Society 74:* 5933.

Pincus, G. and M. C. Chang, 1953. The effects of progesterone and related compounds on ovulation and early development in the rabbit. *Acta Physiologica Latinoamericana 3:* 177-183.

Prenant, A., 1898. La valeur morphologique du corps jaune. Son action physiologique et therapeutique possible. *Revue General Science Pure Applied Bulletin Association of France for Advanced Science 9:* 646-650.

Price, J. H., H. Ismail, R. H. Gorwill, and I. R. Sarda, 1983. Effect of the suppository base on progesterone delivery from the vagina. *Fertility and Sterility 39:* 490-493.

Puech, A., 1942. Menstrual disorder. *Montpellier Medicine 21:* 118.

Rees, L., 1953. The premenstrual tension syndrome and its treatment. *British Medical Journal 1:* 1014-1016.

Rozenbaum, H., 1982. Relationships between chemical structure and biological properties of progestogens. *American Journal of Obstetrics and Gynecology 142:* 719-724.

Rubinow, D. R., P. Roy-Byrne, and M. C. Hoban, 1984. Prospective assessment of menstrually related mood disorders. *American Journal of Psychiatry 141:* 684-686.

Ruble, D. N. and J. Brooks-Gunn, 1979. Menstrual symptoms: A social cognition analysis. *Journal of Behavioral Medicine 2:* 171-194.

Sampson, G. A., 1979. Premenstrual syndrome: A double-blind controlled trial of progesterone and placebo. *British Journal of Psychiatry 135:* 209-215.

Sampson, G. A., 1981. An appraisal of the role of progesterone in the therapy of premenstrual syndrome. In: P. A. van Keep and W. H. Utian (Eds.), *The Premenstrual Syndrome.* MTP Press, Lancaster, England, pp. 51-69.

Slotta, K. H., H. Raschig, and E. Fels, 1934. Reindarstellung der hormone aus dem corpus luteum. *Berichte Chemische Gesellschaft 67:* 1270-1273.

Smith, S. L., 1975. Mood and menstrual cycle. In: E. J. Sacher (Ed.), *Topics in Psychoendocrinology.* Grune & Stratton, New York, NY, pp. 19-59.

Smith, S. L., 1976. The menstrual cycle and mood disturbance. *Clinical Obstetrics and Gynecology 19:* 391-397.

Smith, S. L., J. M. Cleghorn, D. L. Streiner, and E. V. Younglai, 1975. A study of estrogens and progesterone in premenstrual depression. In: *The Family.* 4th International Congress of Psychosomatic Obstetrics and Gynecology, Tel Aviv. Karger, Basel, pp. 538-542.

Spodick, D. H., 1982. The randomized controlled clinical trial: Scientific and ethical bases. *American Journal of Medicine 73:* 420-425.

Stage, S., 1979. *Female Complaints: Lydia Pinkham and the Business of Women's Medicine.* W. W. Norton, New York, NY.

Today Show, 1981. NBC Television, November 20.

Toufexis, A., J. C. Simpson, and S. Wymelenberg, 1981. Coping with Eve's curse. *Time,* July 27, p. 59.

Waxman, D., 1968. Progesterone and premenstrual tension syndrome. *British Medical Journal 4:* 188.

Whitehead, M. I., P. T. Townsend, D. K. Gill, W. P. Collins, and S. Campbell, 1980. Absorption and metabolism of oral progesterone. *British Medical Journal 280:* 825-828.
Widholm, O., M. Frisk, and T. Tenhunen, 1967. Gynecological findings in adolescence. *Acta Obstetrica and Gynecologica Scandinavica (Suppl. 1) 46:* 1-7.
Wintersteiner, O. and W. M. Allen, 1934. Crystalline progestin. *Journal of Biological Chemistry 107:* 321-336.
Witzman, R. F., 1981. *Steroids.* Van Nostrand Reinhold, New York, NY.

SHOULD PREMENSTRUAL SYNDROME BE A LEGAL DEFENSE?

Katharina Dalton, F.R.C.G.P.

University College Hospital
London, England

INTRODUCTION

Before premenstrual syndrome (PMS) can be accepted as a basis for a legal defense, three conditions need to be fulfilled. First, the narrow definition must be recognized, understood, and followed. Second, it must be shown that treatment has diminished the occurrence of criminal acts. Third, effective treatment must be freely available and implemented with adequate supervision to ensure that criminal acts are not repeated during successive premenstra.

DEFINITION

The definition of PMS that has been diagnostically effective in the identification of women whose criminal behavior can be modified by appropriate hormonal intervention is: "The recurrence of symptoms in the premenstruum with complete absence of symptoms in the post-menstruum" (K. Dalton, 1984).

The criteria required to satisfy this definition are threefold:

1. Recurrence of symptoms in every cycle, which, for practical purposes, may be taken as recurrence in at least the last three consecutive menstrual cycles.

2. Limitation of symptoms to the premenstruum or luteal phase; that is, from ovulation until menstruation. The luteal phase cannot be longer than 14 days, even in those women with cycles as long as 35 days. The symptoms may continue during early menstruation, particularly if there is only a slight menstrual loss. Slight bleeding at the beginning of menstruation in such instances, while chronologically menstruation, must be considered physiologically as an extension of the premenstruum.

3. Complete absence of symptoms after true menstruation begins, for a minimum of seven consecutive days. In most cases, we have found that normality is restored for considerably longer, usually for two or three weeks.

In addition, the defendant must be menstruating regularly and not be pregnant, as PMS symptoms characteristically ease during pregnancy. Neither can PMS be implicated in a defense during menopause. As an example, a 57-year-old London housewife charged with shoplifting had not menstruated for five years, and, therefore, was unsuccessful in her claim that her actions were due to PMS.

DIAGNOSIS

We have found that the only positive method of diagnosis is by the menstrual chart, on which the patient records co-instantaneously the presence of symptoms in relation to her menstrual cycle. The diagnosis is then readily made on the basis of the clustering together of the days when the symptoms, or offenses, occur during the premenstrual, post-ovulatory (or luteal) phase of the cycle. The chart is then also used during treatment to ascertain its efficacy as judged by the absence of the previously recurring symptoms. Without these records, no accurate diagnosis can be made, nor can the treatment be evaluated. We have, therefore, found it necessary at the PMS Clinic at University College Hospital, London, where the work has been carried out for 30 years, to discharge any woman who fails to bring her menstrual chart to two consultations. Where the patient is confused or amnesic, the charting can be done by the husband, a parent, or other close observer. Examples of this occurred with three women who committed criminal acts and were diagnosed as having PMS. All three had been initially referred to me because their fathers had observed the relationship between their aberrant behavior in relation to menstruation (K. Dalton, 1980).

Another source of evidence may be personal diaries, where many women keep records of menstruation, although not necessarily noting the dates of their symptoms. Such evidence can be used when combined with other retrospective sources such as police files, hospital admission records for previous suicide attempts or self mutilation, and employer's records of absences or lateness for work. Even a prospective chart starting on the day of the alleged offense and continuing for at least three months while awaiting trial may be helpful in establishing a diagnosis.

At times, the woman herself may be aware that she is cyclically at risk and may even try to arrange her life to minimize the consequences. As an example, consider the part-time community nurse, who worked 10 days per month and chose her duty days with care to avoid the premenstruum, knowing how confused she would then become for one or two days. When a colleague fell ill, she was called to work during her premenstruum. During this time, she stole a prescription form and forged a prescription for appetite suppressants. The administrative nursing officer later gave evidence on her behalf of the meticulous way she calculated her confused days, which were then taken into account when drawing up each month's duty rota. As a criminal offense, the case was dismissed. Progesterone therapy was instituted and was effective in eliminating the confusion (K. Dalton, 1982a).

In other cases, the woman may be unaware of her situation. In the instance of a 47-year-old housewife charged with shoplifting, the husband gave evidence that one day each month, his wife would obtain some inappropriate item from the shops, such as dog food when they had no animals, or baby clothes although their children were almost adults. His wife could never remember how she obtained the items. Knowing that her lapses occurred at predictable intervals, he made great efforts to ensure that the car, cash, and credit cards were not available to her during the days she was at risk. In evidence, he showed his diary of the days when he knew precautions would be required. On the basis of his testimony, the charges against her were dismissed and progesterone treatment was successfully instituted (K. Dalton, 1982a).

We have previously reported the notorious case of the barmaid, Sandie Smith, who was charged with the murder of another barmaid who was her friend (K. Dalton, 1980). The evidence relating this incident to PMS was obtained retrospectively from entries in her prison documents. These showed the precise dates of 30 separate episodes of impulsive behavior, which included trying to set fire to her cell, trying to escape, an attempted strangling, an attempted drowning, smashing windows, cutting her wrist, and committing assault. Statistical analysis of the dates of these episodes of violence while in prison suggested an average cycle length of 29.55 ± 1.45 days, which would accommodate the time between the episodes of violence, and an average cycle length of 29.04 ± 1.47 days, which would accommodate the inter-episode periods for the previous 26 offenses on the basis of which she had been committed to prison (K. Dalton, 1984). The judge accepted this as evidence of PMS, and her sentence was postponed for five months in order to determine whether progesterone therapy would be effective. There were no more episodes of bizarre behavior during that time, and it was further reported that she had become a model prisoner, busy writing poetry and reading one book a day. Therefore, she was released on probation for three years, with the condition that the treatment be continued (K. Dalton, 1980).

In each of the above instances, the circumstances, although highly varied, illustrate the range of expression of PMS. These individual variations are sufficiently instructive to warrant a case history approach rather than a conventional statistical treatment which would obscure the details so important as medical models and legal precedents.

MENSTRUAL DISTRESS

Menstrual distress is NOT PMS. It is the presence of symptoms throughout the months, which increase in severity during the paramenstruum (premenstruum and menstruation). The mere coincidence of an offense being committed during the premenstruum does not constitute PMS. The diagnosis of PMS requires the cyclical recurrence of symptoms which are limited to the premenstruum, as exemplified in the classical description of a PMS woman, which originally put me on the track of PMS: "We have to call a doctor out every month; the only time we don't is when she is pregnant" (K. Dalton, 1955). In contrast, symptoms of menstrual distress are present throughout the menstrual cycle. These may be due to an imbalance of any, some, or none of the menstrual hormones, but do not provide a basis for legal defense at the present time.

Survey data demonstrating the effect of menstruation on such varying events as schoolgirls' work, behavior, and examinations; crime; admissions to hospital for medical, surgical, psychiatric, orthopedic, or infectious fever emergencies; and children's emergency admissions at times of the mother's menstruation may be examples of menstrual distress but not necessarily of PMS (K. Dalton, 1984).

The Moos Menstrual Distress Questionnaire (Moos, 1968) or its modified version (Clare, 1982) are excellent tools for diagnosing menstrual distress, for which they were designed, but they cannot be used for the diagnosis of PMS as they do not specify the complete absence of symptoms in the postmenstruum. Even analyzing the questionnaires quantitatively using sine waves, as suggested by Sampson and Jenner (1977), fails to show the essential complete absence of symptoms in the postmenstruum.

In PMS, symptoms are only present in the luteal phase when progesterone is present in the peripheral blood, and symptoms are absent during the follicular phase of the cycle when no progesterone is present in the peripheral blood. These findings may appear inconsistent since symptoms occur only when progesterone is present in the luteal phase and are absent when no progesterone is present. Why, then, doesn't treatment with progesterone make them worse? We now know that there are cells in the body, particularly in the brain, which require intermittent provision of progesterone in the luteal phase. If there is insufficient progesterone when it is needed, symptoms result. For this reason, prophylactic progesterone must be added to ensure an adequate supply. Symptoms of PMS are also absent during pregnancy, when an additional source of progesterone develops in the form of the placenta. This produces abundant progesterone, rising to some 30 times the maximal level found in a normal menstruating woman at the peak of her luteal phase.

DIAGNOSTIC POINTERS

While the diagnosis of PMS requires a positive menstrual chart, a checklist score can be computed utilizing risk factors associated with the occurrence of PMS. Such a score is not definitive evidence of PMS, but may be quite helpful in initial screening of an individual for possible presence or absence of PMS (K. Dalton, 1982b). Such factors include:

1. Initial onset at the time of a major hormonal event; e.g., puberty, completion of a pregnancy, termination of the use of oral contraceptives, amenorrhea, or sterilization.

2. Increased severity, similarly, occurring at the time of a major hormonal event.

3. Side effects of oral contraceptives, including such symptoms as headaches, depression, weight gain, and nausea. [Since all oral contraceptives today contain artificial progestagens, it should be noted that these lower the blood progesterone level. This is in contrast to natural progesterone, which raises the blood progesterone level, except when taken orally, in which case it is inactivated by the liver (Nillius & Johansson, 1971)].

4. Weight gain in adult life exceeding 12 Kg.

5. Pregnancy complicated by threatened abortion, pre-eclampsia, or postnatal depression.

6. Increased libido in the premenstruum.

7. Altered hunger during the premenstruum.

8. Altered tolerance to alcohol during the premenstruum.

The checklist percentage score can be obtained by multiplying the sum of the positive items by 100 (excluding the non-relevant items) and dividing by the sum of the positive and negative items. If a score exceeding 70% is obtained, it is likely that the menstrual chart will prove positive. However, even a score of 100% is still not diagnostic of PMS without a positive menstrual chart.

Retrospective diagnosis is feasible in Britain because a patient's full medical records are held by the general practitioner, and these records are passed on to the next general practitioner should a patient move. The information in such records can be utilized as legal evidence. For example, in the case of Mrs. English, who was charged with the murder of her lover, the medical records were taken as evidence that she suffered from PMS (*R. v. English*, 1982). She had previously been admitted to the hospital following a premenstrual suicide attempt; she had twice suffered from postnatal depression requiring hospital admission; and she suffered loss of libido when taking oral contraceptives. Furthermore, during her incarceration immediately following the murder, she commented to the police about her increased libido during the premenstruum. She started menstruation 19 hours after the incident. In sum, her checklist score was 100%.

When the medical records of a 34-year-old mother accused of infanticide were examined, several indications of PMS were found. She had previously consulted her doctor about PMS, which was indicated as starting at puberty. Her first pregnancy had been complicated by pre-eclampsia. Her second pregnancy had been followed by postnatal depression, for which she had received a domiciliary visit from a consultant psychiatrist. At the age of 21 years, she developed high blood pressure severe enough to warrant admission to the London Hospital for five days of investigations. As in the case of Mrs. English, her checklist score was 100%. She was acquitted on the charge of infanticide and has since successfully received progesterone, including prophylactic progesterone therapy for postnatal depression, and has another daughter, now 12 months old (K. Dalton, 1985). The greater difficulty in collecting complete medical records in the United States would make retrospective diagnosis more difficult.

BIOCHEMICAL TESTS

There is little diagnostic value to a single measurement of progesterone level in the luteal phase. This is also true for estradiol, FSH, LH, or prolactin, although obtaining serial levels in PMS sufferers and controls for research purposes may reveal differences that could help to unravel etiological factors.

The only biochemical test that we have found useful as an aid in diagnosing PMS is the measurement of sex hormone binding globulin (SHBG). One indicator of the relationship is the finding of a dose-related rise in SHBG when PMS patients are given progesterone (M. E. Dalton, 1981, 1984a). Validity of the SHBG assay was established in a study of 50 women with unequivocal diagnosis of severe PMS, based on their menstrual charts, versus 50 women with complete absence of PMS symptoms (M. E. Dalton, 1981). The result of this study was complete discrimination of these two groups, with low SHBG scores in all the women with PMS (range: 13-49 nmols dihydrotestosterone bound per liter) and no such low scores in the women without PMS (range: 50-80 nmols dihydrotestosterone bound per liter) (M. E. Dalton, 1984a, b). This bimodal clustering is derived through careful selection of the women tested. This was not a full spectrum of normal menstruating women, but two very different samples of women taken from the same hospital or clinic; namely, those with *severe diagnosed* PMS, and those *completely free* from any premenstrual symptoms.

There have been conflicting data reported on the validity of SHBG levels as a diagnostic indicator for PMS. The following methodological variations are suggested as responsible for the negative findings reported by other investigators (Backstrom, Wide, Sodergard, & Cartensen, 1976).

(1) Failure to ensure that the patient is receiving no medication (including self-medication with analgesics) or herbal or vitamin preparations, which can introduce significant uncontrolled variability in both PMS-affected and PMS-unaffected groups.

(2) Unknown variability is also introduced if the definition used for PMS is other than that specified at the outset of this chapter. As indicated above, the SHBG discrimination is specifically valid for differentiating severely affected versus symptom-free individuals.

(3) Methodological congruence is critical. The women must be on no medication, as noted above, nor be suffering from thyroid or liver disease. Neither can they be obese or hirsute. The blood sample must be centrifuged immediately after being taken and stored frozen until assaying. The test itself must be done with the purified two-tier column method of Iqbal and Johnston (1977). (Although at present, this procedure is not performed in the United States, Metpath Laboratories of New York and Los Angeles do fly frozen blood samples to England daily for SHBG estimations at Metpath's London Laboratories.) There is only slight variation during the menstrual cycle and in the same untreated women measured at intervals of 12 or more months. The deviations are measured from the population norm, which in Britain is 50-80 nmols dihydrotestosterone bound per liter.

(4) Lack of agreement among investigators as to the normal range for SHBG for menstruating women *who do not suffer from PMS* can be attributed to several factors. One is the diversity of "control" subjects. When determining the normal range of a new parameter, it is usual for laboratories to recruit volunteers from their staff without necessarily identifying (a) the presence or absence of premenstrual symptoms and normality of menstruation; (b) prescribed or self-medication; and (c) hirsutism, obesity, thyroid, or liver disease. Another factor (as cited above) is lack of uniformity of the assay used. M. E. Dalton (1984b) has presented a comparative study of the checklist scores and the SHBG measurements as diagnostic tools, using a sample of 112 women with PMS, and 102 women referred by their doctor as having PMS but whose diagnosis was not confirmed by subsequent menstrual charts. An additional sample of 42 women, with a double diagnosis of both PMS and another disease, was excluded. The results from the two discrete samples indicated that SHBG discriminated PMS better than the checklist. The only risk factors of significance in differentiating the two groups were intolerance of oral contraceptives, an adult weight change exceeding 12 Kg, and a history of postnatal depressions.

GENETIC FACTORS

A genetic factor appears to be involved in PMS. Sixteen pairs of female twins were all evaluated by this author during 1984. Their diagnoses were by menstrual charts, and all were affected severely enough to require medical treatment. Six of the seven monozygotic pairs exhibited PMS in both sisters, whereas only three of the nine dizygotic pairs had PMS in both sisters. This small sample is not statistically significant but is suggestive, and the study is continuing.

Kantero and Widholm (1971) studied premenstrual *symptoms* (note: NOT premenstrual syndrome) in adolescent daughters and mothers. They noted that 63% of daughters of symptom-free mothers were also symptom-free, but if the mother had premenstrual fatigue or irritability, nearly 70% of the daughters had similar symptoms.

PREMENSTRUAL SYMPTOMS IN A LEGAL PERSPECTIVE

Symptoms alone are not sufficiently indicative of PMS to provide a basis for legal defense. Symptoms which can occur in PMS are highly variable and include recurrent rhinitis, sore throat, asthma, migraine, conjunctivitis, and urethritis (K. Dalton, 1984). Somatic symptoms alone cannot be considered as a legal defense. It is only where there is a recurrent, temporary mood disturbance in the premenstruum, with return to normality afterwards, that PMS can constitute the basis for a legal defense.

It is the psychological symptoms of PMS which have provided a basis for legal defense in Great Britain. These symptoms include psychosis (including delusions, hallucinations, confusions, paranoia), amnesia, loss of control leading to violence, suicidal depression, and nymphomania. In such cases, it remains a matter of chance whether the woman is admitted to a mental hospital or charged with a crime. If she is still confused or deluded at the time she is apprehended, she is more likely to be admitted to the hospital, while if she has returned to normal psychological functioning when the offense is discovered, the chances are that she will be prosecuted. The following examples are illustrations of the importance of the psychological stigmata of the PMS in the legal arena.

A 15-year-old Michigan schoolgirl imagined she was the "Great Goddess." As such, she felt she was so vitally important that she could walk across the road and all traffic would stop, or she could go into a shop, buy to her heart's content, and would not be required to pay. She was admitted to the hospital and tranquilized. Within two days, menstruation started and normal thought processes returned. The next month, she believed she was Adam's wife, and her duty was to procreate the world. She was again admitted to the hospital in her premenstruum. Her parents then recalled previous less severe incidents, all of which occurred premenstrually. With consultation achieved through transatlantic telephone calls, progesterone treatment was organized with her gynecologist and psychiatrist. When seen for follow-up at six months and again two years later, there had been no further incidents.

Another case is the 14-year-old daughter of an education officer in Indiana who became irrationally violent each premenstruum. At such times, she could not be controlled at home and would need hospital admission. The chronological relationship to menstruation is exemplified by the occasion when her flow started while she was awaiting medical attention in the admission ward. Her parents recognized that the emotional turmoil was therefore soon to subside, so they waited a few hours and took her home without treatment or admission. She then had complete amnesia for her violence, as shown by her innocent questions the next day at breakfast: "When are you going to have the door and window mended? How did they get broken?" Progesterone therapy was again arranged through a transatlantic consultation. This young woman has also responded to progesterone therapy (400 milligram suppositories twice daily) and has been well for the last two years.

A 43-year-old housewife from Hertfordshire was charged with shoplifting. She was asked to accompany the plainclothes police officer to the police station, and her disordered thinking then became evident. On the journey, she became convinced that the police officer was a rapist, based on her observations that he wore the same color socks and shoes and was proceeding down the same road reportedly used by a rapist. Her husband and elder daughter confirmed that the defendant had similar strange episodes each premenstruum, but they had not realized appropriate treatment was available. The shoplifting charge was dropped, and progesterone treatment (400 milligram suppositories thrice daily) was started.

Some PMS sufferers have paranoid thoughts recurring only during each premenstruum, with the absence of such thoughts in the postmenstruum. In some cases, paranoid thoughts lead to criminal acts. One example would be the poison pen writers for whom a cyclical pattern often can be easily established using the postage date on the envelope. Others find control of their temper impossible during the immediate premenstruum. In their frustration, they become violent, sometimes resulting in child abuse. A woman, now 51 years old and still menstruating regularly, who abused her 5-year-old daughter in 1961, is still receiving progesterone therapy (400 milligram suppositories twice daily) under my care. Her PMS had developed after severe preeclampsia and resulted in violence each premenstruum.

Premenstrual depression may be so severe that a cry for help is made. The commonest method is a suicidal attempt, but other forms of seeking attention should be recognized as a *cri de coeur*. These include self-mutilation, arson, and telephone hoaxes. An example is an 18-year-old student who was charged with arson (K. Dalton, 1980). Her behavior was exemplary until her menarche at 13 years. By the following year, her behavior had become bizarre. On one occasion, she set fire to the curtains in her bedroom. On another, she shaved off her hair and eyebrows. A few weeks later, she slashed her fingers to the extent that they needed suturing. Finally, she burnt down her father's house and was committed to prison. Retrospective evidence confirmed that these episodes coincided with the premenstruum. She was first treated with progesterone while in prison, and the psychiatrist reported the change in her as "a real miracle." She was released and is now, four years later, in excellent health on progesterone (100 milligram injections daily), and is seeking a Queen's pardon to remove the stigma of criminality from her records.

Another example of this is the case of a 19-year-old unemployed girl who would use the emergency telephone at monthly intervals to report alleged fires, burglaries, or accidents. The police were forced to act on each hoax call. She was warned, placed on probation, and finally committed to prison. Within days of her release, she had again committed the same offense. The monthly cyclicity of the offenses was then recognized, and progesterone therapy started in 1979. She remained well behaved and gradually the dose of her progesterone was reduced from 100-milligram to 25-milligram intramuscular injections daily. One day she returned for her monthly consultation stating that, during the premenstruum, she once again had the urge to enter a telephone box to make a false call, but now she could control the urge. When she was given a higher dose of progesterone (50 milligram injections daily), even these controllable urges disappeared.

CHARACTERISTICS OF PREMENSTRUAL SYNDROME CRIME

There are several characteristics of PMS crime which distinguish it from crime in general. First, the woman always acts alone, not with a gang or in a well organized fashion. The following case is an example of a crime committed during the individual's premenstruum but not attributable to PMS. A 34-year-old vagabond, together with an unemployed man, was charged with murder of an elderly man in his lodgings. They went prepared to burgle the house, and came complete with fire lighting equipment so that they could disguise their crime by setting what would appear to be an accidental fire. This happened during the woman's premenstruum. However, there was no evidence to support her plea of PMS, and it was rejected.

Second, the offense is not premeditated and usually comes as a surprise even to those who were with the defendant shortly before the incident. This was evident in the case of Sandie Smith, who had spent a reportedly happy evening with the barmaid she later murdered. She had even defended her in a quarrel with another couple only minutes before the stabbing.

Third, the action is without apparent motive, such as the arsonist who goes to some distant town and randomly sets fire to a building.

Fourth, there is typically no attempt to escape detection. The telephone hoaxer will stay in the telephone box where she made the call and wait for the police to take her to the station.

Fifth, the action may be a *cri de coeur* manifested as self-mutilation, arson, or an obvious shoplifting offense.

CHARACTERISTICS OF PREMENSTRUAL SYNDROME OFFENDERS

During 1982, the author personally saw 38 women who may be categorized as "PMS offenders;" i.e., individuals who suffer from PMS, who committed a crime during the premenstruum, and who subsequently received progesterone therapy (K. Dalton, 1984). Their crimes (often multiple) included: assault to person (20), arson (7), damage to property (6), theft (6), alcoholic intoxication (6), disorderly conduct (4), school truancy (2), nymphomania (2), hoax telephone calls (2), drugs (2), and homicide (2). They differed from 68 PMS women who admitted to violence in the premenstruum, but were not charged with crimes, in that the "offenders" tended to damage themselves (13%) or other persons (53%), while the "violent" women tended to damage property (94%) and never themselves (0%). The "offenders" were younger, averaging 25 years, as opposed to the "violent" group, averaging 38 years, but they had the usual risk factors of inability to tolerate oral contraceptives and a high incidence of postnatal depression.

During 1982, 22 women with premenstrual psychosis were also treated with progesterone. They, too, were young, 63% being below 35 years, and they had a high incidence of the known hormonal risk factors; i.e., inability to tolerate oral contraceptives containing artificial progestagens which lower progesterone blood level (100%), postnatal depression (94%), and the time of PMS onset occurring at the time of a hormonal event (94%) (K. Dalton, 1984).

ETIOLOGY

The statistical analysis of 1,095 women with PMS treated with progesterone during 1982 supports the hypothesis that PMS, as covered by the narrow definition, is progesterone responsive (K. Dalton, 1984). Exactly where in the metabolic pathway of progesterone the fault lies is unknown, and probably varies across different women. The fault may lie with the neuropeptides or in the hypothalamus, at which level imbalances of endorphins, catecholamines, serotonin, monoamines, and other as yet unknown substances may be significant. "Errors" in secretion of prolactin, adrenalin, renin, aldosterone, thyroid hormone, and pancreatic hormones may all be involved. The output of follicle stimulating hormone (FSH) and luteinizing hormone (LH) from the pituitary may be insufficient. At the ovarian level, not only is estrogen necessary, but FSH receptors are required within the ovarian cells before FSH can be utilized. Before LH from the pituitary can be utilized, it is necessary for LH receptors to be formed within the ovarian cells, and this requires the presence of estradiol, FSH receptors, and FSH. If FSH receptors, FSH, LH receptors, LH, and estradiol are all available, then progesterone can be produced by the Graafian follicle and passed into the peripheral blood. Hormones are carried in the blood stream bound to special protein molecules, which in the case of the sex hormones are known as the sex hormone binding globulins (SHBG). These bind preferentially to dihydrotestosterone, then testosterone, and then estradiol (Vermeulen, 1971).

Before the free progesterone molecules can be used by the tissue cells, progesterone receptors are needed within the cells to transport a free molecule across the cell wall, through the cytoplasm, and into the nucleus where it is metabolized. It is now known that progesterone receptors are plentiful in the cells of the limbic area also known as the midbrain (Greenstein, 1978) and identified as the area associated with rage and violence in animals. They are also found in nasopharyngeal passages, lungs, liver, breasts, eyes, and uterus. All these tissues require intermittent provision of progesterone. Replacement of progesterone in women with PMS relieves all associated symptoms, but progesterone does not relieve all symptoms of menstrual distress.

BLOOD GLUCOSE LEVELS

Sudden irrational behavior, aggression, and violence can result from relative hypoglycemia arising from food deprivation or defects in the regulatory mechanisms associated with blood sugar levels (K. Dalton, 1984). Accordingly, women with moderate or severe PMS should not go for long intervals without carbohydrates. A pattern of eating small amounts frequently (e.g., snacks every three hours) is advisable.

Sandie Smith, who was charged with murder but released after progesterone proved effective in stabilizing her behavior, required daily progesterone injections, which in Britain are given in the home by a community nurse. On one occasion, an administrative error resulted in the district nurse failing to attend for four days and Sandie got herself into trouble again. She randomly threw a brick at a shop window, phoned the police to report the happening, and waited patiently for the police to arrest her. Enquiry showed that not only had the incident occurred when she had missed her progesterone, but also when she had eaten no food for nine hours. She was then released under an order which stated that the nurse's duty each day was not only to give the progesterone injection, but also to ensure that she was eating adequately and frequently. There have been no further problems with her in the last five years. In her case, both progesterone (100 milligram injections daily) and dietary regulation were required.

TREATMENT

All cases of PMS involving a criminal offense should be regarded as severe, and initially progesterone treatment should be given. If daily supervision is required, this can be ensured by administering the progesterone by intramuscular injection, as is done in Great Britain by the community nurse. When progesterone is given orally, it is largely inactivated by the liver and only a very small rise in the blood progesterone level occurs. Progesterone is, therefore, either administered by vaginal or rectal suppository or by deep intramuscular injections. There is a marked difference in the ability of different women to absorb progesterone (K. Dalton, 1984). Some 5-10% of women do not absorb sufficiently from the suppositories and, for this reason, require injections. A nasal preparation has recently been shown to provide good absorption, as evidenced by a rise in blood progesterone level in the follicular phase of normally menstruating women (M. E. Dalton, 1985). Clinical studies of this preparation are now in progress.

Each woman needs individual adjustment of her progesterone regimen. This is not surprising when one appreciates that menstrual cycles vary in duration from 21 to 35 days, the flow may last from 2 to 8 days, and the type and duration of symptoms vary widely. PMS patients have individual progesterone requirements, just as diabetics have individual requirments for insulin. Furthermore, progesterone therapy should be regarded as prophylactic. It therefore should be started at ovulation or at least five days before symptoms are expected.

In order for PMS to be considered as appropriate for medicalization rather than for criminalization, it is necessary to provide assurances that PMS will be adequately treated. It could thus be assured that the criminal act is unlikely to be repeated and the public can be protected.

CLINICAL TRIALS

The ethics of the scientific investigator places a high priority on hypothesis-testing involving double-blind, controlled, crossover studies. However, special problems in regard to clinical trials of progesterone for premenstrual syndrome need to be appreciated. The protocol must contain the precise definition and method of diagnosis as stated in this chapter. The selection of informed volunteers to act as PMS subjects and matching controls must include consideration of the following variables:

1. *Length of normal menstrual cycle.* This varies from 21 to 35 days.

2. *Duration of menstruation.* This varies from 2 to 8 days.

3. *The day of heaviest loss.* Premenstrual symptoms ease only after the full menstruation has been established. In some women, there may be a scanty flow before onset of the full blood loss, in which case premenstrual symptoms may continue during the first few days of apparent menstruation.

4. *Age and parity.* PMS has a higher incidence after age 35, as well as with increasing parity, especially if pre-eclamptic toxemia or postnatal depression has occurred. Controls must not only be matched for ages, but also for these complications of pregnancy.

5. *Differing types of presentation.* Variations include different presentations of a multiplicity of symptoms, as well as differing duration.

6. *Ethnic background.* Janiger, Riffenburgh, and Kersch (1972) studied the cultural differences of 33 common premenstrual *symptoms* (note: not PMS) asking volunteers to evaluate the intensity of their symptoms in the most recent menstruation as none, mild, moderate, or severe. Their sample included 135 American, 100 Japanese, 35 Nigerian, 28 Apache, 51 Turkish, and 50 Greek women. While PMS symptoms were present in all cultures studied, there was considerable variation in the severity and frequency of symptoms. Thus, the Japanese reported relative absence of breast pain and breast engorgement, and the Nigerians reported a high frequency of headaches.

7. *Contraception.* To ensure that a hormonal imbalance is not present in the controls, it is necessary to ensure that they have not taken hormonal contraceptives during the previous six months; are not using an intrauterine device; have not had a bilateral tubal ligation (as this may reduce progesterone level); are not anxious to conceive (as these individuals are likely to disqualify themselves during the 6-month study); and are not infertile (as this may also be due to hormonal problems). This limits the selection of volunteers, and raises the question of whether the individual who has not been excluded for one of the above reasons is indeed sexually and psychologically normal.

If a woman subject to premenstrual outbursts of violence, suicidal attempts, alcoholic urges, epileptic fits, or asthmatic attacks is receiving regular medication to prevent a life threatening event, would it be ethical to stop such medication? If such medication is stopped and a tragedy results, would the event be adequately covered by insurance compensation? Had the obsession with double-blind, controlled trials existed when insulin was first discovered, on whose conscience would lie the death of the placebo-receiving diabetic? The World Medical Association's 1975 Helsinki Declaration states unequivocally that "concern for the interests of the subject must always prevail over the interests of science and society."

CONCLUSIONS

Premenstrual syndrome can constitute a recognizable and treatable condition, appropriate for attention in criminal proceedings, if a specific definition is used; i.e., that posed by the author and presented at the beginning of this chapter. This definition has been derived from extensive clinical experience over a 35-year period with a particular treatment protocol. The diagnosis is largely dependent upon menstrual charts, although a checklist of risk factors can provide reliable corroboration. Assay of sex hormone binding globulin levels provides further documentation of PMS. With the stated definition, the appropriateness of PMS for inclusion in criminal deliberations has been demonstrated in Great Britain. It remains to be seen if PMS will be addressed similarly by the United States courts.

It is important to emphasize that foregoing criminal action in cases of PMS in favor of medical treatment implies the necessity of accessible effective ameliorative measures. In Great Britain, as previously mentioned, the courts have recognized the benefits of progesterone therapy in stabilizing PMS behavior, progesterone treatment is freely available through our National Health Service, and supervision is available through our system of community nurses and probation officers, none of which is yet available in the United States.

Ethical considerations demand that the medical practitioner provide the most effective treatment for the patient. Investigative science has developed procedural conventions such as the double-blind, crossover approach as prerequisite to drawing a conclusion regarding the effectiveness of such treatment even where case histories seem clearly to have established this. In order to reconcile these objectives, the approach that we have used is that of matched controls. Such an approach provides the patient the best treatment available, as determined according to the evidence from the case history method, and at the same time permits clinical scientists to test the inferences on the basis of paired comparisons with a control group where no harm is done by either administering or withholding treatment.

Psychiatrists should consider PMS as a possible diagnosis in those patients admitted as acute emergencies. This is particularly relevant for those who quickly revert to normal with the onset of menstruation. PMS can be a severely disabling condition. Its sufferers deserve compassionate support and assistance from all relevant professionals.

REFERENCES

Backstrom, T. L., L. Wide, R. Sodergard, and H. Cartensen, 1976. FSH, LH, TeBg — capacity, estrogen and progesterone in women with premenstrual tension in the luteal phase. *Journal of Steroid Biochemistry 7:* 473-476.

Clare, A. W., 1982. Psychiatric and social aspects of premenstrual complaint. *Psychological Medicine (Monograph Supplement) 4:* 1-58.

Dalton, K., 1955. Discussion on the Premenstrual Syndrome. *Proceedings of the Royal Society of Medicine 50:* 415-417.

Dalton, K., 1980. Cyclical criminal acts in premenstrual syndrome. *The Lancet 2:* 1070-1071.

Dalton, K., 1982a. Legal implications of PMS. *World Medicine,* April 17, pp. 93-94.

Dalton, K., 1982b. An overview — premenstrual tension. In: R. Friedman (Ed.), *Menstruation and Behaviour.* Marcel Dekker, New York, Chapter 11.

Dalton, K., 1984. *Premenstrual Syndrome and Progesterone Therapy* (second edition). Year Book Publishers, Chicago; and William Heinemann Medical Books, London.

Dalton, K., 1985. Progesterone prophylaxis used successfully in Postnatal Depression. *The Practitioner 229:* 507-508.

Dalton, M. E., 1981. Sex hormone binding globulin binding capacity in women with severe premenstrual syndrome. *Postgraduate Medical Journal 57:* 560-561.

Dalton, M. E., 1984a. The effect of progesterone administration on sex hormone binding capacity in women with severe premenstrual syndrome. *Journal of Steroid Biochemistry 20:* 437-439.

Dalton, M. E., 1984b. The diagnostic value of sex hormone binding globulin in women with premenstrual syndrome. Paper presented at the 15th International Congress of the International Society for Psychoneuroendocrinology, Vienna, June.

Dalton, M. E., 1985. Nasal absorption of progesterone. Paper presented at the International Premenstrual Syndrome Symposium, Los Angeles, CA, June.

Greenstein, B. D., 1978. Evidence of specific progesterone receptors in rat brain cortisol. *Journal of Endocrinology 79:* 327-338.

Iqbal, M. J. and M. Johnston, 1977. Study of steroid protein binding by a novel "two-tier" column employing ciba-cron blue F3GA Sepharose 4B I-sex hormone binding globulin. *Journal of Steroid Biochemistry 8:* 977-985.

Janiger, O., R. Riffenburgh, and R. Kersch, 1972. Cross cultural study of premenstrual symptoms. *Psychosomatics 13:* 226-235.

Kantero, R. L. and C. Widholm, 1971. The age of menarche in Finnish girls in 1969. *Acta Obstetrica and Gynecologica Scandinavica Supplement 14:* 7-18.

Moos, R. H., 1968. The development of a Menstrual Distress Questionnaire. *Psychosomatic Medicine 30:* 853-867.

Nillius, S. J. and E.D.B. Johansson, 1971. Plasma levels of progesterone after vaginal, rectal or intramuscular administration of progesterone. *American Journal of Obstetrics and Gynecology 110:* 470-477.

Sampson, G. A. and F. A. Jenner, 1977. Studies of daily recordings from the Moos Menstrual Distress Questionnaire. *British Journal of Psychiatry 130:* 265-271.

Vermeulen, A., 1971. Capacity of testosterone binding globulin in human plasma and influence of specific binding of testosterone on its metabolic clearance rate. *Journal of Clinical Endocrinology and Metabolism 33:* 759.

PREMENSTRUAL SYNDROME: CHARACTERIZATION, THERAPIES, AND THE LAW

Gwyneth A. Sampson, D.P.M., M.R.C.Psych.

Whiteley Wood Clinic
Sheffield, United Kingdom

INTRODUCTION

Premenstrual syndrome (PMS) is a global term which implies changes in mood, behavior, and physical characteristics in relation to the menstrual cycle, usually with an increase in intensity of symptoms premenstrually and a diminution of intensity with the onset of menstruation. Within the medical profession, there are as many definitions as authors of scientific papers, but the essence of all definitions is periodicity, and the relationship between symptoms and the time of onset of menstruation. Complaints in relation to the paramenstruum have presumably been present since Eve and were well recorded by Soranus of Ephesus in 100 A.D. It is only in the last 50 years that these complaints have been accorded a "disease" status and have been proffered to the medical profession as a disease process requiring treatment. Having been presented with PMS, we must develop means of rating the symptoms and their effects, in order to assess the existence, nature, incidence, and epidemiology of PMS.

The majority of early reports of the effects of any therapy on PMS symptoms, and many recent reports as well, have been based on studies which simply (1) asked a woman, "Do you have PMS?"; (2) imposed one or two months of the treatment; and (3) then asked again, "Is your PMS better?" However, as with other conditions, a complaint to a practitioner of a specific disorder is not a very accurate basis for diagnosis. "I have PMS, Doctor" might mean the patient has premenstrual syndrome, or it could indicate premenstrual "vulnerability," dysmenorrhea, an unhappy, anxious life, or periodic edema.

In clinical research, ethical considerations require first that subjects are referred as potential participants only after complaining of PMS themselves in order to be referred; and second, to have to consent to accept whatever therapy is offered. Such ethical considerations will mean treatment studies must acknowledge and accommodate stereotypic beliefs about the psychological concomitants of menstruation. If this is done, medical attention can be addressed to the alleviation of premenstrual symptoms without committing the potential errors of inappropriate paternalism and dangerous stigmatization. (These are fully discussed elsewhere in the present volume; e.g., chapters by Macklin and Ruble.)

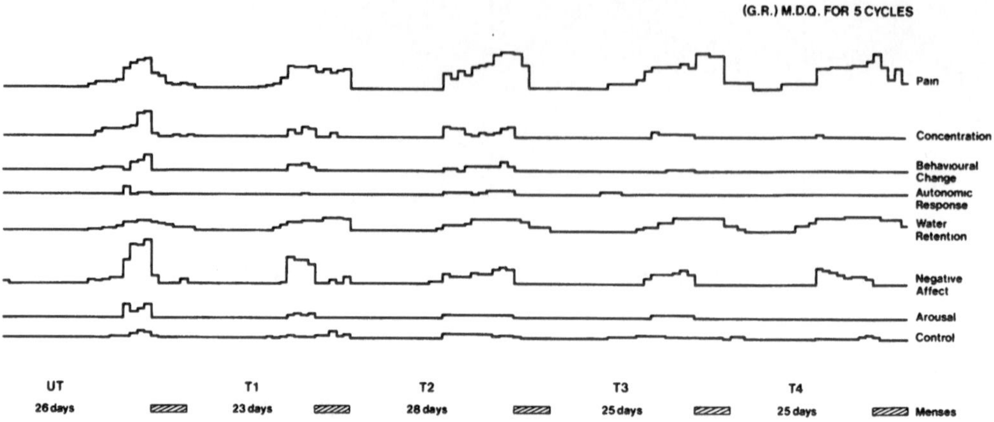

Fig. 1. Daily scores from the Moos Menstrual Distress Questionnaire (MDQ) subdivided into symptom clusters and plotted to show five consecutive menstrual cycles in one subject.

A further ethical concern regarding the scientific evaluation of medical treatment is that conducting a crossover control study (assessing symptom alleviation with administration of an active agent versus placebo) will deprive patients of earliest accessibility to an available therapy. This is less of an actual concern in assessing treatment efficacy for PMS than for other conditions because, as will be detailed later, there is a very substantial placebo effect in treating PMS. Thus, it is not true that the crucial crossover studies should not be conducted because of the clinical ethical principle that every patient deserves the most effective therapy available.

THE ASSESSMENT OF SYMPTOMS

Studies by Altman, Knowles, and Bull (1941), May (1976), McCance, Luff, and Widdowson (1937), and Sampson (1981) identify the discrepancies between recalled data and information obtained daily throughout the menstrual cycle. Retrospective ratings may be affected by the mood of the subject on the day on which rating is undertaken. Further problems develop if symptoms are recorded only once or twice in the cycle, as clear specification of a baseline is essential, against which to assess any premenstrual increase in symptoms. Among the several ways of assessing symptoms, prospective daily ratings provide the most accurate information, although even this approach presents difficulties (Parlee, 1974).

There is much debate as to what should be recorded and studied in a clinical situation. Recording behavior is difficult. It can be assessed by independent raters, but this is costly, and nevertheless remains individually subjective unless a structured rating scale is used. Observable discrete events (suicide attempts, child abuse) are rare. While such rarity is fortunate in terms of human concerns, it is unfortunate that the incidence is too low to use changes in frequency of these events to evaluate symptom changes. Self-rating is the commonest means of daily prospective recording. There are several rating scales; the most widely used is the Moos Menstrual Distress Questionnaire (MDQ; Moos, 1977). This is a list of 47 symptoms, each of which is rated for presence and severity on a 1-6 scale. The 47 symptoms have been factor-analyzed and subdivided into symptom clusters described as Pain,

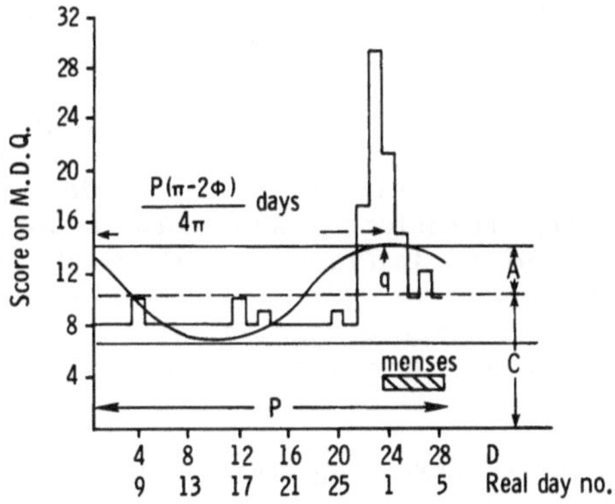

Fig. 2. Data showing the scores for the Negative Affect Scale of the Moos Menstrual Distress Questionnaire over one cycle. The least mean square fitted sine wave is also shown, and the significance of the various constants is illustrated. The sine wave is the one for which the sum of the squares of the deviation of the sine wave from the raw data is minimal. [Also see Appendix to this chapter.]

Concentration Difficulties, Behavioral Change, Autonomic Reaction, Water Retention, Negative Affect, and a "control" set of questions. As we use it, women are asked to complete a questionnaire every evening to describe how they have felt during the previous 24 hours. The daily questionnaires can be scored according to individual symptoms or the symptom clusters, as is shown in Figure 1.

Having obtained daily, or at least frequent, scores measuring mood and other symptoms, an assessment must be made of the periodicity of these symptoms. First, one has to assess whether there are any significant changes in symptom occurrence or intensity with time; and second, where in the menstrual cycles these changes occur. If all women had the same length menstrual cycle with no inter- or intra-personal variance, and if hormonal events proceeded in a known consistent pattern in every cycle, these determinations would be less problematic. One method of accommodating cycle length variation involves subdividing the menstrual cycle into phases. Scores are summed for each phase to detect any significant difference between phases in relationship to menstruation.

Unfortunately, different authors identify differing cycle phases, and there are real problems in adjusting phases to a cycle length that varies from 21 to 37 days. This author has previously described a method using a least mean square method of fitting sine waves, which allows for varying cycle length and gives quantitative figures for the magnitude of the symptoms and the time of maximum occurrence (Sampson & Jenner, 1977; Fig. 2; see also the Appendix to this chapter). Utilizing a statistical method providing adjustment for cycle lengths, PMS can be defined as the presence of significant "A" values in at least three of the MDQ's symptom clusters, where "A" is an estimate of the amplitude of symptom severity which is maximal between the 23rd day after the onset of the preceding menses and the third day after the onset of the next menses. A reduction of "A" in a later cycle would correspond to a reduction in symptom severity. The data for a single cycle are then compared with consecutive cycles in the same patient or with single cycles in other individuals; there are several methodological ways of doing this (Sampson & Prescott, 1981): In comparing different cycles in one individual, it may be presumed that the baseline level of symptoms is reasonably constant and that she rates her symptoms consistently (e.g., a headache which is rated at 3 is worse than one rated at 2). With differing individuals, their baseline symptom scores and the way they rate symptoms will differ. Several authors standardize scores to a scale with a mean of zero and a standard deviation of one; for example, Moos (1977) transforms MDQ raw scores into standard scores with a mean of 50 and a standard deviation of 10 for each scale. This transformation makes it possible to compare scales with each other within one phase, to compare scales across different phases, and to compare women with each other across scales.

ASSESSING AND REPORTING THE RESPONSE OF SYMPTOMS TO THERAPY

There have been many reports of therapeutic success with PMS since Frank first described and gave medical respectability to the syndrome in 1931. In uncontrolled studies, most therapies appear effective. For example, Block (1960) reported Vitamin A as having a "good effect" in 60 percent of patients and a moderate improvement of symptoms for a further 30 percent, leaving only 10 percent unimproved. The majority of double-blind, controlled trials comparing pharmacologically-active agents against identical inert placebos demonstrates a high placebo response (e.g., Jordheim, 1972; Mattson & Schoultz, 1974; Sampson, 1979).

It is important to record at least one untreated baseline cycle to act as baseline from which to compare other cycles, and thereby verify the presence of PMS. The subjects of a treatment study need to be defined; a woman who sees herself as "ill" and identifies herself as a "patient" by consulting a doctor is likely to differ in many variables from a "volunteer" to a research investigation. Age, parity, personality, and concurrent stresses should all be documented so comparisons can be made across differing studies. In our studies, we only consider a woman a "patient" if she has symptoms which, in her own assessment, interfere with her home, work, or social life.

Women are very different from each other (as are men), and there are so many factors influencing each individual that it is a highly complex task to evaluate what is being measured in a "treatment" study. To evaluate a PMS therapy, one should assess the effect of treatment over at least four cycles. Including a control cycle, this comprises six calendar months of an individual's life. The problem of controlling and allowing for other variables within this six months [including universal variables such as holidays (e.g., Christmas) and health changes (e.g., the common cold)] increases the difficulty of assessing the effect on the "treatment." For these reasons, it is important to use the individual woman as her own control in a crossover study design; i.e., each subject receives placebo and active treatment at different times in the study, so that the effect of treatment versus placebo can be made within each subject as well as across multiple subjects. It could be possible that the effect of one treatment will carry over into the following menstrual cycle. In a crossover design, the sequence of treatments should be arranged so that these "carry over" or "residual" effects are balanced relative to the main treatment effects. For example, the response in the second treated cycle for an individual receiving the sequence of treatments A.P.P.A. is due to the main effect of placebo (P) given in that cycle and the residual effect of the active drug (A) given during the preceding cycle. Figure 3 is an example of a completely balanced design for two treatments, arranged so that the main effects of the treatments are orthogonal to the residual effects. It is a

Patient \ Cycle	1	2	3	4
1	A	P	P	A
2	A	A	P	P
3	P	A	A	P
4	P	P	A	A

Fig. 3. A balanced design for two treatments, allowing examination of direct treatment effects and residual treatment effects separately. A = active drug; P = placebo.

crossover design since each patient receives each treatment twice and each treatment is given the same number of times during each cycle. The basic design involves four patients and should be replicated using additional sets of four patients as many times as predictable. All treatment studies should be double blind as the doctor's belief in an agent can affect the subject.

In all reported studies of any therapeutic agent for PMS against indistinguishable placebo, there has been a high placebo response. It can be as high as 60 percent, which is the level found in studies comparing psychotropic agents against placebo (Jenner, 1977). With such a high placebo response, there are difficulties in assessment of statistical significance of treatment effect. This may constitute one reason that the majority of treatment studies comparing therapeutic agents against placebo have not found the therapeutic agent to be significantly better than placebo, particularly in double-blind, crossover studies.

Claims for effective therapy based mainly on clinical observation or non-blind studies without placebo are not scientifically valid. These claims are often widely reported in the media, and the public is often misled because the media and the general population do not distinguish between anecdotal claims of therapeutic efficacy and scientific reports accepted as valid by the medical profession, the Food and Drug Administration in the United States, or the Committee of Safety on Medicines in the United Kingdom (CSM-UK). A recent example involves the massive publicity in the United Kingdom for B vitamins, claiming great efficacy in treatment for PMS. The vitamins were often manufactured and marketed by companies who were not members of the Association of the British Pharmaceutical Industry (ABPI), and who therefore did not comply with ABPI regulations. Furthermore, the B vitamins were not approved by the CSM-UK for the treatment of PMS; yet the majority of books, articles, and other media coverage claimed they were effective in treating PMS. The preparations were expensive, but could be brought over-the-counter in pharmacies or health food shops, and they became widely used. Then, many women developed secondary anxieties following a TV program listing side effects of vitamins. The predicament was: They had utilized as a treatment something the media had initially presented as "safe and effective" but later reported as "unsafe." Many women seeking help for PMS continue to be misled, spending money and time on products that are at least ineffective and perhaps even harmful. It is often difficult for the general population to distinguish between a media report stating, "Dr. X says it works because he has tried it in five patients," and another media report stating, "Many doctors say it works because they have completed careful studies of many patients in many centers." Perhaps improved collaboration between scientists and the media would allow presentation of

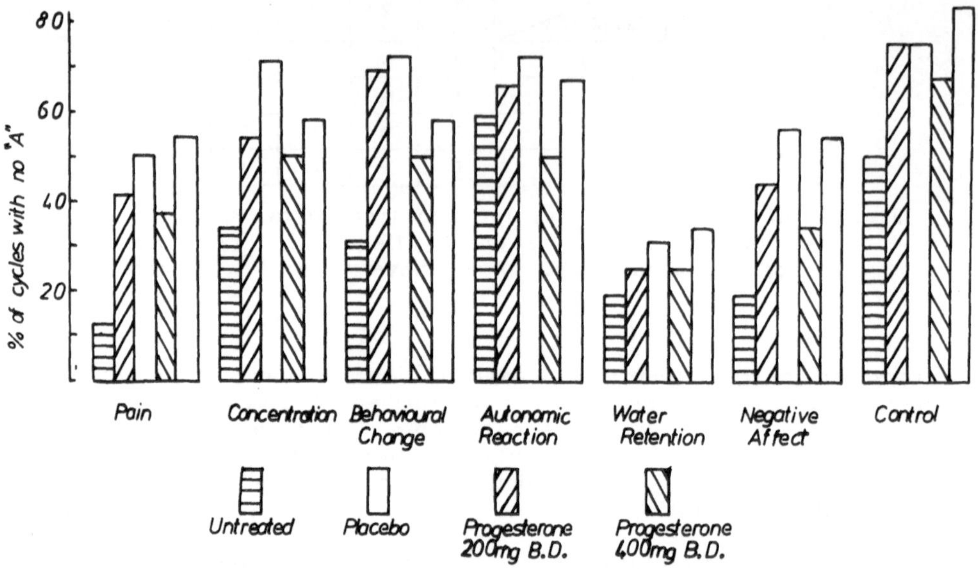

Fig. 4. The percentages without "A" (the measure of symptom severity in relation to menstruation) for each scale of the Moos Menstrual Distress Questionnaire, in untreated, progesterone-treated, and placebo-treated cycles.

clinical data in a more balanced and less dramatic form (also see Parlee, this volume).

STUDIES OF PROGESTERONE AND DYDROGESTERONE

Having been impressed by the claims of Dalton (1977) and the results of treatment in our uncontrolled study (Sampson, 1981), we undertook a double-blind, crossover study comparing progesterone pessaries/suppositories with identical placebo pessaries/suppositories. The latter were made of the same base as the active agents, but without the addition of progesterone (Sampson, 1979). Subjects were chosen from women attending the Sheffield Premenstrual Syndrome Clinic. They were assessed clinically, and completed daily Moos MDQs for at least one untreated menstrual cycle. From each daily chart, the scores of individual questions were marked in Moos' symptom clusters, and a graph showing daily scores for each of the seven symptom clusters plus appetite change was plotted for each cycle. A best fit sine wave was then determined giving a value "A" (a measure of symptom severity) and a value "q" (an indication of the timing of symptoms in relation to menstruation; see Fig. 1). The criterion for a subject's inclusion in the study was a significant increase in symptoms premenstrually ("A") in at least three of the negative symptom groups (Pain, Behavioral Change, Concentration, Autonomic Reaction, Water Retention, Negative Affect). Subjects also reported their symptoms retrospectively when seen at each monthly visit. Progesterone (200 milligrams twice daily) and placebo (twice daily) were given in the first half of the study, with the dose of progesterone increased to 400 milligrams twice daily in the second half. Both the patients' own retrospective assessments and their daily ratings showed that for Autonomic Reaction and Water Retention, neither progesterone nor placebo cycles were significantly different from untreated cycles. Progesterone—400 milligram twice daily cycles were

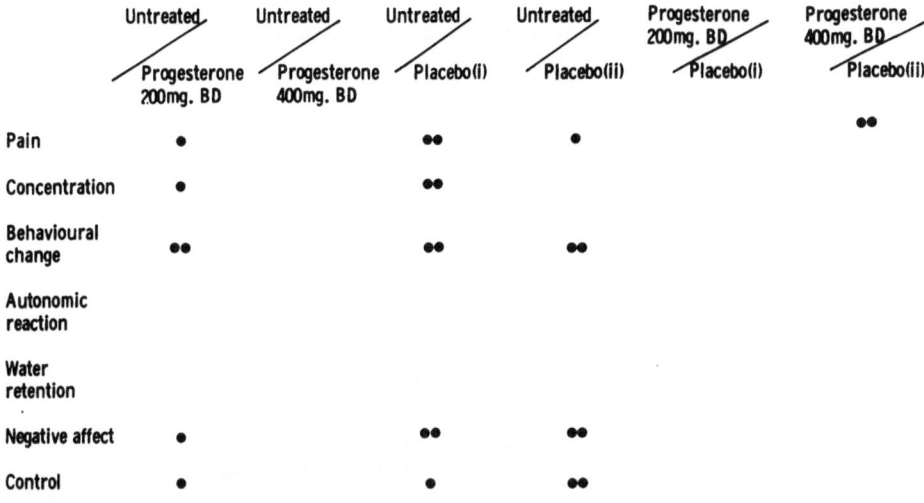

	Untreated / Progesterone 200mg. BD	Untreated / Progesterone 400mg. BD	Untreated / Placebo(i)	Untreated / Placebo(ii)	Progesterone 200mg. BD / Placebo(i)	Progesterone 400mg. BD / Placebo(ii)
Pain	•		••	•		••
Concentration	•		••			
Behavioural change	••		••	••		
Autonomic reaction						
Water retention						
Negative affect	•		••	••		
Control	•		•	••		

SIGNIFICANT DIFFERENCE BETWEEN CYCLES COMPARING NUMBER OF "A" (CHI SQUARE)

• = $p<0.05$ •• = $p<0.01$

Fig. 5. Significant differences between untreated versus placebo-treated or progesterone-treated cycles for symptom severity in relation to menstruation; symptom severity being measured by "A."

never significantly better than untreated cycles. Significant improvement was shown from the untreated cycle to both progesterone-200 milligram treated and placebo cycles for the Pain, Behavioral Change, Concentration, Negative Affect, and Control scales (Figs. 4 and 5). Therefore, although progesterone appeared to be an effective treatment for some symptoms, placebo was at least equally effective. (In fact, placebo was usually even more effective, although this difference did not reach statistical significance.) Smith (1975) also reported a comparison of progesterone with placebo, with no difference in effectiveness between the two.

We have recently completed a double-blind, crossover study of dydrogesterone (6-dehydroretroprogesterone) — an orally active progestagen — against identical placebo. In an attempt to assess inter-patient variables, we accessed subjects through two centers: the hospital-based PMS Clinic utilizing medical referral, and a self-referral Family Planning Association Clinic. Two hundred patients were assessed, with 108 entering the study. Twelve who were entered were later excluded, as their untreated cycle data did not meet the criterion of significant "A" values in at least three of the MDQ negative symptom groups. Data from 64 patients were used for final analysis of treatment response, which was performed using a crossover design balanced for carry-over effects, as described earlier. Dydrogesterone was given in a dose of 10 milligrams twice daily from days 12 to 26 of a cycle, with the timing adjusted for cycle length.

The MDQs were analyzed as for the progesterone study presented above. The doctor's assessment, the patient's recall of individual symptoms, and her own assessment of the effect of her symptoms on home, work, and social life were also analyzed. The MDQ analysis indicates significant improvement in all negative symptom clusters when

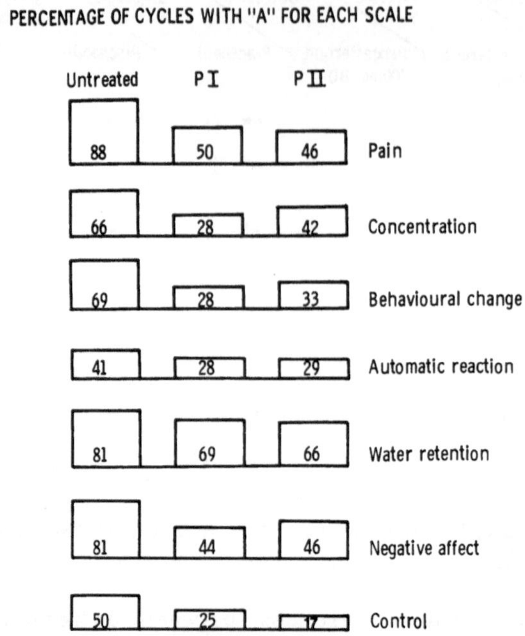

Fig 6. The percentage of untreated and placebo (PI, PII) cycles in which there is a significant change in "A" (the measure of symptom severity in relation to menstruation) for each scale of the Moos Menstrual Distress Questionnaire. There are significant differences ($p < .05$) between untreated cycles and PI on the Pain, Concentration, Behavior Change, and Negative Affect Scales, and between untreated cycles and PII for the Behavior Change, Negative Affect, and Control Scales. There are also significant differences ($p < .01$) between untreated cycles and PI for the Control Scale, and untreated cycles and PII for the Pain Scale.

treated cycles are compared with the untreated cycle. However, there is no significant difference between the response to dydrogesterone and the response to placebo.

The analysis of patients' recall of the severity and duration of individual symptoms showed two significant findings. First, there was a significantly lower score for severity and frequency of pain during menstruation with dydrogesterone compared with placebo; and second, there was a significantly higher frequency of breast tenderness with dydrogesterone than placebo. These findings suggest that, while breast symptoms were not alleviated by dydrogesterone and could be aggravated by this medication, dydrogesterone is an effective treatment for dysmenorrhea. There were further differences between the hospital and the self-referral populations in that patients at the hospital (i.e., medical referrals) presented with greater loss of energy, difficulty concentrating, depression, and irritability.

Our studies comparing progesterone and dydrogesterone with placebo were double-blind, and showed that each treatment — whether placebo, progesterone, or dydrogesterone — is very effective. Our studies highlight the importance of assessing the placebo response of pharmacologic treatments for PMS (Fig. 6). The non-pharmacologic aspects of intervention also may contribute to the placebo effect.

In a retrospective survey inquiring what aspects of their management had been helpful, patients reported that all of the following activities were beneficial: Completing self-rating questionnaires; having an interested person take a case history; being able to tell their partner and family they had been to a "specialist at a PMS Clinic;" and and receiving simple education and counselling.

One difficulty in assessing the response of PMS symptoms to a particular endocrine agent is the assumption that a medication would have a similar endocrine/biochemical effect in each cycle. No consistent obvious endocrine difference has been found between women complaining of premenstrual syndrome and those who do not; differing authors often report conflicting findings (Backstrom, Wide, Sodergard, & Carstensen, 1976; Reid, 1985; Taylor, 1979). The effects of administered dydrogesterone and progesterone on the naturally-occurring hormones of the menstrual cycle are still being evaluated. For example, in work undertaken since the above-described dydrogesterone trial was completed, Lenton (1984) has shown that giving the same dose of dydrogesterone at different times in the menstrual cycle produces marked changes in hormonal profiles. When given before ovulation, the mid-cycle gonadotropin surge was either abolished or markedly diminished. Dydrogesterone given after ovulation did not produce any alteration in endocrine profiles.

In an assessment of those patients at the Sheffield Clinic who responded dramatically to progesterone, it was determined that the treatment had been given almost continuously or in very high doses of over 1000 milligrams daily and often suppressed menstruation (Sampson, 1981). Such data may be used to argue that both progesterone and dydrogesterone could be more effective than placebo if given in a different dosage regime. This should not distract from the fact that symptoms of PMS respond significantly and often dramatically to placebo.

IS PREMENSTRUAL SYNDROME A DISEASE?

During the 14 years that the Sheffield PMS Clinic has been functioning, there have been marked changes in the attitude of society and the medical profession to PMS, changes contributed to by the media and the women's rights movement. Thus, many women come to the Clinic with such comments as: "I didn't know I had PMS, but I read an article describing feelings I have and it said these were symptoms of PMS." Not all women, however, wish to give PMS disease status, and others are open to alternative explanations of why they feel irritable and tense at a certain time.

I have been asked to provide court reports on women who have committed offenses and who report having PMS. For the majority, careful history-taking and charting of symptoms reveal that the premenstruum was only one of the many factors involved in the occurrence of the offense. This is generally recognized by the woman herself, and the report usually becomes general psychiatric/social evaluation rather than a specific statement for a PMS-based defense.

The women who attend both the Sheffield Clinics (those who are medically referred and those who self-refer) appear to be closer to a neurotic/stressed group than to the general population "norm" on the basis of several variables. Data analysis on 162 consecutive patients with a mean age of 34.7 found a mean score for neuroticism (Eysenck Personality Inventory Neuroticism or N Score; Eysenck & Eysenck, 1964) of 15.8, which is in the anxiety neurotic range; their E (Extraversion Score) in the same test is low and is similar to the group described by

Eysenck and Eysenck as "neurotic-hysteric" (Eysenck & Eysenck, 1964). Only 10 percent of the combined Clinic population had N scores at or below the mean for a normal population. A high proportion — over 30 percent — of the group had time away from school or work with menstrual problems during their teen years. Over 58 percent had received tranquilizers at some time, and 13 percent had made a suicide gesture. Sixty percent had seen a gynecologist. [In the United Kingdom, a visit to a gynecologist implies a referral for a second medical opinion; primary gynecological care (e.g., cervical smear and routine examination) is undertaken by general practitioners.] Data on their personal history included 41 percent reporting parental conflict when they were children; being born to older mothers (mean age of mother at patient's birth: 28 years); and 35 percent reporting their mothers as being "unsympathetic." Their current relationships were often reported as unstable; and in 22 percent, it was in a worse state than two years earlier. These and other data imply that the group coming to the Clinic may simply be a group generally at increased risk for psychological or physical distress at any time of the month. However, 75 percent of this group had a significant increase in symptomatology premenstrually in at least three of the Moos negative symptom scales; although some symptoms may be present throughout the month, there is a significant increase in the symptoms premenstrually.

Our data could be interpreted as supporting a concept of premenstrual increase in vulnerability to neurotic symptoms which are already present, and either evident or under control during the follicular phase of the cycle but which manifest themselves or are exacerbated premenstrually. This concept of increased vulnerability is consistent with reported findings (d'Orban & Dalton, 1980) that women who commit crimes of violence are significantly more likely to do so during the premenstruum. These women may be described as having a premenstrual increase in vulnerability to criminal action.

It seems necessary that we discard any simplistic view of PMS, and, instead, assess at least two distinct areas in future studies. First, there appears to be reasonable evidence that some percentage of the female population is vulnerable premenstrually to physical or psychological changes; and we need to identify the affected women and ascertain the reasons for their vulnerability. Second, these vulnerable women attract professional attention in many different guises: as a patient complaining specifically of PMS; as a prisoner convicted of a violent, premenstrual crime; as a woman with menstrual migraine, etc. We need to understand each individual woman, including those personality features which are clearly evident only during the premenstruum, as they are controlled and hidden at other times. The distinction of these two aspects can be crucial in the medico-legal assessment: In a clinical setting, a woman's tendency to develop migraine rather than other symptoms is a different consideration than why she only experiences particular symptoms premenstrually.

CONCLUSIONS

Premenstrual syndrome is a real but complex phenomenon. The women who complain of premenstrual symptoms need ongoing assessment, with daily recording in order to ascertain definitively the presence and extent of any premenstrual worsening of symptoms. As documented here and by others, purported placebo actually provides a significantly effective therapy ($p < .05$), and no formal therapies subjected to the requisite double-blind, crossover study have been shown more effective than placebo. Psychological factors are likely contributors to this placebo response, and clearly warrant further research. In the meantime, we see that neither progesterone nor dydrogesterone is significantly better than placebo, and therefore cannot be considered the ultimate form of treatment. Such a simplistic view of PMS is inappropriate. Each case should have a complete assessment of the many functional systems and individual characteristics which comprise the whole woman, as well as an assessment of whether she is more likely to experience particular problems premenstrually.

REFERENCES

Altman, M., E. Knowles, and H. D. Bull, 1941. A psychosomatic study of the sex cycle in women. *Psychosomatic Medicine 3:* 199-225.

Backstrom, T., L. Wide, R. Sodergard, and H. Carstensen, 1976. FSH, LH, TeBg — capacity, estrogen and progesterone in women with premenstrual tension during the luteal phase. *Journal of Steroid Biochemistry 7:* 473-476.

Block, E., 1960. The use of vitamin A in premenstrual tension. *Acta Obstetrica et Gynecologica Scandinavica 39:* 586-592.

Dalton, K., 1977. *The Premenstrual Syndrome and Progesterone Therapy.* William Heinemann Medical Books, Ltd., London.

d'Orban, P. T. and K. Dalton, 1980. Violent crime and the menstrual cycle. *Psychological Medicine 10:* 353-359.

Eysenck, H. J. and S.B.G. Eysenck, 1964. *Eysenck Personality Inventory and Manual.* Hodder and Stoughton, London.

Frank, R., 1931. The hormonal causes of premenstrual tension. *Archives of Neurology and Psychiatry 26:* 1053-1057.

Halberg, G., Y. L. Tong, and E. A. Johnson, 1965. Circadian system phase — an aspect of temporal morphology: Procedures and illustrative examples. In: *The Cellular Aspects of Biorhythms* (Symposium on Rhythmic Research sponsored by the VIIIth International Congress of Anatomy, Wiesbaden, 8-14 August 1965). Springer-Verlag, Berlin.

Jenner, F. A., 1977. Some of the problems and difficulties associated with clinical studies of antidepressant agents. *British Journal of Clinical Pharmacology 4:* 1995-2085.

Jordheim, O., 1972. The premenstrual syndrome — clinical trials of treatment with a progestagen combined with a diuretic compared with both progestagen alone and a placebo. *Acta Psychiatrica Scandinavica (Supplement) 51:* 77-80.

Lenton, E. A., 1984. The effect of dydrogesterone on the midcycle gonadotrophin surge in regularly cycling women. *Clinical Endocrinology 20:* 129-135.

Mattson, B. and B. V. Schoultz, 1974. A comparison between lithium, placebo and a diuretic in premenstrual tension. *Acta Psychiatrica Scandinavica (Supplement) 225:* 75-84.

May, P. R., 1976. Mood shifts and the menstrual cycle. *Journal of Psychosomatic Research 20:* 125-130.

McCance, R. A., M. C. Luff, and E. H. Widdowson, 1937. Physical and emotional periodicity in women. *Journal of Hygiene (London) 37:* 571-611.

Moos, R. H., 1977. *Menstrual Distress Questionnaire Manual.* Stanford University School of Medicine, Stanford, CA.

Parlee, M. B., 1974. Stereotypic beliefs about menstruation: A methodological note on the Moos Menstrual Distress Questionnaire and some new data. *Psychosomatic Medicine 36:* 229-240.

Reid, R. L., 1985. The endocrinology of premenstrual syndrome. In: M. Y. Dawood, J. L. McGuire, and L. M. Demers (Eds.), *Premenstrual Syndrome and Dysmenorrhea.* Urban and Schwarzenberg, Baltimore, MD, pp. 51-66.

Sampson, G. A., 1979. Premenstrual syndrome — a double-blind controlled trial of progesterone and placebo. *British Journal of Psychiatry 135:* 209-215.

Sampson, G. A., 1981. An appraisal of the role of progesterone in the therapy of premenstrual syndrome. In: P. A. Van Keep and W. H. Utian (Eds.), *The Premenstrual Syndrome.* MTP Press, London.

Sampson, G. A. and F. A. Jenner, 1977. Studies of daily recordings from the Moos Menstrual Distress Questionnaire. *British Journal of Psychiatry 130:* 265-271.

Sampson, G. A. and P. Prescott, 1981. The assessment of symptoms of premenstrual syndrome and their response to therapy. *British Journal of Psychiatry 138:* 399-405.

Smith, S. L., 1975. Mood and the menstrual cycle. In: E. J. Sachar (Ed.), *Topics in Endocrinology.* Grune and Stratton, New York, NY.

Solberger, A., 1965. *Biological Rhythm Research.* Elsevier, Amsterdam.

Taylor, J. W., 1979. Plasma progesterone, estradiol 17-beta and premenstrual symptoms. *Acta Psychiatrica Scandinavica 60:* 70.

APPENDIX

APPENDIX:

SCORING THE MENSTRUAL DISTRESS QUESTIONNAIRE

The score for each symptom cluster is obtained by adding together the scores (1 to 6) for each of the relevant symptoms. Each subject then has, for every day, eight scores plus one further score for any "Appetite Change." The first five days were used as practice days to enable the subject to get used to the forms. The results from these five days were discarded. Data from day 6 of one cycle to day 5 of the next cycle (inclusive) were used in order to include the menstrual bleed following a premenstrual phase in the same cycle.

It is well known that (a) the mathematics of fitting sine waves to data of unknown phase is simple compared to that of fitting other wave forms, but (b) that the implied assumption of a sinusoidal curve introduces errors. Nevertheless, with caution, the method is fairly robust and seems suitable for our purposes.

Sine waves were fitted by a least mean square method (Solberger, 1965). The quantitative values of the constants A, Ø, and C of $Y = A \sin(2\pi D/p + \emptyset) + C$ are calculated. The number of days between the onset of the menses included in the data and the onset of the previous menses is P; i.e., it is the period length. The number of the day of the menstrual cycle is D. We, in fact, called day 6 of the actual menstrual cycle day 1 for reasons of computation, and the following days up to the number P were numbered sequentially. The phase in the menstrual cycle for the symptoms is indicated by Ø of the fitted curves. The mesor, or the mean value of the measures throughout the whole cycle from the fitted curve is C, while A is the amplitude of the best fit sine wave and is a measure of the variation of complaining due to the menstrual cycle. The acrophase q is the time of the maximum value of the best fit curve compared to the onset of menses. This is assessed from Ø and can be converted from radians to days for an individual. Alternatively, the mean acrophase in radians for a group of persons can be converted to the equivalent day of a standardized 28-day cycle for the group.

Statistical significance of a fit for a cycle of a person was assessed from the following equations.

$$\text{The confidence limits of } A = t\sqrt{\frac{2\sigma^2}{P}}$$

$$\text{and of } \emptyset = t\sqrt{\frac{2\sigma^2}{PA^2}}$$

Student's t is found for the selected P value required with (P-3) degrees of freedom. The variance from the best fit curve of the crude data is σ^2. If $A < t\sqrt{\frac{2\sigma^2}{P}}$ then the fit can be accepted at the value of P used to determine t. The above is taken from Halberg, Tong, and Johnson (1965) and is almost the same as applying the so-called cosinor method. Figure 2 shows a least mean square fitted sine wave applied to data from one subject for the Negative Affect Scale. This subject's premenstrual score is unusually high.

The tendency to complain, irrespective of the menstrual cycle, is best assessed from the mean value of the crude data at times other than the premenstrual and menstrual period. The "Average Non-Menstrual Score" is an average of the scores on each scale from day 6 to ovulation, which we calculated as 14 days preceding the next bleed.

For some purposes, the premenstrual syndrome might be defined as a statistically significant A value with an acrophase occurring within a defined number of days of the onset of menses. The severity might be taken as the value of A, and a statistically significant reduction of A in the treated cycle is evidence of efficacy.

CONTROVERSIES IN PREMENSTRUAL SYNDROME: ETIOLOGY AND TREATMENT

P.M.S. O'Brien, M.D., M.R.C.O.G.

Academic Department of Obstetrics and Gynaecology
The Royal Free Hospital
Hampstead, London
England

INTRODUCTION

It may be premature to discuss the ethical implications of the premenstrual syndrome (PMS) when the scientific foundations of the disorder are so poorly established. There are virtually no conclusive data available concerning its diagnosis or measurement; or specifying the precise endocrine and biochemical changes involved; nor are there any reliable studies enabling us to offer adequate treatment to patients. The present chapter attempts to identify some of the major deficiencies in our understanding of PMS and to assess the efficacies of the treatments available. Much of the discussion will center around the failure of the majority of research studies to arrive at strict definitions and the inadequate means of characterizing and quantifying PMS when attempting to diagnose individuals and when trying to measure the day-to-day changes in symptoms. Two other important problems relate to etiology: the as yet unproven theories relating to progesterone deficiency, and the frequently reiterated phenomenon of water retention, which has, to date, not been shown to be a consistent component of PMS. Probably one of the most common and fundamental shortcomings in the study of PMS is the failure to include placebo controls in studies of therapy. This is surprising in a syndrome where the placebo effect of any therapy usually has been 40-50 percent, and occasionally greater (Sampson, 1979).

For the scientist investigating the etiology(ies) of PMS, these uncertainties demand further investigation. Ethically, it is the responsibility of the scientist to ensure that testable hypotheses are generated, and that the methodologies for testing these are adequate and do not expose the persons to be tested to unacceptable risks. For the clinician, whose responsibility is to provide optimum treatment for each patient based on the best knowledge available, there is the imperative of keeping abreast of the field in order to exercise an informed judgment. Where the clinician is also the investigator, these objectives may not be congruent as, for example, when the investigative method mandates a double-blind trial involving a placebo, but as clinician, he/she is convinced that the treatment being tested is effective, and is therefore reluctant to relinquish control over the regime to be imposed on the patient. At the same time, it is easy for the clinician to be prematurely convinced when the placebo response is so high; accordingly, it may be considered unethical to promote the use of inadequately assessed treatment regimes.

Unfortunately, despite our incomplete knowledge of PMS, the subject has caught the imagination of writers, not just in medical, gynecological, and psychiatric journals, but also those of the lay media, particularly women's magazines. The surge of interest has led to many sequelae. First, women are being actively encouraged to seek "aggressive" treatment regardless of whether they are experiencing a severely disabling condition, as appears to be the case for some, or whether they are merely experiencing functionally trivial symptoms. Second, members of both the medical profession and the pharmaceutical industry are jumping on the PMS "bandwagon." Both pharmacologic and non-medical treatments of PMS present a potentially lucrative market, especially when one considers the large number of women who purportedly have PMS according to some of the broader definitions of the syndrome (including self-diagnosis). Finally, and not surprisingly, PMS is increasingly being introduced or considered as a defense in the criminal courts, although, as yet, this is in no way universally accepted. It appears that this is being encouraged by lawyers as they pursue the client advocacy which characterizes their professional role.

DEFINITION OF THE PREMENSTRUAL SYNDROME

Although many vague definitions of PMS have appeared in earlier research studies, the majority now adhere fairly closely to that proposed by Dalton (1977). The essentials of the definition are: (a) that the character of the symptoms is not strictly important (although there are certain typical symptoms, such as irritability, bloatedness, headache, breast tenderness, aggression, depression, and anxiety); (b) that the timing of symptoms is diagnostically important, and although varying symptom patterns are seen, essentially they must occur in the premenstrual week; (c) that symptoms must resolve completely by the end of menstruation, and there must be a symptom-free week between menstruation and ovulation; and (d) some others add that symptoms should be of sufficient severity either to interfere with work or social activity, or to require the patient to seek treatment.

The variations in definition of PMS sufferers is highlighted by the range of prevalence reports in the literature (Table 1). Rees (1953) described patients in a psychiatric clinic, and using very strict criteria, reported an incidence of only 5 percent. Pennington (1957) reported a sample of 1,000 women, predominantly middle class and well educated, and stated that 95 percent complained of at least one PMS symptom. It is generally considered that the incidence ranges between 30-50 percent of women in their reproductive years when the criteria used are the ones stated above, as adapted from Dalton.

Table 1. Variability of Prevalence Reports in Premenstrual Syndrome.

Rees (1953)	Psychiatric Clinic	5%
Bickers & Wood (1951)	Factory Workers	36%
O'Brien (1979)	Hospital Staff	43%
Clare (1983)	General Practitioners	75%
Pennington (1957)	Mainly Housewives	95%

> "A woman suffers from premenstrual syndrome if she complains of cyclically recurring physical or somatic symptoms specifically during the luteal phase of the cycle. It is essential that she has a symptom-free week following menstruation. The symptoms should be of sufficient severity to either disrupt work or social activities or cause the patient to seek treatment."
>
> — K. Dalton (1977)

It is thus the timing rather than the specific nature of the symptoms which is important, although there are key symptoms (such as irritability and/or bloatedness) which invariably are present. A vast number of other symptoms have been reported (Table 2).

CHARACTERIZATION AND QUANTIFICATION OF PREMENSTRUAL SYNDROME

A second fundamental problem is the lack of an objective measure of PMS. This is highlighted by a recent study from Nottingham, England, in which weight and abdominal diameters failed to show any increase premenstrually while *subjective* assessment of bloatedness and body image increased markedly (Faratian, Gaspar, O'Brien, Johnson, Filshie, & Prescott, 1984). There are, as yet, no blood tests which can be used to separate affected from asymptomatic women. No differences in estrogen, progesterone, prolactin, or gonadotrophins have proved to be of diagnostic value. Dalton (1981) has reported significantly lower levels for sex hormone binding globulin (SHBG) in PMS, but this has yet to be assessed for clinical use, and it contradicts the findings of previous workers (Backstrom, Wide, Sodergard, & Carstensen, 1976). In the absence of objective indicators of PMS, both clinical and research assessments become entirely dependent upon self-reporting by the patient. For research purposes, specific visual analog scales or the Moos Menstrual Distress Questionnaire (Moos, 1977) are appropriate. For clinical purposes, a full history and a simple menstrual chart will pinpoint the timing (essential for diagnosis) and character (essential for treatment) of the symptoms, but not the severity. Recording of weight will also define the subgroup of women who do actually gain weight and may help to exclude those with idiopathic edema. However, it is important to realize that the production of weight *loss* cannot be considered an adequate means of assessing therapy, since even male subjects will lose weight when given a diuretic.

With this nebulous background, it is not surprising that we have a poor understanding of PMS etiology. Nevertheless, it seems highly probable that PMS symptoms are related to the cyclical changes of ovarian hormones, although even this association has never been conclusively established. The theory that a progesterone deficiency is the key factor has been widely popularized (Dalton, 1977), but there are as many studies showing no differences or higher progesterone levels as there are studies showing low progesterone levels in association with the symptoms. The problem cannot be as simple as one of progesterone deficiency or increase of estrogen/progesterone ratio, since progesterone is lowest (and the ratio is highest) in the *first* half of the cycle (i.e., the "postmenstruum"), when PMS symptoms are absent.

The most convincing data relating the cyclical hormonal variations of the menstrual cycle to symptoms have used analogs of gonadotrophin releasing hormone (GnRH), which essentially produces a temporary "medical oophorectomy" (Muse, Cetal, Futterman, & Yen, 1984). This treatment has, in a small number of women, produced complete

Table 2. The Range of Symptoms Reported in Premenstrual Syndrome.

Psychological	Somatic
Aggression	Accident prone
Agitation	Acne
Anorexia	Asthma
Anxiety	Bloatedness (actual)
Argumentative	Bloatedness (feeling of)
Confusion	Blurred vision
Crying bouts	Breast swelling
Decreased alertness	Breast tenderness
Decreased libido	Clumsiness
Depression	Constipation
Diminished self esteem	Diarrhea
Drowsiness	Diminished activity
Emotional lability	Diminished efficiency
Energetic	Diminished performance
Fatigue	Dizziness
Food craving	Edema
Hopelessness	Epilepsy
Housebound	Finger swelling
Hunger	Flushes
Hypersomnia	Fornication
Impulsive behavior	Headache
Increased libido	Joint pain
Insomnia	Mastodyna
Irritability	Migraine
Lack of inspiration	Muscle pain
Lack of volition	Nausea
Lethargy	Oligura
Listlessness	Pain — iliac fossa
Loss of attention to appearance	Pain — lower abdomen
Loss of concentration	Pain — pelvic
Loss of confidence	Polyuria
Loss of judgment	Poor coordination
Loss of self control	Premenstrual dysmenorrhea
Malaise	Pruritis
Moody — Sadness	Puffiness
Pessimism	Rhinorrhea
Social isolation	Sinusitis
Suicidal tendency	Skin lesions
Tension	Sore eye
Thirst	Sweating
Violence	Vaginal discharge
	Vertigo
	Vomiting
	Weakness
	Weight increase (feeling of)
	Weight increase (true)

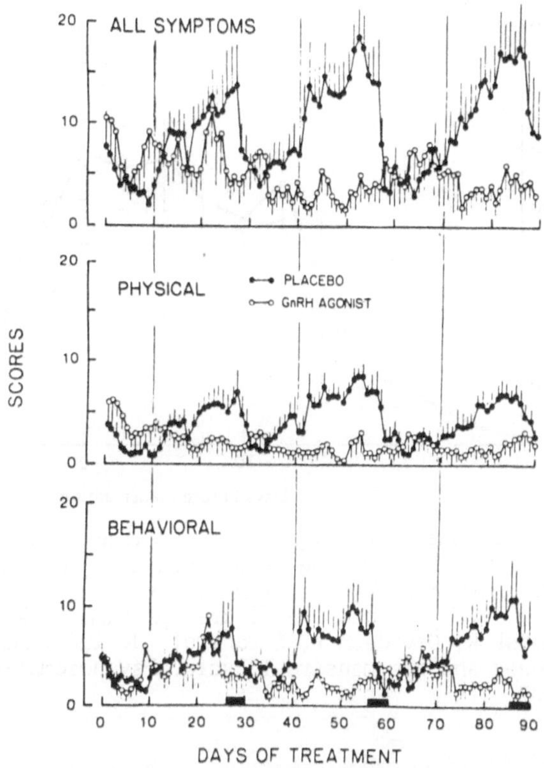

Fig 1. Suppression of the ovarian cycle and symptoms of premenstrual syndrome using gonadotropin releasing hormone. From: Muse et al. (1984). [Reproduced by permission of *New England Journal of Medicine*, and the figure is from Muse K, Cetel N, Futterman, L & Yen S. 1984 The Premenstrual Syndrome: effects of "medical oophorectomy" NEJM 311, 1345 - 49.]

suppression of the cyclical hormonal changes of the cycle, with parallel suppression of PMS symptoms (Fig. 1). Criteria for inclusion in the study were strict, and therapy was compared with placebo throughout. Unfortunately, it is unlikely that this preparation will be useful for long-term therapy because it leads to the development of an estrogen deficiency which could produce menopausal symptoms, which may include side effects such as osteoporosis.

PROGESTERONE DEFICIENCY THEORY

The most popular etiological concept regarding PMS is that of progesterone deficiency or an imbalance between estrogen and progesterone, and one may be forgiven for believing this to be an established fact since both scientific and lay publications continue to reiterate the concept.

In 1931, Frank implied that estrogen excess caused PMS, and Israel (1938) later suggested that it was due to an imbalance between estrogen and progesterone; i.e., an increase in estrogen/progesterone ratio.

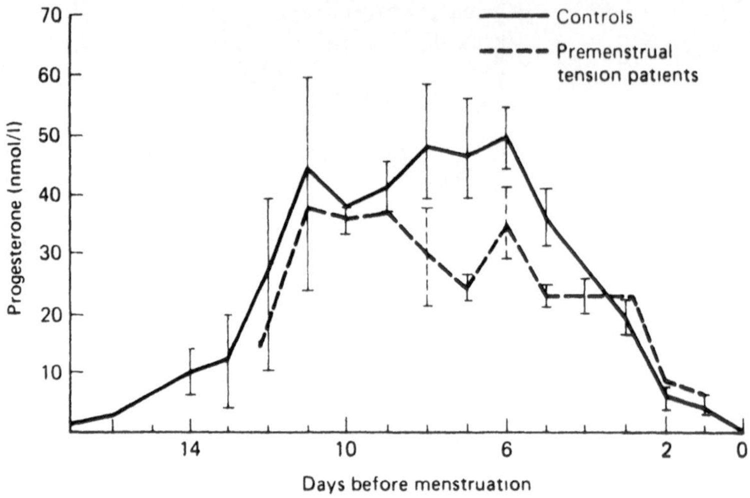

Fig. 2. Mean plasma progesterone values in women with premenstrual syndrome and controls. From: Munday (1977). [Reproduced by permission of *Current Medical Research and Opinion*. and the figure is from Backstrom T, Sanders D, Leask R, Davidson P, & Bancroft J. 1983. Mood, sexuality, hormones and the menstrual cycle. Psychosomatic Medicine 45; 503-507

Later, Dalton (1964) applied these concepts to therapy and began treating patients with progestagens and progesterone. One of the first studies in which hormonal changes were actually measured showed progesterone levels to be significantly lowered on days 4-6 prior to menstruation (Backstrom & Carstensen, 1974). This study presents the best data supporting the progesterone hypothesis and is often quoted. However, the lower levels are only seen during a short phase of the cycle and are not adequate to account for the usual duration of

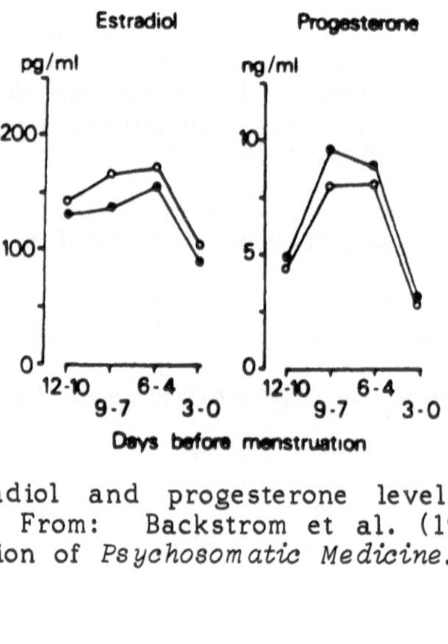

Fig. 3. Mean estradiol and progesterone levels in premenstrual syndrome. From: Backstrom et al. (1983). [Reproduced by permission of *Psychosomatic Medicine*.]

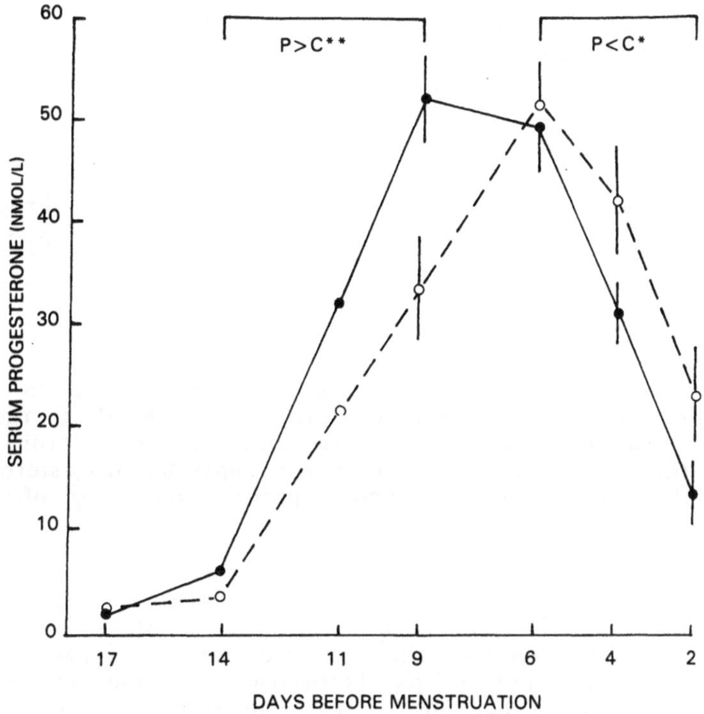

Fig. 4. Mean serum progesterone concentrations in ten patients with PMS (●—●) and eight control subjects (o---o). The bars indicate standard errors in results which are normally distributed: the median is shown for non-parametric data. Degrees of significance between patients (P) compared with controls (C), * $p < .05$; ** $p < .01$. From: Butt et al. (1983). [Reproduced by permission of Medical News Tribune, Ltd.]

symptoms. Two further studies have reported lower plasma levels of progesterone (Munday, 1977) (Fig. 2) and lower urinary pregnanediol levels in association with PMS (Dennerstein, Spencer-Gardner, & Burrows, 1984). Another study, often quoted as confirming the hypothesis, shows significantly lower levels on the day prior to menstruation only, with no significant difference being shown on other days of the cycle (Smith, 1975). Andersch, Abrahamsson, Wendestam, Ohman, and Hahn (1979) found no differences in progesterone levels associated with any part of the luteal phase of the cycle. Backstrom and co-workers have reported a more recent and better controlled study in which no differences could be seen in progesterone levels between severely affected women and controls, thus contradicting their earlier work (Backstrom, Sanders, Leask, Davidson, Warner, & Bancroft, 1983) (Fig. 3). In 1942, Gillman reported the simulation of PMS-like symptoms following the intramuscular injection of progesterone. A 1979 study showed progesterone levels to be higher and to peak earlier than in controls (O'Brien, Craven, Selby, & Symonds, 1979), and a more recent study (Butt, Watts, & Holder, 1983) again showed a marked early peak of progesterone (Fig. 4). It is

Table 3. Typical Reports of Placebo Response in the Treatment of Premenstrual Syndrome.

Smith (1975)	57%	Progesterone
Day (1979)	43%	Dydrogesterone
Sampson (1979)	43–60%	Progesterone
Haspels (1981)	53%	Dydrogesterone
Studd & Magos (1983)	75%	Hormone Implants

difficult to account for these diverse findings; and to date, no firm conclusions can be drawn relating progesterone levels to the pathogenesis of PMS. The studies based on measures of progesterone levels would indicate that the problem cannot be as simple as progesterone deficiency, despite the claims that exogenous progesterone may often relieve the symptoms.

There have, of course, been many other causes postulated for this syndrome, including endorphin deficiency, vitamin deficiency (particularly vitamin B6), alterations of prostaglandin metabolism, and excesses of prolactin, renin, angiotensin, or aldosterone. PMS has also been considered to be purely psychosomatic, or due to "menotoxin," to hypoglycemia, or to hormone allergy (in Tonks, 1975). There is little or no empirical evidence to support any of these theories.

TREATMENT

Of all the controversial aspects of PMS, treatment poses the greatest uncertainty. The main contribution to this confusion is the vast number of reports which fail to include placebo therapy controls. As the placebo effect is generally reported to be 40-60 percent (Sampson, 1979), it is clearly inadequate to undertake or report studies which do not include placebo controls (Table 3).

Treatments that do not involve medications include such diverse approaches as isolation in menstrual huts, yoga, aerobic, homeopathy, masturbation, electrical vaginal stimulation, hypnosis, psychotherapy, music therapy, and acupuncture. Treatments involving medications have ranged from psychotropic drugs (such as diazepam, anti-depressants, and lithium) to vitamins (such as A and B6) to diuretics. Endocrine manipulation has been attempted with estrogens, progesterone, progestagens, testosterone, combined oral contraceptives, bromocriptine, danazol, and prostaglandin synthetase inhibitors (for a full review, see O'Brien, 1982).

Of all the available treatments, the use of progesterone or progestagens has received the most publicity and almost fanatical support. The rationale is based on the progesterone deficiency theory, and, as we have documented, this has as yet an unproven basis.

Dalton (1984) has treated many women over many years, and her reports, although entirely anecdotal and without placebo-controlled trials, appear very convincing. There are only a few studies reported in the literature with adequate trial designs. Smith (1975) reported the use of progesterone and showed it to be ineffective, but unfortunately he used much lower doses than in most other investigations. Sampson

(1979) conducted a double-blind, controlled trial of progesterone administered via suppositories and pessaries, and showed no advantage of drug compared with placebo. Recently, Haspels (1981) has shown the progestagen, dydrogesterone, to be more effective than placebo for some symptoms. But it remains that there is no clear evidence to implicate progesterone in the pathogenesis of PMS, and despite the positive case history reports, the available scientifically controlled studies (e.g., using placebo in double-blind, crossover procedures) of progesterone therapy are not convincing. Progesterone does, however, have a diuretic action which may make patients symptomatically better. In addition, progesterone has a depressant effect on the central nervous system, and hence it may be effective purely by its tranquilizing action.

SUGGESTED APPROACHES TO THERAPY

In the absence of a confirmed scientific basis on which to treat patients, the following approaches to management might aid the clinician confronted with a PMS patient.

First, it is inadvisable to see patients in a busy gynecological outpatient clinic. Time is required for discussion and reassurance, and the "psychotherapeutic" impact of talking to the patient cannot be overemphasized. A full history, including analysis of symptoms peculiar to each patient, will give the best guide to treatment. Full examination of the pelvis (including cervical smear) and the breasts is important both for specific diagnosis and to allay "cancer-phobia." It is also important to distinguish PMS patients from those with primary psychiatric disorders and those with endometriosis and pelvic inflammatory disease (especially where premenstrual pelvic pain occurs). The problem must also be distinguished from dysmenorrhea and the menopause; both patients and doctors confuse these. A large but difficult group to exclude are those women who are relying on the PMS label to rationalize social, sexual, or psychological inadequacies. There are, of course, several psychological tests available which may assist in the exclusion of this group; these tend to be too complex and time-consuming for routine clinical use.

Blood tests are of no diagnostic value, although progesterone estimation may designate the sub-group of women with low progesterone. Prolactin levels should be measured in women experiencing swelling and tenderness of the breasts, and in whom bromocriptine is anticipated for therapy. Estimates of thyroid function will identify the occasional patient whose anxiety or irritability symptoms are due to thyrotoxicosis. Gonadotrophin estimation in the middle-aged woman will assist in the exclusion of the woman whose symptoms are due to the peri-menopause. Urea and electrolytes should be monitored when the use of spironolactone is anticipated in order to detect the rare possibility of hyperkalemia.

Of the treatment regimens above, a few have been evaluated scientifically and provide a stronger basis for choice of drug therapy than simply anecdotal reports. This choice will depend on age, the desire for future pregnancy, the co-existence of menstrual with other disorders, the patient's preferences, and the specific nature of her symptoms. The first step is to determine whether discussion and education will be sufficient to alleviate symptoms, or if specific drug therapy is necessary.

For a woman under 35 who does not smoke and currently does not wish to become pregnant, an oral contraception which combines estrogen and progestagen is the best first approach, although it must be cautioned that a small group of women experience worsening of symptoms using this regime. For these, predominantly progestagenic pills may be better (Cullberg, 1972). If oral contraception is not suitable, several other approaches are possible. Vitamin B6 (pyridoxine) has been reported to be of some value (albeit in uncontrolled studies), particularly for women whose symptoms are predominantly psychological (Day, 1979). It is possible, of course, that vitamin B6 is no more than an effective placebo. A progestagen is indicated in patients with multiple symptoms or those who *also* have irregular cycles, dysmenorrhea, or heavy periods. Dydrogesterone (10 milligrams twice daily) given from days 12 to 26 of the menstrual cycle is the progestagen usually prescribed, and of the few trials available, the one (progestagen) which has been best assessed (Haspels, 1981). There is much anecdotal support for the use of progesterone pessaries or suppositories, but, as we have seen, the few controlled studies have shown them to be no more effective than placebo. Because of the promotion and media reporting, many women will request this therapy and, in this situation, it is reasonable to prescribe progesterone; side effects are few, even on long-term therapy, although some authors report suppression of ovulation (see chapter by Bell, this volume, for consideration of long-term side effects).

If there is proven weight increase, or if physical symptoms predominate, spironolactone (100 milligrams daily) should be given three days before the expected onset of symptoms until the onset of menstruation. It will also improve psychological symptoms in many women (O'Brien et al., 1979). Unlike the regime required by many diuretics, potassium supplements must *not* be given.

Many women experiencing severe breast symptoms benefit from bromocriptine despite normal plasma prolactin levels (Benedek-Jaszmann, Lequin, & Sternthal, 1975). Bromocriptine (5 milligrams daily) is effective when given from days 10 to 26 of the cycle. Side effects such as nausea, vomiting, and dizziness can be avoided by administering at night. Danazol is also useful for the alleviation of breast symptoms (Mansel, Wisbey, & Hughes, 1979). It would also be expected that suppression of the ovarian cycle would be accompanied by improvement of other symptoms, but this can only be reported as an anecdote. It should be noted that virilizing side effects have been reported when the daily dose exceeds 400 milligrams.

Evening primrose oil is another treatment which has been recently popularized by the press. It appears effective in cyclical breast pain (Preece & Mansel, 1981). Reports of double-blind treatments for other symptoms are awaited, although single-blind studies show a beneficial effect on most PMS symptoms (Brush, 1983).

Prostaglandin synthetase inhibitors (such as mefenamic acid) have been shown to improve most symptoms, but particularly pain (Wood & Jakubowicz, 1980). In women approaching the menopause, estrogen implants with intermittent progestagen are of value, but the use of implants appears to have one of the highest placebo effects (Studd & Magos, 1983) (Table 3).

Using this armamentarium of approaches, the majority of patients will achieve significant improvement in most of their symptoms. If response to treatment is not achieved, the diagnosis should be re-evaluated. If the diagnosis is confirmed, then the clinician will have to resort to a more empirical approach until the successful drug or combination of drugs is achieved.

CONCLUSIONS

Although premenstrual syndrome poses many problems for the clinician and the investigator, these difficulties will be overcome when adequate objective methods of assessment become available, when drug assessment studies include placebo therapy, and when precise definitions and criteria for diagnosis are utilized. These factors will afford credibility for studies of PMS and for its "disease status." In the meantime, the clinician is advised to scrutinize studies of PMS carefully and interpret them with caution.

REFERENCES

Andersch, B., L. Abrahamsson, C. Wendestam, R. Ohman, and L. Hahn, 1979. Hormone profile in premenstrual tension: Effects of bromocriptine and diuretics. *Clinical Endocrinology 11:* 657-664.

Backstrom, T. and H. Carstensen, 1974. Estrogen and progesterone in plasma in relation to premenstrual tension. *Journal of Steroid Biochemistry 5:* 257-260.

Backstrom, T., D. Sanders, R. Leask, D. Davidson, P. Warner, and J. Bancroft, 1983. Mood, sexuality, hormones, and the menstrual cycle: Hormone levels and their relationship to the premenstrual syndrome. *Psychosomatic Medicine 45:* 503-507.

Backstrom, T., L. Wide, R. Sodergard, and H. Carstensen, 1976. FSH, LH, TeBG — capacity, estrogen and progesterone in women with premenstrual tension during the luteal phase. *Journal of Steroid Biochemistry 7:* 473-476.

Benedek-Jaszmann, L. J., R. N. Lequin, and V. Sternthal, 1975. Treatment of the premenstrual syndrome with Bromocriptine. *Acta Endocrinologica (Supplement 193):* 29.

Bickers, W. and M. Wood, 1951. Premenstrual tension: Rational treatment. *Texas Reports on Biology and Medicine 9:* 406.

Brush, M. G., 1983. The significance of pyridoxine and gamma-linolenic acid in premenstrual syndrome. In: R. W. Taylor (Ed.), *Premenstrual Syndrome.* Proceedings of the Workshop at Royal College of Obstetricians and Gynaecologists. Medical News Tribune, Ltd., London, pp. 57-62.

Butt, W. R., J. F. Watts, and G. Holder, 1983. The biochemical background to the premenstrual syndrome. In: R. W. Taylor (Ed.), *Premenstrual Syndrome.* Proceedings of the Workshop at Royal College of Obstetricians and Gynaecologists. Medical News Tribune, Ltd., London, pp. 16-24.

Clare, A. W., 1983. Psychiatric and social aspects of premenstrual complaints. *Psychological Medicine (Monograph Supplement) 4:* 1-58.

Cullberg, J., 1972. Mood changes and menstrual symptoms with different gestagen/oestrogen combinations. *Acta Psychiatrica Scandinavica (Supplement):* 236.

Dalton, K., 1964. *The Premenstrual Syndrome.* William Heinemann Medical Books, Ltd., London.

Dalton, K., 1977. *The Premenstrual Syndrome and Progesterone Therapy.* William Heinemann Medical Books, Ltd., London.

Dalton, K., 1981. Sex hormone-binding globulin concentrations in women with severe premenstrual syndrome. *Postgraduate Medical Journal 57:* 560-561.

Dalton, K., 1984. *The Premenstrual Syndrome and Progesterone Therapy* (second edition). William Heinemann Books, Ltd., London.

Day, J. B., 1979. Clinical trials in the premenstrual syndrome. *Current Medical Research Opinion 6 (Supplement 5):* 40-45.

Dennerstein, L., C. Spencer-Gardner, and G. D. Burrows, 1984. Mood and the menstrual cycle. *Journal of Psychiatric Research 18:* 1-12.
Faratian, B., A. Gaspar, P.M.S. O'Brien, I. R. Johnson, G. A. Filshie, and P. Prescott, 1984. Weight, abdominal size and perceived body image in premenstrual syndrome. *American Journal of Obstetrics and Gynecology 150:* 200-204.
Frank, R. T., 1931. The hormonal causes of premenstrual tension. *Archives of Neurology and Psychiatry 26:* 1053-1057.
Gillman, J., 1942. The nature of subjective reactions evoked in women by progesterone with special reference to the problems of premenstrual tension. *Journal of Clinical Endocrinology and Metabolism 2:* 157-160.
Haspels, A. A., 1981. A double-blind, placebo-controlled, multicentre study of the efficacy of dydrogesterone (Duphaston). In: *Proceedings of the Sixth International Congress of Psychosomatic Obstetrics and Gynaecology, Berlin.* MTP Press, Lancaster, England, pp. 81-92.
Israel, S. L., 1938. Premenstrual tension. *Journal of the American Medical Association 110:* 1721.
Mansel, R. E., J. R. Wisbey, and L. E. Hughes, 1979. The use of Danazol in the treatment of painful benign breast disease: Preliminary results. *Postgraduate Medical Journal 55* (Supplement 5): 51.
Moos, R. H., 1977. *Menstrual Distress Questionnaire Manual.* Stanford University School of Medicine, Stanford, CA.
Munday, M., 1977. Progesterone and aldosterone levels in the premenstrual tension syndrome. *Current Medical Research and Opinion 4:* 16-22.
Muse, K., N. Cetel, L. Futterman, and I. S. Yen, 1984. The premenstrual syndrome: Effects of "medical ovariectomy." *New England Journal of Medicine 311:* 1345-1349.
O'Brien, P.M.S., 1979. Endocrine Changes in Premenstrual Syndrome. M.D. Thesis, University of Wales.
O'Brien, P.M.S., 1982. The premenstrual syndrome: A review of the present status of therapy. *Drugs 24:* 140-151.
O'Brien, P.M.S., D. Craven, C. Selby, and E. M. Symonds, 1979. Treatment of premenstrual syndrome by spironolactone. *British Journal of Obstetrics and Gynaecology 86:* 142-147.
Pennington, V. M., 1957. Meprobamate (Miltown) in premenstrual tension. *Journal of the American Medical Association 164:* 638-640.
Preece, P. E. and R. E. Mansel, 1981. Management of breast pain using Efamol. Paper presented at the First Symposium on the Clinical Uses of Efamol and Essential Fatty Acids, London.
Rees, W. L., 1953. Psychosomatic aspects of the premenstrual tension syndrome. *Journal of Mental Science 99:* 62.
Sampson, G. A., 1979. Premenstrual syndrome: A double-blind controlled trial of progesterone and placebo. *British Journal of Psychiatry 135:* 209-215.
Smith, S. L., 1975. Mood and the menstrual cycle. In: E. J. Sachar (Ed.), *Topics in Psychoendocrinology.* Grune & Stratton, New York, NY, pp. 19-58.
Studd, J.W.W. and A. L. Magos, 1983. Management of the premenstrual syndrome by subcutaneous implants of oestradiol. *Proceedings of the 23rd British Congress of Obstetricians and Gynaecologists, Birmingham,* p. 66.
Tonks, C. M., 1975. Premenstrual tension. *British Journal of Psychiatry, Special No. 9:* 399-407.
Wood, C. and D. Jakubowicz, 1980. The treatment of premenstrual symptoms with mefenamic acid. *British Journal of Obstetrics and Gynaecology 87:* 627-630.

PATHOPHYSIOLOGY AND TREATMENT OF PREMENSTRUAL SYNDROME

Robert L. Reid, M.D., F.R.C.S.(C)

Division of Reproductive Endocrinology
Department of Obstetrics and Gynaecology
Queen's University
Kingston, Ontario, Canada

INTRODUCTION

The premenstrual syndrome (PMS) is a complex psychoneuroendocrine disorder that results in recurrent temporary disruption of the personal and professional lives of a substantial number of women throughout their reproductive years (Reid & Yen, 1981a). PMS is now recognized as an important factor contributing to marital discord, social isolation, and work inefficiency or absenteeism (Bickers & Wood, 1951; Dalton, 1964). Suicidal and psychotic behavior (Dalton, 1959; Endo, Daiguji, Asano, Yamashitu, & Takahashi, 1978; Glass, Heninger, Lansky, & Talan, 1971; Janowski, Gorney, Castelnuovo-Tedesco, & Stone, 1969; Mandell & Mandell, 1967; Tanks, Rach, & Rose, 1968), accidents requiring admission to the hospital (Dalton, 1960; MacKinnon & MacKinnon, 1956), and criminal activities including child battering, theft, and murder (Dalton, 1961, 1966, 1980; d'Orban & Dalton, 1980) are all reported as occurring with increased frequency in the premenstrual week, indicating that the adverse effects of PMS on both the individual and on society in general may be far-ranging. Conflicting theories about the pathophysiology of PMS and a host of alleged but unproven remedies have both confused and frustrated practitioners faced with the reality of treating affected individuals. The dissatisfaction and skepticism that this has generated among physicians has, in general, resulted in a disinterest in PMS which is mirrored by the paucity of information on this subject in most texts on obstetrics and gynecology. In a recent detailed review, this author has examined many of the controversies, both social and scientific, surrounding the topic of PMS (Reid, 1985).

DEFINITION

The term *premenstrual syndrome* (PMS) refers to the cyclic recurrence in the luteal phase of the menstrual cycle of a combination of distressing physical, psychological, and behavioral changes of sufficient severity to result in deterioration of interpersonal relationships and/or interference with normal activities. Recurrent midcycle pain (Mittelschmertz) and dysmenorrhea (painful menstruation, which may be primary or secondary) are not features of PMS, although these conditions may coexist in some individuals. In addition, the existence of a symptom-free interval lasting for at least one week following menses is important to avoid confusing PMS with other chronic conditions such as idiopathic edema, fibrocystic breast disease, endogenous depression, or anxiety neurosis, all of which may show a premenstrual exacerbation. The term "premenstrual tension" is imprecise because it refers to only one possible presentation of PMS, and should therefore be abandoned.

INCIDENCE

Up to 90% of the women of reproductive age are aware of at least some symptoms in the latter part of their cycle which indicate that menstruation is approaching. Self-report studies revealed that 20-40% of the women sampled perceive their symptoms to be of sufficient severity to temporarily interfere with their social interactions and/or work performance (Abraham, 1980). Recent data collected by a neighborhood census among a free-living population (i.e., not institutionalized) of North American women revealed that PMS was mild to moderate in 40% and severe in an additional 10% of women in their reproductive years (Woods, Most, & Dery, 1982). PMS occurs in both ovulatory and anovulatory cycles, and the incidence of PMS correlates neither with age nor parity (Greene & Dalton, 1953). This condition may be present from puberty or may become apparent as premenstrual symptoms worsen insidiously over a number of years. In some women, PMS appears abruptly in the first menstrual cycle following pregnancy (Greene & Dalton, 1953).

In contrast, dysmenorrhea is said to occur in 50% of menstruating women and to cause significant impairment in 5% (Dawood, 1983). Dysmenorrhea is generally associated with ovulatory cycles, and its incidence bears a negative correlation with parity. Although PMS and dysmenorrhea often coexist, the variable nature of this association suggests that different pathophysiological mechanisms are involved.

CLINICAL MANIFESTATIONS

The symptoms experienced by most women will fall into one of four temporal patterns based on the onset and duration of symptoms, with the vast majority experiencing pattern A or B (Fig. 1). Careful questioning will reveal a common progression of symptoms in relation to the phase of the menstrual cycle, although specific components of the syndrome (e.g., depression, irritability) may predominate in any given individual.

As early as 7-10 days prior to menses, affected women may notice painful breast enlargement, lower abdominal distension, and constipation sufficient to necessitate a change to looser clothing as the menses approach. Although this sensation of swelling is often perceived by affected individuals as evidence of a generalized fluid retention, only a minority of women with PMS show actual weight gain or edema. A dramatic increase in appetite and unusual cravings for chocolate or salty foods are frequently noted in the premenstrual week, with the result that binge eating is common at this time (Melody, 1961). For most women, these symptoms represent minor annoyances that are well tolerated in the absence of other psychological and behavioral aspects of PMS.

Variable degrees of fatigue, emotional lability, and depression may appear up to two weeks prior to menses. Women troubled by these changes find that they sleep longer, have less energy to devote to their usual routines, and may cry or have emotional outbursts over relatively trivial matters. More severely affected individuals may become completely withdrawn from family and friends, choosing to physically isolate

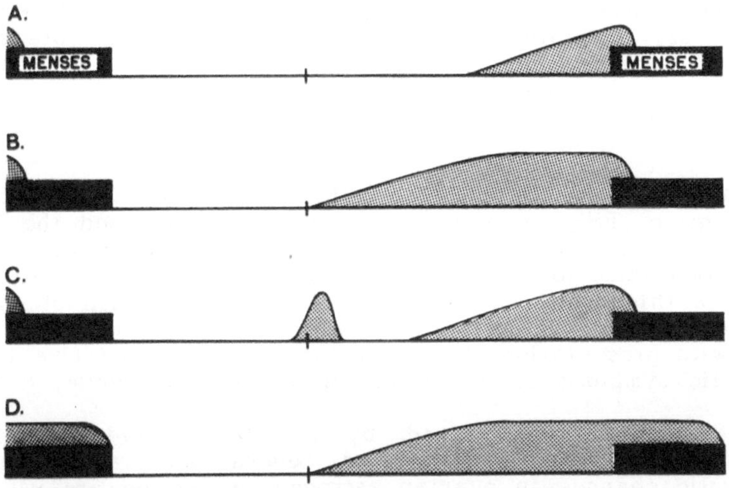

Fig. 1. Schematic diagram showing variability in the onset and duration of premenstrual symptoms. Most patients experience patterns A or B. From Reid and Yen (1983). [Reproduced by permission of *Clinical Obstetrics and Gynaecology.*]

themselves and to cancel any social commitments. Uncommonly, recurrent suicidal thoughts or behavior may be present.

As the menses approach, anxiety, inward tension, and anger develop, leading to physical unrest, insomnia, irritability, and combativeness. Some women find that this inward tension is accompanied by a burst of energy in the 2-3 days before menses which allows them to complete any neglected responsibilities, while others describe associated confusion, inability to concentrate, and forgetfulness which frustrate any efforts to organize their time effectively. Frequent angry confrontations over matters of minor importance are often the first clue to other family members that it is "that time of the month" again. Deterioration of interpersonal relationships and work efficiency often precipitate feelings of personal inadequacy, hopelessness, and guilt. Alcohol consumption may increase substantially in the premenstruum (Melody, 1961). Some women have difficulty concentrating and may purposely avoid driving the car, while others, believing that their judgment is impaired, may postpone important decisions until the days following menstruation. Sexual drive may show a marked increase or decrease depending on whether feelings of tension or depression predominate. Sensations of awkwardness or motor incoordination and a susceptibility to accidents are sometimes reported in the final days of the cycle. Some women will report recurrent cold chills or night sweats as the menses approach. The appearance of acne and the onset of headaches usually precede menstruation by 1-2 days, while the onset of crampy low back pain and the passage of a loose stool signal that the menses are imminent. Although some women report the dramatic "lifting" of the inward tension and irritability several hours before the onset of menstrual flow, most experience relief from premenstrual psychological distress during the first or second days of menstruation. Somatic symptoms, particularly headaches, may persist for a further 1-2 days. Premenstrual pelvic pain is seldom a feature of PMS and is more likely the result of endometriosis or dysmenorrhea. Where these conditions coexist with PMS, they may prolong or intensify the perceived summation of premenstrual and menstrual distress.

PATHOPHYSIOLOGY

Although many theories have been advanced to explain the pathophysiology of PMS, none has satisfactorily explained the heterogeneous clinical manifestations of this disorder. It seems clear that PMS is intimately related to cyclic function of the hypothalamic-pituitary-ovarian axis, for this condition begins only after activation of the ovaries at puberty and ceases following surgical or natural menopause. Hysterectomy alone, with preservation of ovarian function, is ineffective in eradicating the cyclic symptoms of this condition (Backstrom, Boyle, & Baird, 1981).

The precise role played by gonadal steroids in effecting this syndrome remains poorly understood. Several observations have suggested that cyclic changes in ovarian estrogen production are important in the pathophysiology of PMS. Characteristic changes of PMS may occur shortly before menarche at a time when estrogen levels begin to rise and fall coincident with earliest development and atresia of ovarian follicles (Greene & Dalton, 1953), and PMS is known to increase in intensity when a prolonged anovulatory cycle occurs (Woods et al., 1982). Some women experience recurrence of PMS-like symptoms each month as estrogen levels rise and fall precipitously at ovulation (Fig. 1, pattern C)(Reid, 1983) and oophorectomized women (i.e., with surgical removal of the ovaries) are known to experience PMS-like symptoms following injection of large doses of estrogen (Morton, 1950). These findings, together with the observation that symptoms frequently intensify as progesterone levels fall prior to menstruation, have caused several groups to propose *estrogen excess or progesterone deficiency* as the cause of PMS (Greene & Dalton, 1953; Morton, Addison, Addison, Hunt, & Sullivan, 1953). As a result, progesterone replacement therapy has been widely promoted by PMS clinics in Britain and the United States, and is now enthusiastically sought by many women who desperately seek relief from PMS. This theory about the causation of PMS has been challenged on several accounts (Sampson, 1981). Although several investigators have reported slight differences in the estrogen/progesterone ratios of PMS sufferers versus controls, others have documented apparently normal gonadal steroid production in women with PMS. The doses of progesterone used in the many uncontrolled clinical trials with this agent are much greater than that needed to achieve normal luteal phase progesterone levels; hence, it seems likely that any positive effects attributed to this agent are more the result of some pharmacological action of progesterone than an effect of correcting slight discrepancies in the estrogen/progesterone ratio. Until now, the only controlled trial (albeit small and short term) comparing progesterone to identical non-medicated placebo suppositories for the treatment of PMS showed both to have a beneficial effect with neither treatment being superior (Sampson, 1979). In view of the known high initial placebo response rate in PMS (Reid & Yen, 1981a), protagonists of progesterone therapy have argued that a longer trial period might have shown a beneficial effect of progesterone following abatement of any positive placebo response. Although it seems likely that changing levels of estrogen and/or progesterone incite other neuroendocrine changes leading to premenstrual symptomatology, there is presently insufficient data to allow any firm conclusions about the relationship between the estrogen/progesterone ratio and the type or severity of premenstrual complaints. In a long-term double-blind, placebo-controlled trial, we found no significant difference in the benefits afforded by progesterone (200 milligrams per vagina twice daily) and identical non-medicated polyethylene glycol placebo suppositories (Maddocks, Moller, Hahn, & Reid, 1986). We believe this raises a serious challenge to the continued promotion of this costly and unproven treatment (progesterone) for PMS.

A generalized *fluid retention* was proposed as the cause of PMS over 40 years ago (Greenhill & Freed, 1941) and widespread acceptance of this hypothesis has resulted in the frequent use of diuretics in the treatment of PMS. There are several clear accounts in the literature of women with recurrent premenstrual weight gain and edema, and even one report of recurrent pulmonary edema in a woman with underlying heart disease (Edeiken & Griffith, 1940). However, careful studies have shown that most women with premenstrual breast swelling and abdominal bloating lack evidence of fluid retention as determined by serial determinations of weight, total exchangeable sodium, and total body water (Reid & Yen, 1981a). It is likely therefore that these symptoms are the result of local changes within the breast and bowel, respectively. While diuretics may alleviate these specific complaints through a process of generalized dehydration, they afford little relief for the other symptoms of PMS. Efforts to identify a specific etiologic agent in cases of true premenstrual fluid accumulation have not yet been rewarded. A variety of hormones (including estrogen, progesterone, angiotensin, aldosterone, catecholamines, prolactin, and vasopressin) have all been suggested as possible causes for fluid retention in PMS, but none have been clearly implicated to date (Reid & Yen, 1981a). Sudden increments in the carbohydrate and salt content of the diet (occasioned by cravings for sweets and salty foods) may induce substantial actual weight gain in some women (MacGregor, Roulston, Markandu, de Wardener, & Jones, 1979) (Fig. 2).

Vitamin B6 (pyridoxine) deficiency has been suggestsed as the cause of PMS (Janowski et al., 1969), although objective proof for this hypothesis is lacking. Pyridoxal phosphate acts as a coenzyme in the final step of biosynthesis of the brain monoamines, dopamine, and serotonin, which play an important role in the regulation of mood and behavior. The clinical response to pyridoxine in controlled trials has been variable, with reports of improvement (Abraham & Hargrove, 1980) and no change (Stokes & Mendels, 1972).

Hypoglycemia has been suggested as the cause of PMS (Morton et al., 1953), based on reports that glucose tolerance curves were flattened with evidence of delayed hypoglycemia late in the luteal phase. Gonadal steroid-induced changes in insulin action have been suggested as the explanation for these findings (Bertoli, de Pirro, Fusco, Grecco, Magnatta, & Lauro, 1980). However, we have been unable to confirm any menstrual cycle-related abnormalities in glucose metabolism in women with premenstrual syndrome and alleged premenstrual "hypoglycemic" attacks (Reid, Greenaway-Coates, & Hahn, 1986). Although hypoglycemia may be a feature of this disorder, it is not the cause of PMS, for PMS does not exist solely at the times when blood sugar is low and is not relieved merely by the ingestion of food (Reid & Yen, 1981a).

Hyperprolactinemia has been suggested as the cause of PMS based on case reports of increased prolactin levels in some affected individuals (Halbreich, Ben-David, Assael, & Bornstein, 1976) and on the premise that prolactin may cause fluid retention in man as it does in other species (Cole, Everend, Horrobin, Manku, Mtabaji, & Nassar, 1975). The uncommon association of hyperprolactinemia and PMS observed by most investigators and the lack of a demonstrable osmoregulatory effect of prolactin in many suggest that, contrary to previous assertions, these disorders are not causally related (Reid & Yen, 1981a). Moreover, in

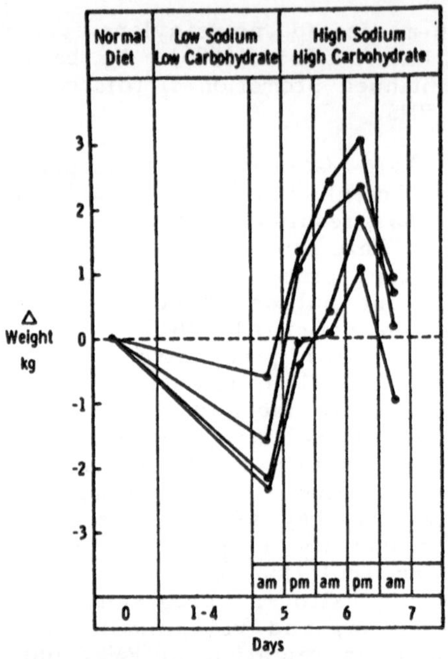

Fig. 2. Patterns of premenstrual syndrome. Changes with weight in four normal young women upon changing from their normal diet to a low sodium, low carbohydrate diet and then to a high sodium, high carbohydrate diet. From MacGregor et al. (1979). [Reproduced by permission of *The Lancet.*]

controlled trials, prolactin suppression with the dopaminergic agonist, bromocriptine, alleviated discomfort of the breast (a prolactin target organ), but had equivocal effects on other symptoms of PMS (Anderson & Larsen, 1979).

Rare individuals may show recurrent premenstrual oral and vulvar ulcers which are thought to result from an *allergy to an endogenous hormone* (progesterone) (Berger, 1955). The postulate that PMS results from the manifestations of a similar hypersensitivity to progesterone or one of its metabolites at multiple gonadal steroid target sites (Zondek & Bromberg, 1947) is inconsistent with the observation that PMS may occur both in ovulatory and anovulatory cycles and contradicts many of the tenets of allergic disease.

The failure to explain the complex changes that make up the PMS have led numerous investigators to postulate a *psychogenic* origin. One author (Suarez-Murias, 1953) has suggested that the woman with PMS is "unconsciously utilizing her menstrual function to express distress about pressing environmental situations, difficult interpersonal relationships and her own attitudes concerning being a woman." Others have reported a correlation between PMS and disturbed attitudes toward menarche and the menses, guilt feelings over sexual temptations, severe medical and gynecologic histories, poor sexual and martial adjustments, and high neuroticism scores. For male skeptics, this has provided a satisfactory way to "understand" the unusual behavior of women with PMS; while for women who have never (yet) experienced PMS, it provides a convenient way to isolate themselves from their "less stable" counterparts whom they may perceive as a threat to the movement for equality for women. In a provocative paper entitled, "Alleged psychogenic disorders in women — a possible manifestation of sexual prejudice," which was written prior to our understanding of the primary role of prostaglandins in the pathogenesis of dysmenorrhea, it was charged that the acceptance of a psychogenic origin of dysmenorrhea had delayed scientific study of the problem, resulting in an irrational and ineffective approach to the management (Lennane & Lennane, 1973). Statements to the effect that dysmenorrhea "occurred more frequently in the high strung, nervous or neurotic female than in her more stable sister," or was the result of "faulty outlook — leading to exaggeration of minor discomfort as an excuse to avoid doing something that is disliked," and that "pain was always secondary to an emotional problem" were, in fact, a form of sexual prejudice. Furthermore, by delaying investigation into the cause and cure of dysmenorrhea, these erroneous conclusions were actually perpetuating a treatable disorder while identifying the symptoms of affected women as "indisputable proof" of male-female inequality. When prostaglandins were subsequently implicated in the pathophysiology of dysmenorrhea and dramatic relief accompanied the use of prostaglandin synthetase inhibitors, even the most skeptical observers were forced to reconsider the role of psychogenic factors in dysmenorrhea (Dawood, 1983).

Despite compelling evidence which suggests that PMS is hormonally mediated, there are many who, for a variety of reasons, continue to argue that PMS is a psychogenic disorder. The parallels with the controversy about dysmenorrhea in the 1970's are obvious. The many studies which have supported a psychogenic origin of PMS have been critically reappraised and have been found deficient in numerous respects (Ganon, 1981), and it is clear that there is a need for continuing scientific scrutiny of this problem in an effort to delineate the underlying pathophysiology. Those who would argue that the recognition of PMS as a true hormonal disorder threatens equality for women should consider how many more women might enjoy a happy family life or excel in a career once the cause and cure for PMS are known.

ENDOGENOUS OPIATE HYPOTHESIS

A new hypothesis about the pathophysiology of PMS has been formulated based on recent discoveries about the neuroendocrine regulation of the menstrual cycle. Temporary "addiction" to high central levels of endogenous opiates during the luteal phase with subsequent opiate withdrawal as central opiate peptide levels fall prior to menstruation have been proposed as the central neuroendocrine events that ultimately precipitate the other manifestations of PMS (Fig. 3) (Reid & Yen, 1981a).

The endogenous opiate peptides (termed *endorphins* as an abbreviation for *endogenous morphine)*, when first discovered, were enthusiastically welcomed as possible potent non-addicting natural pain killers. It was soon found that temporary exposure to elevated levels of exogenous (Wei & Loh, 1976) or endogenous (Christie & Chester, 1982) endorphins could lead to addiction similar to that seen with other natural and synthetic opiates. Widely distributed throughout the body, endorphins are known to have a variety of effects in addition to analgesia, including such diverse actions as modulation of hormone secretion, mood, behavior,

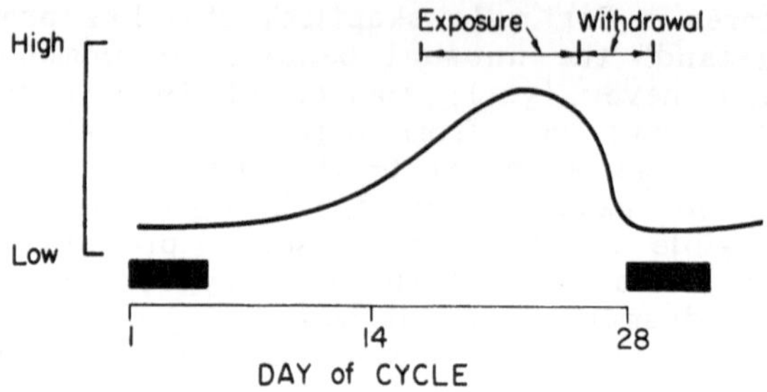

Fig. 3. Schematic diagram showing proposed cyclic changes in levels of endogenous opiate activity throughout the menstrual cycle. Maximal opiate exposure which occurs in the mid-luteal phase is followed by acute opiate withdrawal prior to the onset of menstruation (shown by the shaded boxes). From Reid and Yen (1983). [Reproduced by permission of *Clinical Obstetrics and Gynaecology.*]

appetite, and bowel function. The possibility that cyclic changes in central endogenous opiate activity occur during the human menstrual cycle was first suggested in 1980 by the demonstration that the opiate receptor antagonist, naloxone, elicited increments in the circulating levels of luteinizing hormone (which is normally suppressed by opiates) in the luteal (high estrogen, high progesterone) phase but not in the early follicular or menstrual (low estrogen, low progesterone) phase of the cycle (Quigley & Yen, 1980). This finding suggested that estrogen and progesterone, acting either alone or in combination, could increase central endogenous opiate activity. Support of this concept is the recent observation in the non-human primate (which has a 28-day cycle like humans) that the concentration of β-endorphin entering the pituitary stalk blood from the brain peaks during the luteal phase and falls to undetectable levels at the onset of menstruation (Wehrenberg, Wardlaw, Frantz, & Ferin, 1982). Indeed, blood levels of β-endorphin in the pituitary stalk hypophyseal portal system (the direct vascular connection between the hypothalamus and the pituitary) become undetectable following oophorectomy and rise once again during sequential replacement therapy with estrogen and progestin (Wardlaw, Wehrenberg, Ferin, Antunes, & Frantz, 1982).

Neurons which contain norepinephrine and dopamine (neurotransmitters which have important functions in the regulation of mood and behavior) are known to have presynaptic opiate receptors (Llorens, Martres, Bandry, & Schwartz, 1978)(Fig. 4). Activation of these receptors at times of increased endogenous opiate activity (e.g., during the luteal phase) may result in fatigue and depression by decreasing the amount of norepinephrine and dopamine reaching the postsynaptic receptor. Central injections of endorphin have recently been shown to cause satiated animals to resume vigorous eating (Grandison & Guidotti, 1977); hence, increased endorphin activity within the hypothalamus may explain the profound increase in appetite observed by some women during the luteal phase. Endorphins have been found throughout the small bowel in the human and are known to diminish both muscular propulsive activity and fluid secretion into the lumen. A temporary increase in endorphin levels within the bowel during the luteal phase may account for the constipation and delayed gastrointestinal transit that are known to occur in the premenstruum (Wald, Van Thiel, Hoechstetter, Gavaler, Egler, Verm, Scott, & Lester, 1981). Endorphins are present in

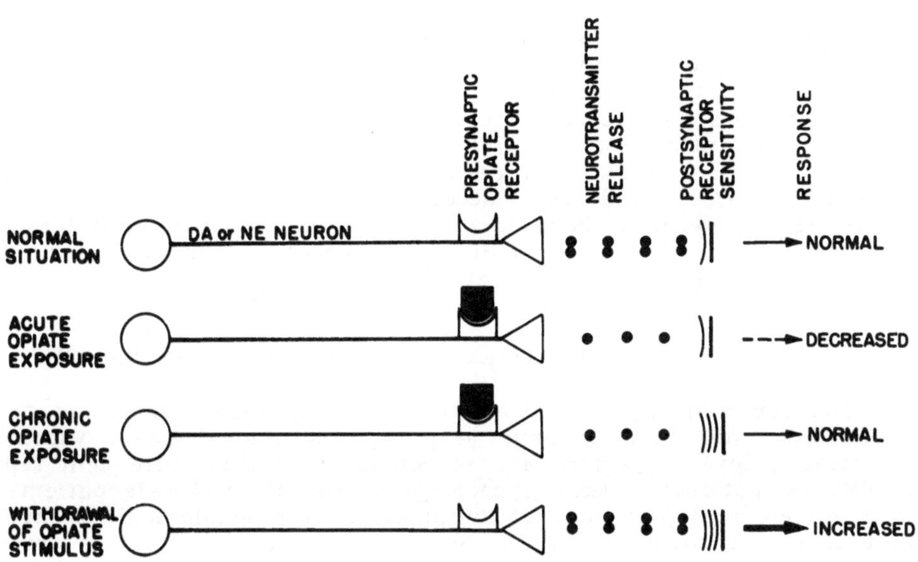

Fig. 4. Model depicting the effects of endogenous opiates on the function of aminergic neurons. Occupation of the presynaptic opiate receptor secondary to increased endogenous opiate activity (second panel) results in decreased release of neurotransmitter compared to the normal situation (first panel). During continuous exposure to increased endogenous opiate activity, accommodation to this decreased level of neurotransmission results from increasing receptor sensitivity (third panel). Persistence of this postsynaptic receptor supersensitivity following a return to normal levels of neurotransmission as endogenous opiate levels decline elicits an increased response following activation of aminergic systems (fourth panel). Modified with permission from Llorens et al. (1978). From Reid and Yen (1983). [Reproduced by permission of *Clinical Obstetrics and Gynaecology.*]

pancreatic islets, and injections of β-endorphin into humans have been shown to induce sustained hyperglycemia with hyperinsulinism (Reid & Yen, 1981b). The participation of endorphins in the altered gluco-regulation of the luteal phase of the cycle is currently under investigation.

The development of tolerance to opiates (both endogenous and exogenous) results from increasing sensitivity of the receptors for dopamine and norepinephrine, such that less of these neurotransmitters is needed to effect the same response (Fig. 4). When the opiate inhibition of neurotransmission is suddenly removed (i.e., with falling endorphin levels prior to menstruation), rebound hyperactivity of these pathways may result in irritability, anxiety, tension, aggression, and the burst of energy experienced by some women as the menses approach (Gianutsos & Lal, 1978; Lal & Puri, 1972). These same behavioral changes have been produced in normal human volunteers in whom endorphin activity has been suddenly blocked by the administration of the opiate antagonist naloxone (Cohen, Cohen, Pickar, Weingartner, Murphy, & Bunney, 1981).

These symptoms, which are characteristic of acute opiate withdrawal in humans, are known to vary in intensity depending on the degree and duration of exposure and the rapidity of withdrawal; hence, differences in these factors may account for the variable severity of PMS from month to month (Gianutsos & Lal, 1978; Lal & Puri, 1972). Severe dopaminergic hyperfunction is a well known cause of psychosis (Ellinwood, Sudilovsky, & Nelson, 1973), and may account for unusual cases of recurrent premenstrual psychotic behavior. Diarrhea and disordered temperature regulation, which are both features of opiate withdrawal, are common complaints just prior to the onset of menstruation.

IDENTIFYING THE PATIENT WITH PREMENSTRUAL SYNDROME

The reported high incidence of PMS may seem surprising to many physicians who claim to have seen only occasional cases within their practices. Several factors are responsible for this infrequent reporting of PMS by patients. Most gynecologists and their female patients alike tend to view mild premenstrual symptoms as a physiological inconvenience that is part of being a woman. As a result, these complaints are seldom elicited by the physician or volunteered by the patient during the medical history. In cases where these changes eventually become sufficiently troublesome to constitute PMS, affected women (many of whom have never heard of PMS) are often afraid to discuss their curious or distressing symptoms with their doctors. A common fear expressed by these women is that they are "going crazy;" and all too often, this belief is reinforced by hostile comments from a frustrated spouse or by a hasty psychiatric referral from a disinterested physician. Other women fear that symptoms such as clumsiness, binge eating, or altered sexual drive may be evidence of a personal idiosyncrasy or will be a source of embarrassment or ridicule. Some PMS sufferers determine to put "mind over matter," and may endure severe symptoms for years. Most women with PMS develop feelings of guilt and personal inadequacy as, over the years, their PMS leads to progressive deterioration of interpersonal relationships and/or work performance. Only careful direct questioning of these women will identify those with violent or suicidal tendencies, or those who believe that their judgment, concentration (i.e., driving a car), or work performance is temporarily impaired.

TAKING THE HISTORY

A few moments should be routinely taken when obtaining the menstrual history to ascertain the sequence and severity of premenstrual symptoms in women of reproductive age. Asking the patient what symptoms indicate to her that her menstrual period is approaching will frequently elicit only the response that "I retain fluid" or "My breasts get sore and my slacks don't fit." Further direct questioning about energy levels, changes in mood or temperament, changes in appetite or cravings, and alterations in bowel function or sexual drive will almost invariably elicit additional information. A more valid appraisal of the patient's premenstrual experience may be obtained if questions are posed in a fashion that would invite a response relating unusual as well as positive and negative symptomatology. Such questioning reassures the patient that other women have similar changes and lends an air of legitimacy to premenstrual symptoms which frequently sets the stage for an educational discussion. To document the chronology of premenstrual symptoms and to confirm the symptom-free interval following menstruation, it is essential to have the patient maintain a record of symptoms on a codified menstrual calendar such as the *Prospective Record of the Impact and Severity of Menstrual Symptoms* (PRISM calendar, Fig. 5).

PRISM
CALENDAR

Name ______________________

Baseline Weight On Day 1. ________ lbs. or kg. (circle one)

Day of Menstrual Cycle / BLEEDING / Month: Date:	1	2	3	4	5	6	7	8	9	10	11	12	13	14	15	16	17	18	19	20	21	22	23	24	25	26	27	28	29	30	31	32	33	34	35	36	37	38	39	40	41	42	43	44	45	46	47	48	49
WEIGHT CHANGE																																																	
SYMPTOMS																																																	
Irritable																																																	
Fatigue																																																	
Inward Anger																																																	
Labile Mood (crying)																																																	
Depressed																																																	
Restless																																																	
Anxious																																																	
Insomnia																																																	
Lack of Control																																																	
Edema or rings tight																																																	
Breast Tenderness																																																	
Abdominal Bloating																																																	
Bowels: const (c) loose (l)																																																	
Appetite. up↑ down↓																																																	
Sex Drive: up↑ down↓																																																	
Chills (C) /Sweats (S)																																																	
Headaches																																																	
Crave: sweets, salt																																																	
Feel Unattractive																																																	
Guilty																																																	
Unreasonable Behaviour																																																	
Low self image																																																	
Nausea																																																	
Menstrual Cramps																																																	
LIFESTYLE IMPACT																																																	
Aggressive towards others: Physically																																																	
Aggressive towards others: Verbally																																																	
Wish to be alone																																																	
Neglect Housework																																																	
Time off work																																																	
Disorganized, distractable																																																	
Accident Prone/Clumsy																																																	
Uneasy about driving																																																	
Suicidal Thoughts																																																	
Stayed at Home																																																	
Increased use of Alcohol																																																	
LIFE EVENTS																																																	
Negative Experience																																																	
Positive Experience																																																	
Social Activities																																																	
Vigorous Exercise																																																	
MEDICATIONS																																																	

INSTRUCTIONS FOR COMPLETING THIS CALENDAR

1 On the first day of menstruation prepare the calendar: Considering the first day of bleeding as day 1 of your menstrual cycle enter the corresponding calendar date for each day in the space provided below
2 Each Morning: Take weight after emptying bladder and before breakfast. Record **WEIGHT CHANGE** from baseline.
3 Each Evening: At about the same time complete the column for that day as described below.

BLEEDING: Indicate if you have had bleeding by shading the box above that days date ■, for spotting use an ☒
SYMPTOMS: If you do not experience any symptoms leave the corresponding square blank If present indicate severity.

MILD 1 (noticeable but not troublesome)
MODERATE. 2 (interferes with normal activity)
SEVERE. 3 (temporarily incapacitating)

LIFESTYLE IMPACT: If the listed phrase applies to you that day enter an ☒
LIFE EVENTS: If you experienced one of these events that day enter an ☒
Experiences: For positive (happy) or negative (sad or disappointing) experiences unrelated to your symptoms specify the nature of the events on the reverse side of this form
Social Activities imply events such as a special dinner, show or party etc involving family or friends
Vigorous Exercise implies participation in a sporting event or exercise programme lasting more than 30 minutes
MEDICATION: In the bottom 3 rows list medications if any and indicate days when taken by entering an ☒

Fig. 5. A calendar for recording the pattern and severity of symptoms in relation to the menstrual cycle (developed by R. L. Reid and S. Maddocks). Using such a calendar, PMS can be readily differentiated from symptoms unrelated to the menstrual cycle (e.g., no PMS). From Reid (1985). [Reproduced by permission of Year Book Medical Publishers, Inc.]

When the history reveals that troublesome premenstrual symptoms exist, it is important to determine the extent of physical and psychological impairment. Do fatigue and depression cause the patient to neglect housework or take "sick-days" from work? Does she spend time alone avoiding social interactions with family and friends? Does she have suicidal thoughts or plans? Does she have frequent emotional outbursts or angry confrontations over trivial matters? Is physical violence ever directed towards her children or spouse? Does she make decisions or manifest behavior in the premenstrual period that she later regrets? Is she accident prone or forgetful? Does she feel reluctant to drive the car?

It may be useful to have the patient complete a self-rating scale such as that designed by Steiner, Haskett, and Carroll (1980a) (Fig. 6). A premenstrual score greater than 15 on this scale with low intermenstrual scores usually indicates a significant degree of premenstrual impairment.

MANAGEMENT OF PREMENSTRUAL SYNDROME

To date, there has been no single scientifically established medical therapy for PMS. Of the many studies performed to assess various treatment modalities, few have given sufficient consideration to the striking placebo response in this disorder, and as a result, unsubstantiated remedies abound. [The belief that a response to placebo is indicative of a psychosomatic disorder must be re-evaluated in view of recent evidence which suggests that placebos may, in fact, exert beneficial effects by causing release of endogenous opiates (Gowdey, 1983)]. Given the pathophysiological uncertainties, it would seem prudent at the present time to manage PMS with liberal amounts of education and reassurance and the judicious use of medications. Termination of cyclic ovarian function by oophorectomy should be considered only in the most extreme cases when PMS is unresponsive to other measures or when a surgical approach is indicated due to coexisting pelvic pathology.

EDUCATION AND REASSURANCE

Education and reassurance begins with the taking of a careful history documenting the onset, pattern, type, and severity of premenstrual complaints. A description of the way that PMS is related to cyclic production of ovarian steroids and reassurance that many other women experience similar symptoms is frequently all that is needed to convince the patient that this disorder is not "all in her head."

In addition, it may prove useful to explain the patient's specific symptoms in terms of the endogenous opiate hypothesis because most women can readily grasp the similarities between symptoms of PMS and those resulting from opiate exposure (fatigue, depression, constipation, increased appetite) and withdrawal (irritability, aggression, cold chills, diarrhea, headache). It is equally important to the patient that family members understand the nature of the disorder, and it is therefore helpful to discuss the problem in the presence of the spouse or to provide the patient with some literature which she may take home. A helpful patient guide entitled *Good News About Premenstrual Blues* can be obtained from the publishers of Drug Therapy, 800 Second Avenue, New York, NY 10017. Support groups, such as Premenstrual Syndrome Action, provide another useful source of informative literature for the affected woman.

SELF-RATING SCALE FOR PREMENSTRUAL SYNDROME

Name: **Date:**

Instructions: The following questions are concerned with the way you feel or act today.

Please answer *all* questions by circling YES or NO as indicated.

1. Do you find yourself avoiding some of your social commitments? YES NO
2. Have you gained 5 or more pounds during the past week? YES NO
3. Is your coordination so poor that your are unable to use kitchen utensils, garden tools or unable to drive? YES NO
4. Do you feel more angry than usual ? YES NO
5. Do you avoid family activities and prefer to be left alone? YES NO
6. Do you doubt your judgement or feel that you are prone to hasty decisions? YES NO
7. Do you feel more irritable than usual? YES NO
8. Is your efficiency diminished? YES NO
9. Do you feel tense and restless? YES NO
10. Do you feel a marked change in your sexual drive or desire during the last week? YES NO
    If YES, is it *increased* or *decreased*? ↑ ↓
11. Are your present physical symptoms causing so much pain and discomfort that you are unable to function? YES NO
12. Have you recently cancelled previously scheduled social activities? YES NO
13. Do you feel as if you were unable to relax at all? YES NO
14. Do you feel confused? YES NO
15. Do you suffer from painful or tender breasts? YES NO
16. Do you have an increased desire for specific kinds of food (e.g. cravings for candy, chocolate, etc.)? YES NO
17. Do you scream/yell at family members (friends, colleagues) more than usual? Are you "short-fused"? YES NO
18. Do you feel sad, gloomy, and hopeless most of the time? YES NO
19. Do you feel like crying? YES NO
20. Do you have difficulty completing your daily household/job routine? YES NO
21. Was there a marked change in your sexual drive with definite change in your sexual behavior during the last week? YES NO
    If YES, is it *increased* or *decreased?* ↑ ↓
22. Do you find yourself being more forgetful than usual or unable to concentrate? YES NO
23. Do you happen to have more "accidents" with your daily housework/job (cut fingers, break dishes, etc.)? YES NO
24. Have you noticed significant swelling of your breasts and/or ankles and/or bloating of your abdomen? YES NO
25. Does your mood change suddenly without obvious reason? YES NO
26. Are you easily distracted? YES NO
27. Do you think that your restless behavior is noticeable by others? YES NO
28. Are you clumsier than usual? YES NO
29. Are you obviously negative and hostile towards other people? YES NO
30. Are you so fatigued that it interferes with your usual level of functioning? YES NO
31. Do you tend to eat more than usual or at odd irregular hours (sweet, snacks, etc.)? YES NO
32. Do you become more easily fatigued than usual? YES NO
33. Is your handwriting different (less neat than usual)? YES NO
34. Do you feel jittery or upset? YES NO
35. Do you feel sad or blue? YES NO
36. Have you stopped calling or visiting some of your best friends? YES NO

Adapted from: Steiner M., Haskett R.F., Carroll B.J.; Acta psychiat Scand. 62:177, 1980

Fig. 6. Self-rating scale for premenstrual syndrome. From Steiner et al. (1980a). [Reproduced with permission of *Acta Psychiatrica Scandinavica.*]

MEDICATION FOR PREMENSTRUAL SYNDROME

An ideal treatment for PMS would be a medication that corrects all aspects of the disorder by correcting the underlying pathophysiology. To date, the pathophysiology of this disorder is uncertain, and none of the many therapeutic agents that have been tried have afforded such global relief. Therapy for PMS continues to rely largely upon medication with proven efficacy for specific PMS symptoms and other less certain placebo benefits. In selecting medication for the treatment of PMS, it is wise to (1) avoid the use of multiple drugs, and (2) exercise caution when prescribing medication during the luteal phase if the possibility of pregnancy exists.

In general, *oral contraceptive steroids* have not proven superior to placebo for the treatment of PMS (Cullberg, 1972), and, in fact, some women first experience severe PMS while taking these agents. Some women, however, report a definite improvement in PMS when started on this medication, making contraceptive steroids a reasonable choice of therapy for the woman under 40 years of age who also requires birth control. At times, the relief from dysmenorrhea afforded by contraceptive steroids causes a significant decrease in the perceived premenstrual and menstrual distress, making this a highly effective therapy. *Prostaglandin synthetase inhibitors* have not proven beneficial for treatment of PMS *per se* (Wood & Jakubowicz, 1980), but, unlike contraceptive steroids, may cause a significant reduction in overall menstrual distress in some women because of their effectiveness in preventing dysmenorrhea.

Simple *analgesics* such as aspirin or acetominophen, with or without codeine, may be sufficient to relieve the headaches and minor musculoskeletal pains that accompany the PMS. There is now compelling evidence that menstrual migraine may result from falling estradiol levels (Somerville, 1972), and preliminary data indicate that subcutaneous estradiol implants may effectively alleviate this condition (Magos, Zilkha, & Studd, 1983).

The routine use of *diuretics* in the treatment of PMS should be abandoned. Breast tenderness and abdominal bloating are rarely manifestations of a generalized fluid retention, and probably result from local fluid shifts within the breast and bowel. Through a process of generalized dehydration, diuretics may make these symptoms less noticeable and temporarily improve the woman's self image; however, diuretics may actually precipitate fluid retention in some cases if taken intermittently because of the activation of the renin angiotensin-aldosterone axis which they induce (MacGregor et al., 1979). Dietary manipulation aimed at reducing the intake of refined carbohydrates and salt may be sufficient to eliminate swelling and weight gain in those women with true premenstrual fluid accumulation. Only if these measures fail and physical symptoms remain a major component of PMS should the use of diuretics be considered. *Spironolactone* (100 mg orally in single or divided doses) is the drug of choice because it prevents the hypokalemia and the tendency toward secondary aldosteronism associated with other diuretics (O'Brien, Craven, Selby, & Symonds, 1979).

Bromocriptine (2.5 milligrams by mouth twice daily) (Anderson & Larsen, 1979) and *danazol* (100-200 milligrams by mouth twice daily) (Day, 1979) both relieve breast swelling and tenderness in PMS, but are of limited value as far as other symptoms are concerned. The expense and potential troublesome side effects of these medications should preclude their routine use for long-term treatment of PMS.

Perhaps the least progress has been made toward the treatment of the distressing psychological changes of PMS. Severely depressed women with suicidal thoughts, those who exhibit violent or psychotic behavior, and women who may have an associated alcohol problem should have the benefit of a complete psychiatric evaluation to rule out or treat any underlying chronic psychiatric illness. In most cases, however, women with cyclic premenstrual recurrence of these symptoms respond poorly to conventional psychiatric treatments. Psychotherapy alone has proven ineffective in the treatment of PMS. *Tricyclic antidepressants*, such as amitryptyline or desipramine (75 to 150 milligrams by mouth daily) have a delayed onset of action which make their use for short-term treatment both inappropriate and ineffective. When administered chronically, these drugs seldom relieve premenstrual depression; yet, they have the potential to exacerbate premenstrual manic behavior. Therefore, these agents should be reserved for individuals who have endogenous depression that worsens during the premenstrual period. *Minor tranquilizers* of the benzodiazepine family, such as diazepam, may be useful when prescribed sparingly in individuals in whom symptoms of anxiety, irritability, tension, or restlessness predominate. Both antidepressants and anxiolytic agents may cause drowsiness and should be prescribed with caution in women whose work requires them to be alert.

Pyridoxine (50-100 milligrams by mouth twice daily) (throughout the month) has been shown to improve mood in depressed oral contraceptive users (Adams, Rose, Folkard, Wynn, Seed, & Strong, 1973), but has produced variable results in women with PMS (Abraham & Hargrove, 1980; Stokes & Mendels, 1972). At higher doses, this medication may have adverse effects; hence, patients must be cautioned about the possibility of overdosing (Schaumburg, Kaplan, Windebank, Vick, Rasmus, Pleasure, & Brown, 1983). A trial over several months is useful to determine whether pyridoxine will afford benefit in individual cases.

Lithium carbonate (600-1800 milligrams/day orally) is effective in controlling recurrent psychotic or cyclothymic behavior in severely affected individuals (Glick & Stewart, 1980; Steiner, Haskett, Osmun, & Carroll, 1980b). Troublesome side effects and the need for careful monitoring of renal function and serum lithium levels make this therapy unsuitable for all but the most severely affected individuals.

Progesterone has received wide acclaim for its effectiveness in treating PMS, although clear scientific proof of its superiority to placebo is lacking. Although progesterone by vaginal suppository (200-400 milligrams twice daily) appears to be safe, even if pregnancy should occur, the expense of this medication, the tendency for desperate individuals to try anything that offers a chance for cure, and the lack of efficacy in every controlled clinical trial to date are sufficient reasons to raise a serious challenge to the perpetuation of this therapy.

FUTURE DIRECTIONS IN THE MANAGEMENT OF PREMENSTRUAL SYNDROME

Several new therapies are currently under investigation for the treatment of PMS based on the intriguing possibility that cyclic gonadal steroid-induced changes in endogenous opiate levels may be implicated in the pathogenesis of this disorder. Long-acting luteinizing-hormone releasing-hormone (LHRH) agonists are able to induce temporary cessation of cyclic ovarian function by diminishing pituitary sensitivity to LHRH through a process of receptor down-regulation (Yen, 1983). The constant low ovarian steroid concentrations afforded by this treatment would eliminate the major fluctuations in central endogenous opiate activity that characterize a normal menstrual cycle. This treatment has been shown to provide relief from cyclic symptoms of PMS (Muse, Cetel, Futterman, & Yen, 1984).

Narcotic antagonists are known to cause a marked reduction in appetite (Grandison & Guidotti, 1977), and it is possible that orally active preparations such as naltrexone could effectively counteract other features of PMS if these are, in fact, the result of excessive exposure to endogenous opiates during the luteal phase. In the event that certain changes of PMS can be linked to withdrawal of endogenous opiates, these symptoms are attenuated by the α_2-adrenergic agonist, clonidine, which is currently being used to prevent signs and symptoms of opiate withdrawal in addicts undergoing detoxification (Gold, Pottash, Sweeney, & Kleber, 1980). By preventing the excessive noradrenergic activity that may follow a precipitous premenstrual decline of endogenous opiate activity, this agent may attenuate the pronounced psychological and behavioral manifestations of PMS.

To avoid the addition of more unproven remedies to the already cumbersome therapeutic armamentarium, more basic research and adequate testing in controlled clinical trials are needed before these medications (LRF agonists, naltrexone, and clonidine) can be recommended for the treatment of PMS.

MEDICAL-LEGAL CONSIDERATIONS ABOUT PREMENSTRUAL SYNDROME

The legal implications of PMS and the manner in which PMS, like temporary insanity, may alter the legal assessment of mental competence and criminal responsibility have long been of interest to the legal community. As far back as 1845, a maid was acquitted on a charge of murdering her employer's child on the grounds of insanity due to "obstructed menstruation" (d'Orban, 1981). The novel legal problems that PMS poses when considering the criminal and civil responsibility of women were raised again in relation to automobile accidents occurring in the premenstruum in the 1950's (Perr, 1958; Stewart, 1957a, b). More recently, attention has been refocused on this issue by several highly publicized trials abroad. In England, the successful pleas of diminished responsibility or mitigating circumstances on behalf of three PMS sufferers charged with manslaughter, arson, and assault (Dalton, 1980) triggered widespread public debate about the validity of PMS as a basis for a defense (d'Orban, 1981). In Canada, PMS has already been cited as a mitigating circumstance resulting in reduced sentences in cases of assault and shoplifting (Gray, 1981). In the United States, cases of premenstrual child battering and manslaughter have been before the courts (Chambers, 1982; Gray, 1981).

The charge that accepting PMS as a mitigating circumstance is tantamount to providing a "free hand" to women with criminal tendencies is not unexpected; yet this form of emotional argument certainly denies the fact that some individuals affected with PMS may act in an irrational or impulsive manner if sufficiently provoked at times of severe psychological distress. Obviously, many factors are important in assessing criminal responsibility, including the patient's history, personality, mental state at the time of the act, and the circumstances of the offense. The timing of the offense in relation to menstruation (or similar episodes in the past) and documentation of the type and severity of premenstrual symptoms provide additional important information which may help to determine whether PMS, on the balance of probabilities, may have acted as a triggering factor for the commission. Clear precedents are yet to be established in such cases; however, it seems certain that legal opinion about this issue is likely to continue to evolve as further scientific information about PMS becomes available.

ETHICAL CONSIDERATIONS

> "In its highest form medical controversy provides the energy for inquiry and progress. When controversy descends from the intellectual to the emotional plane, participants become more the advocates of belief than the seekers of truth."
>
> — Samuel O. Thier (1977)

As with most controversial subjects, the ethical issues seem to be shaped as much by the nature of current involvement as they are by the past perspectives of the various participants. For some, the major ethical issue of the PMS controversy revolves around the dangers inherent in accepting reports of adverse premenstrual experience as evidence that PMS is a legitimate medical condition. For others, the primary focus has been on the injustice of a male-dominated medical profession allowing the perpetuation of a unique, potentially treatable female disorder either due to the skepticism or indifference of those charting current research directions.

There is, perhaps, only one thing more destructive to the woman with severe PMS than insight into the devastating consequences of her condition on family and career, and that is the frequent aspersions cast by some members of the very medical community from which she must seek help. Judgmental positions adopted by other special interest groups with admittedly little or no exposure to affected women in a clinical setting have served to intensify this dichotomy by castigating concerned physicians for medicalizing a "normal" phenomenon and vilifying those who seek help for causing irreparable damage to the cause of achieving male:female equality. Embittered by these recriminations, and frustrated by the collective failure of medicine over the past 50 years to direct sufficient energy and resources toward the understanding and treatment of PMS, affected women have assumed a new militancy with the formation of organizations like Premenstrual Syndrome Action, Inc. The lay press has championed such a movement, giving wide coverage to every imaginable theory of causation and treatment of premenstrual syndrome, making this disorder clearly the cause célèbre of women's health of the 1980's. Front line physicians caught up in busy clinical practices, and lacking the time, expertise, or financial resources to conduct effective clinical research programs of their own, are often at a loss to provide concise, reliable information or proven therapies to their patients. Uncertainty about the precise definition and lack of a clear biochemical test for premenstrual syndrome have further confounded the efforts of conscientious physicians who are often presented with a confusing array of psychiatric, social, and behavioral disorders under the guise of premenstrual syndrome. The anecdotal and contradictory nature of the literature emanating from such a setting have kindled new doubts within the scientific community about the validity of PMS as a clinical entity. The few clinicians/scientists with the interest and wherewithal to make a concerted effort to address many of the unresolved issues about premenstrual syndrome are faced, on one hand, with the concern that their peers will not accord their research proposals sufficient priority to ensure funding at times of government cutbacks and, on the other hand, with the fear that editors of first-rate scientific journals may ultimately refuse to publish the results of research on PMS for fear that this quasi-scientific "quality of life" issue might not conform to the rigid scientific standards expected by their readership. Finally, the legal community, by prematurely introducing PMS as a consideration in the determination of legal responsibility of women, may have created a backlash against PMS sufferers by generating fears that, in the absence of a biochemical test for PMS, sexual assignment alone might contribute sufficient reason to argue diminished capacity (see Fig. 7).

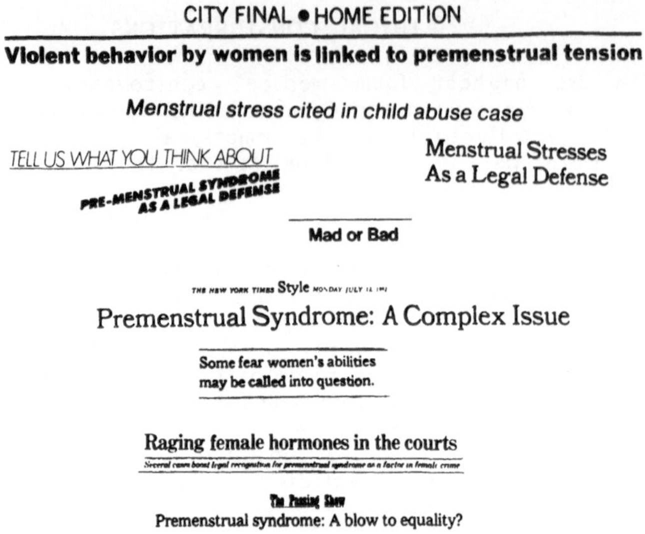

CITY FINAL • HOME EDITION

Violent behavior by women is linked to premenstrual tension

Menstrual stress cited in child abuse case

TELL US WHAT YOU THINK ABOUT
PRE-MENSTRUAL SYNDROME AS A LEGAL DEFENSE

Menstrual Stresses
As a Legal Defense

Mad or Bad

Style

Premenstrual Syndrome: A Complex Issue

Some fear women's abilities
may be called into question.

Raging female hormones in the courts

Premenstrual syndrome: A blow to equality?

Fig. 7. The lay press has made "PMS" a household word. Recent headlines have addressed the social and legal implications of accepting PMS as a defense for criminal behavior.

How do we chart a course through these troubled waters and wherein lies the truth about premenstrual syndrome? It is time that clinicians dealing with women who claim to have cyclic premenstrual symptomatology heed the exhortations of many psychologists that we be exacting in our evaluation of these women, cognizant of the impact of attitudes and expectations on actual experiences, sensitive to the importance of co-existing life stresses, and cautious in the attribution of symptoms to biochemical changes which could then potentially be extrapolated to the entire female population. Psychologists, on the other hand, must cross into the camp of the clinician and come face-to-face with women who experience these dramatic time-limited changes in mood and behavior in order to appreciate that, for some women at least, menstrual cycle-related illness is a very real phenomenon. Only by employing rigorous scientific methodology, and the expertise of interdisciplinary teams, will the clinician/scientist gain the respect of his colleagues and thereby accord the whole issue of menstrual cycle-related illness a fair trial in the scientific forum. The lay press, while having a responsibility to inform, has an equal responsibility to educate. This implies that they must be sensitive to the adverse impact of sensational articles based more on conjecture than on scientific fact. At the very minimum, it must be the responsibility of this group to identify to their readership the reliability of their information source and whether such information represents hypothesis or fact. While the legal profession may perceive it to be their responsibility to defend their client by whatever means available, they must realize that the use of "premenstrual syndrome" as a defense before this condition has established a sound foundation in the realm of science may further polarize opinion on this issue. Ultimately, this may hinder the rational formulation of the true impact, if any, of PMS on criminal behavior.

The one major windfall of this resurgence of interest in PMS has been the renewed efforts of clinical scientists to study and define the normal menstrual cycle and its variations. Only through the development of a clear understanding of normal processes will we achieve the proper scientific foundation upon which to advance our knowledge of abnormal menstrual experience.

CONCLUSIONS

Current concepts relating to the pathophysiology and management of premenstrual syndrome have been re-evaluated in light of recent developments in the field of reproductive neuroendocrinology. A unifying hypothesis based on known menstrual cycle-related changes in central endogenous opiate activity has been advanced and future research directions discussed.

ACKNOWLEDGMENTS

I wish to acknowledge the continuing encouragement that I receive from Dr. Samuel S.C. Yen, whose enthusiasm for, and insight into, the field of psychoneuroendocrinology of reproduction have kindled my interest in menstrual cycle-related mood and behavioral disorders. My thanks also to Denise From for her diligent help in the preparation of this manuscript.

REFERENCES

Abraham, G. E., 1980. Premenstrual tension. *Current Problems in Obstetrics and Gynecology 3:* 10.

Abraham, G. E. and J. T. Hargrove, 1980. Effect of Vitamin B6 on premenstrual symptomatology in women with premenstrual tension syndromes: a double blind crossover study. *Infertility 3:* 155-165.

Adams, P. W., D. P. Rose, J. Folkard, V. Wynn, M. Seed, and R. Strong, 1973. Effect of pyridoxine hydrochloride (Vitamin B6) upon depression associated with oral contraception. *The Lancet 1:* 897-904.

Anderson, A. N. and J. F. Larsen, 1979. Bromocriptine in the treatment of premenstrual syndrome. *Drugs 17:* 383-388.

Backstrom, C. T., H. Boyle, and D. T. Baird, 1981. Persistence of symptoms of premenstrual tension in hysterectomized women. *British Journal of Obstetrics and Gynaecology 88:* 530-536.

Berger, H., 1955. Ulcerative stomatitis caused by endogenous progesterone. *Annals of Internal Medicine 42:* 205-208.

Bertoli, A., R. de Pirro, A. Fusco, A. V. Greco, R. Magnatta, and R. Lauro, 1980. Differences in insulin receptors between men and menstruating women and influence of sex hormones on insulin binding during the menstrual cycle. *Journal of Clinical Endocrinology and Metabolism 50:* 246-250.

Bickers, W. and M. Woods, 1951. Premenstrual tension — rational treatment. *Texas Report on Biological Medicine 9:* 406-419.

Chambers, M., 1982. Menstrual stresses as legal defenses. *New York Times*, May 29, p. 46.

Christie, M. J. and G. B. Chester, 1982. Physical dependence on physiologically released endogenous opiates. *Life Sciences 30:* 1173-1177.

Cohen, M. R., R. M. Cohen, D. Pickar, H. Weingartner, D. L. Murphy, and W. Bunney, Jr., 1981. Behavioural effects after high dose naloxone administration to normal volunteers. *The Lancet 2:* 1110.

Cole, E. N., D. Everend, D. F. Horrobin, M. S. Manku, J. P. Mtabaji, and B. A. Nassar, 1975. Is prolactin a fluid and electrolyte regulating hormone in man? *Journal of Physiology (London) 252:* 54P.

Cullberg, J., 1972. Mood changes and menstrual symptoms with different gestagen estrogen combinations. *Acta Psychiatrica Scandinavica 236:* 1-86.

Dalton, K., 1959. Menstruation and acute psychiatric illnesses. *British Medical Journal 1:* 148-149.

Dalton, K., 1960. Menstruation and accidents. *British Medical Journal 2:* 1425-1426.
Dalton, K., 1961. Menstruation and crime. *British Medical Journal 2:* 1752-1753.
Dalton, K., 1964. The influence of menstruation on health and disease. *Proceedings of the Royal Society of Medicine 57:* 18-20.
Dalton, K., 1966. The influence of mother's menstruation on her child. *Proceedings of the Royal Society of Medicine 59:* 1014-1016.
Dalton, K., 1980. Cyclical criminal acts in premenstrual syndrome. *The Lancet 2:* 1070-1071.
Dawood, M. Y., 1981. Dysmenorrhea. *American College of Obstetricians and Gynecologists Technical Bulletin No. 68,* March.
Day, J., 1979. Danazol and the premenstrual syndrome. *Postgraduate Medical Journal 55:* 87-89.
d'Orban, P. T., 1981. Premenstrual syndrome: a disease of the mind. *The Lancet 2:* 1413.
d'Orban, P. T. and K. Dalton, 1980. Violent crime and the menstrual cycle. *Psychological Bulletin 10:* 353-359.
Edeiken, J. and J. Q. Griffith, Jr., 1940. Cyclic pulmonary edema at menses in mitral stenosis. *Journal of the American Medical Association 115:* 287-289.
Ellinwood, E. H., A. Sudilovsky, and L. M. Nelson, 1973. Evolving behaviour in the clinical and experimental amphetamine (model) psychosis. *American Journal of Psychiatry 130:* 1088.
Endo, M., M. Daiguji, Y. Asano, I. Yamashitu, and S. Takahashi, 1978. Periodic psychosis recurring in association with the menstrual cycle. *Journal of Clinical Psychiatry 39:* 456-466.
Ganon, L., 1981. Evidence for a psychological etiology of menstrual disorders: A critical review. *Psychological Reports 48:* 287-294.
Gianutsos, G. and H. Lal, 1978. Narcotic analgesics and aggression. *Modern Problems in Pharmacopsychiatry 13:* 114-138.
Glass, G. S., G. R. Heninger, M. Lansky, and K. Talan, 1971. Psychiatric emergency related to the menstrual cycle. *American Journal of Psychiatry 128:* 705-711.
Glick, I. D. and D. Stewart, 1980. A new drug treatment for premenstrual exacerbation of schizophrenia. *Comprehensive Psychiatry 21:* 281-287.
Gold, M. S., A. C. Pottash, D. R. Sweeney, and H. D. Kleber, 1980. Opiate withdrawal using clonidine, a safe, effective and rapid nonopiate treatment. *Journal of the American Medical Association 243:* 346-353.
Gowdey, C. W., 1983. A guide to the pharmacology of placebos. *Canadian Medical Association Journal 128:* 921-925.
Grandison, L. and A. Guidotti, 1977. Stimulation of food intake by muscimol and Beta-endorphin. *Neuropharmacology 16:* 533-536.
Gray, C., 1981. Raging female hormones in the courts. *McLeans Magazine,* June 15, pp. 46-49.
Greene, R. and K. Dalton, 1953. The premenstrual syndrome. *British Medical Journal 1:* 1007-1014.
Greenhill, J. P. and S. C. Freed, 1941. The electrolyte therapy of premenstrual distress. *Journal of the American Medical Association 117:* 504-506.
Halbreich, U., M. Ben-David, M. Assael, and R. Bornstein, 1976. Serum-prolactin in women with premenstrual syndrome. *The Lancet 2:* 654-656.
Janowski, D. S., R. Gorney, P. Castelnuovo-Tedesco, and C. B. Stone, 1969. Premenstrual-menstrual increases in psychiatric hospital admission rates. *American Journal of Obstetrics and Gynecology 103:* 189-191.
Kerr, G. D., 1977. The management of the premenstrual syndrome. *Current Medical Research Opinion 4* (Suppl.): 29-34.

Lal, H. and S. K. Puri, 1972. Morphine withdrawal aggression: role of dopaminergic stimulation. In: J. M. Singh, I. Miller, and H. Lal (Eds.), *Drug Addiction: Experimental Pharmacology.* Futura Publishing Co., Mount Kisco, New York, pp. 301-310.
Lennane, K. J. and R. J. Lennane, 1973. Alleged psychogenic disorders in women — possible manifestation of sexual prejudice. *The Lancet 1:* 288-292.
Levine, J. D., N. C. Gordon, and H. L. Fields, 1978. The mechanism of placebo analgesia. *The Lancet 2:* 654-657.
Llorens, C., M. P. Martres, M. Bandry, and J. C. Schwartz, 1978. Hypersensitivity to noradrenaline in cortex after chronic morphine: relevance to tolerance and dependence. *Nature 274:* 603-605.
MacGregor, G. A., J. E. Roulston, N. D. Markandu, H. E. de Wardener, and J. C. Jones, 1979. Is "idiopathic" edema idiopathic? *The Lancet 1:* 397-400.
MacKinnon, P.C.B. and I. L. MacKinnon, 1956. Hazards of the menstrual cycle. *British Medical Journal 1:* 555.
Maddocks, S., F. Moller, P. Hahn, and R. L. Reid, 1986. A double-blind, placebo-controlled trial of progesterone vaginal suppositories in the treatment of premenstrual syndrome. *American Journal of Obstetrics and Gynecology,* in press.
Magos, A. L., K. J. Zilkha, and J.W.W. Studd, 1983. Treatment of menstrual migraines by oestradiol implants. *Journal of Neurology, Neurosurgery & Psychiatry 46:* 1044-1046.
Mandell, A. J. and M. P. Mandell, 1967. Suicide and the menstrual cycle. *Journal of the American Medical Association 200:* 792-793.
Melody, G. F., 1961. Behavioural implications of premenstrual tension. *Obstetrics and Gynaecology 17:* 439-441.
Morton, J. H., 1950. Premenstrual tension. *American Journal of Obstetrics and Gynecology 60:* 343-352.
Morton, J. H., H. Addison, R. G. Addison, I. Hunt, and J. J. Sullivan, 1953. A clinical study of premenstrual tension. *American Journal of Obstetrics and Gynecology 65:* 1182-1191.
Muse, K. N., N. S. Cetel, L. A. Futterman, and S.S.C. Yen, 1984. The premenstrual syndrome: Effects of "medical ovariectomy." *New England Journal of Medicine 311:* 1345-1349.
O'Brien, P.M.S., D. Craven, C. Selby, and E. M. Symonds, 1979. Treatment of premenstrual syndrome by spironolactone. *British Journal of Obstetrics and Gynaecology 86:* 142-147.
Perr, I. N., 1958. Medical, psychiatric, and legal aspects of premenstrual tension. *American Journal of Psychiatry 115:* 211-219.
Quigley, M. E. and S.S.C. Yen, 1980. The role of endogenous opiates on LH secretion during the menstrual cycle. *Journal of Clinical Endocrinology and Metabolism 51:* 179-181.
Reid, R. L., 1983. Endogenous opioid activity in premenstrual syndrome. *The Lancet 2:* 786.
Reid, R. L., 1985. Premenstrual syndrome. *Current Problems in Obstetrics, Gynecology, and Fertility 8:* 1-57.
Reid, R. L., 1986. Clinical opinion. Premenstrual syndrome: A time for introspection. *American Journal of Obstetrics and Gynecology,* in press.
Reid, R. L., A. Greenaway-Coates, and P. M. Hahn, 1986. Oral glucose tolerance during the menstrual cycle in normal women (NW) and women with alleged premenstrual "hypoglycemic" attacks (PMHA): Effects of Naloxone. *Journal of Clinical Endocrinology and Metabolism,* in press.
Reid, R. L. and S.S.C. Yen, 1981a. Premenstrual syndrome. *American Journal of Obstetrics and Gynecology 139:* 85-104.
Reid, R. L. and S.S.C. Yen, 1981b. β-endorphin stimulates the secretion of insulin and glucagon in human. *Journal of Clinical Endocrinology and Metabolism 52:* 592-594.

Reid, R. L. and S.S.C. Yen, 1983. The premenstrual syndrome. *Clinical Obstetrics and Gynaecology 26:* 710-718.
Sampson, G. A., 1979. Premenstrual syndrome: A double-blind controlled trial of progesterone and placebo. *British Journal of Psychiatry 135:* 209-215.
Sampson, G. A., 1981. An appraisal of the role of progesterone in the therapy of premenstrual syndrome. In: P. A. van Keep (Ed.), *The Premenstrual Syndrome.* MTP Press Ltd. (Falcon House International Publishers), Lancaster, England, pp. 51-69.
Schaumburg, H., J. Kaplan, A. Windebank, N. Vick, S. Rasmus, D. Pleasure, and M. J. Brown, 1983. Sensory neuropathy from pyridoxine abuse. *New England Journal of Medicine 309:* 445-448.
Somerville, B. W., 1972. The role of oestradiol withdrawal in the etiology of menstrual migraine. *Neurology (Minneapol.) 22:* 355-365.
Steiner, M., R. F. Haskett, and B. J. Carroll, 1980a. Premenstrual tension syndrome: The development of research diagnostic criteria and new rating scales. *Acta Psychiatrica Scandinavica 62:* 177-190.
Steiner, M., R. F. Haskett, J. M. Osmun, and B. J. Carroll, 1980b. Treatment of premenstrual tension with lithium carbonate: A pilot study. *Acta Psychiatrica Scandinavica 61:* 96-102.
Stewart, N. L., 1957a. Psychotic aspects of premenstrual tension. *Cleveland-Marshall Law Review 6:* 410-427.
Stewart, N. L., 1957b. Premenstrual tension in automobile accidents. *Cleveland-Marshall Law Review 6:* 17-30.
Stokes, J. and J. Mendels, 1972. Pyridoxine and premenstrual tension. *The Lancet 1:* 1177-1178.
Suarez-Murias, E. L., 1953. The psychophysiologic syndrome of premenstrual tension with emphasis on the psychiatric aspect. *International Record of Medicine 166:* 475-486.
Tanks, C. M., P. H. Rach, and M. J. Rose, 1968. Attempted suicide and the menstrual cycle. *Journal of Psychosomatic Research 11:* 319-323.
Thier, S. O., 1977. Breast cancer screening: A view from outside the controversy. *New England Journal of Medicine 297:* 1063.
Wald, A., D. H. Van Thiel, L. Hoechstetter, J. S. Gavaler, K. M. Egler, R. Verm, L. Scott, and R. Lester, 1981. Gastrointestinal transit: The effect of the menstrual cycle. *Gastroenterology 80:* 1497-1500.
Wardlaw, S. L., W. B. Wehrenberg, M. Ferin, J. L. Antunes, and A. G. Frantz, 1982. Effect of sex steroids on β-endorphin in hypophyseal portal blood. *Journal of Clinical Endocrinology and Metabolism 55:* 877-881.
Wehrenberg, W. B., S. L. Wardlaw, A. G. Frantz, and M. Ferin, 1982. β-Endorphin in hypophyseal portal blood variations throughout the menstrual cycle. *Endocrinology 111:* 879-881.
Wei, E. and H. Loh, 1976. Physical dependence on opiate-like peptides. *Science 193:* 1262-1263.
Wood, C. and D. Jakubowicz, 1980. The treatment of premenstrual symptoms with mefenamic acid. *British Journal of Obstetrics and Gynaecology 87:* 627-630.
Woods, N. F., A. Most, and G. K. Dery, 1982. Prevalence of perimenstrual symptoms. *American Journal of Public Health 72:* 1257-1264.
Yen, S.S.C., 1983. Clinical applications of gonadotropin releasing hormone and gonadotropin releasing hormone analogs. *Fertility and Sterility 39:* 257-266.
Zondek, B. and Y. M. Bromberg, 1947. Clinical reactions of allergy to endogenous hormones and their treatment. *British Journal of Obstetrics and Gynaecology 54:* 1-19.

DYSPHORIC PREMENSTRUAL CHANGES:
ARE THEY RELATED TO AFFECTIVE DISORDERS?

Uriel Halbreich, M.D.* and Jean Endicott, Ph.D.**

*Department of Psychiatry, SUNY
462 Grider Street, K-Annex
Buffalo, New York 14215

**New York Psychiatric Institute
New York, New York

INTRODUCTION

Some investigators hope to study premenstrual changes (PMC) as a model for more severe affective disorders. The use of premenstrual depression as a model for affective disorder is supported by studies that have found: (1) a differential and positive relationship between premenstrual depressive changes and a lifetime diagnosis of affective disorder, as compared with a lifetime diagnosis of no mental disorder or some other mental disorders (Coppen, 1965; Diamond, Rubinstein, Dunner, & Fieve, 1976; Kashiwagi, McClure, Reich, & Wetzel, 1976; Schuckit, Daly, Herrman, & Hineman, 1975; Wetzel, Reich, McClure, & Wald, 1975); (2) that some women experience a depressive syndrome during the premenstrual period severe enough to seek treatment for the condition (reviewed by Halbreich & Endicott, 1985a); (3) that suicide attempts and admissions to psychiatric hospitals for depressive episodes are associated with the paramenstrual period (Abramowitz, Backer, & Freischer, 1982); and (4) that premenstrual exacerbation of depressive syndromes is seen in those with depressive disorders.

In the current chapter, we will summarize the methods applied by us to the assessment of PMC, the nature of these changes, and data which support the hypothesis that dysphoric PMC are associated with more severe depressive disorders. The implications of such an association and some practical aspects that may issue from it will be discussed (see also Endicott, Halbreich, Schacht, & Nee, 1981; Halbreich & Endicott, 1985a, b; Halbreich, Endicott, & Nee, 1982, 1983).

DEFINITION OF PREMENSTRUAL CHANGES (PMC)

A review of the literature as well as our own work (Endicott et al., 1981; Halbreich et al., 1982, 1983) clearly indicates that premenstrual changes can be classified into distinguishable typological categories and dimensional measures. The typological categories or dimensional measures are not independent and there are varying degrees of overlap and intercorrelation between them. However, as is the case with affective disorders in which depression is a dominant feature and in which psychotic features are highly correlated with, and overlap with, endogenous features, an effort to look at the differential correlates of even the premenstrual dysphoric changes yields independent variables.

An unbiased survey of various groups of women reveals that some women have positive changes premenstrually; e.g., increased energy, increased sex drive, or increased feelings of affection. Hence, we believe the rubric "premenstrual changes" (PMC) is more suitable than "premenstrual tension syndrome" (PMTS) because it more accurately describes the diversity of premenstrual changes, positive as well as negative. In addition, bipolarity of some of the main PMC has been demonstrated (Halbreich et al., 1982). For example, combining data from women who have decreased activity premenstrually with data from women whose activity is increased, or women who sleep less with those who sleep more, or women with increased appetites with those whose appetite is decreased, is almost certain to obscure correlations with other variables. Delineation of the subtype or the dimension of PMC to be studied or treated is essential. In this sense, "premenstrual changes" is an umbrella term. One may refer to a specific subtype, or a cluster of premenstrual symptoms as a "syndrome," with the understanding that PMC include a variety of premenstrual syndromes (PMS).

AN OPERATIONAL DEFINITION OF PREMENSTRUAL CHANGES

There is a need for an agreed-upon definition of PMC, for the sake of standardization of clinical observation and replication of results. We suggest the following definition:

> Symptom(s) are considered as PMC if there is a cyclic recurrent change in intensity of symptom(s) measured from the second week of the menstrual cycle compared to the peak intensity of the symptom(s) during the late luteal phase (one to seven days prior to onset of menses).

THE ASSESSMENT OF PREMENSTRUAL DYSPHORIC CHANGES

In order to study PMC as putative diversified clusters of phenomena, we developed the Premenstrual Assessment Form (PAF)(Halbreich et al., 1982), which allows for flexibility and lends itself to three different ways of scoring PMC: (1) on the basis of specific criteria for categorical subtypes of premenstrual changes; (2) using summary scale scores based upon sets of unipolar dimensional scales (percentage of maximal possible severity on each cluster of symptoms or complaints); and (3) on the basis of dimensional measures for bipolar continua (e.g., between a maximum increase and a maximum decrease of a specific activity or change). A page of the PAF is illustrated in Figure 1.

The PAF's 95 items measure premenstrual change from usual state and provide an index of severity of changes of mood and physical condition in single items as well as in the dimensional scales. Additional measures of severity are provided by two other sets of items describing impaired social functioning and impaired physical and mental functioning ("organic syndrome").

The initial criteria for PAF subtypes of premenstrual changes were developed to be comparable to current psychiatric diagnostic criteria of the *Diagnostic and Statistical Manual* (DSM—III) and the Research Diagnostic Criteria (RDC). The items may also be clustered according

PAF

1 - Not applicable, not present at all, or no change from usual level,
2 - Minimal change, 3 - Mild change, 4 - Moderate change,
5 - Severe change, 6 - Extreme change

Changes Present During Premenstrual Period	Usual Level of Change During Last 3 Premenstrual Periods	
Have rapid changes in mood (e.g., laughing, crying, angry, happy, etc.) all within the same day.	1 2 (3) 4 5 6	215
Have decreased energy or tend to fatigue easily	1 2 3 4 5 (6)	216
Have decreased ability to coordinate fine movements, poor motor coordination or clumsiness	1 (2) 3 4 5 6	217
Feel anxious or more anxious	(1) 2 3 4 5 6	218
Sleep too much or have difficulty getting up in the morning or from naps	1 2 3 4 (5) 6	219
Have a feeling of malaise (i.e., general, non-specific bad feeling or vague sense of mental or physical ill-health)	(1) 2 3 4 5 6	220
Feel jittery or restless	1 (2) 3 4 5 6	221
Have loss of appetite	(1) 2 3 4 5 6	222
Have pain, tenderness, enlargement, or swelling of breasts	1 2 3 4 (5) 6	223
Have headaches or migraines	1 (2) 3 4 5 6	224
Be more easily distracted (i.e., attention shifts easily and rapidly)	(1) 2 3 4 5 6	225
Tend to have accidents, fall, cut self, or break things unintentionally	1 2 3 (4) 5 6	226
Have nausea or vomiting	(1) 2 3 4 5 6	227
Show physical agitation (e.g., fidgeting, hand wringing, pacing, can't sit still)	(1) 2 3 4 5 6	228
Have feelings of weakness	1 (2) 3 4 5 6	229
Feel that you just "can't cope" or are overwhelmed by ordinary demands	1 2 (3) 4 5 6	230
Feel insecure	1 (2) 3 4 5 6	231
Have "flare-ups" of allergy, breathing difficulties, stuffy feeling, or watery discharge from the nose (specify)	(1) 2 3 4 5 6	232
Feel depressed	1 2 3 4 (5) 6	233
Have periods of dizziness, faintness, vertigo, (room spinning), ringing in the ears, numbness, tingling of skin, trembling, lightheadedness (specify)	(1) 2 3 4 5 6	234
Tend to "nag" or quarrel over unimportant issues	1 2 (3) 4 5 6	235
Think of what it would be like to do something to self, like crash the car, wish to go to sleep and not wake up, or have thoughts of death or suicide	1 2 (3) 4 5 6	236
Feel less desire to talk or move about (it takes an effort to do so)	1 2 3 (4) 5 6	237
Become more forgetful	(1) 2 3 4 5 6	238
Feel dissatisfied with personal appearance	1 (2) 3 4 5 6	239

Fig. 1. A page of the Premenstrual Assessment Form (PAF).

to criteria specific to a given study as will be defined by the investigators. Mathematical procedures may be used to develop additional or complementary scores. Some PAF subtypes are described in Table 1. The PAF item content of unipolar summary scale scores used by us is shown in Table 2. The items that were paired to express manifestations of opposite roles for the seven bipolar continua are listed in Table 3. Figure 2 shows an example of computerized analysis of PAF.

The data are based upon retrospective reports; and as such, the PAF is used for initial screening. The same items may be used for a state measurement twice a month with a slight change of the instructions. The existence and severity of symptoms and complaints only during the premenstrual period (new formation or a marked change in intensity — at least two points on a 6-point scale), and their disappearance during other phases of the menstrual cycle should be confirmed by use of the PAF daily ratings, a form which monitors 20 items descriptive of mood and behavior over one or more menstrual cycles. Examples of confirmation and disconfirmation of a report over time are shown in Figure 3.

THE NATURE OF PREMENSTRUAL DYSPHORIC CHANGES

For the study of premenstrual dysphoric changes, we focused on the typological category of PAF Full Depressive Syndrome and its six, non-mutually-exclusive subtypes listed in Table 4 (Halbreich et al., 1982): Endogenous features, Atypical features, Hysteroid features, Anxious-agitated features, Hostile features, and Withdrawn features.

Most investigators who studied PMC as a model for depression were looking for premenstrual endogenous depressive syndrome [e.g., sadness, lack of reactivity, guilt feelings, psychomotor retardation, and terminal insomnia (i.e., early morning awakening)]. When this syndrome was not found, some investigators reached the disappointing conclusion that PMC cannot be studied as a model for affective disorders. Given that many depressed patients do not have an "endogenous" syndrome, the study of premenstrual depressive features is warranted based on the following findings (Halbreich et al., 1983):

Among a group of 335 women, 145 women met PAF criteria for Full Depressive Syndrome. None of these women met typological criteria for endogenous features, thus confirming previous reports. However, 63% of that group had "Atypical" Depressive features (mood swings or rapid mood changes, hypersomnia, increased appetite and craving for specific foods, in addition to meeting criteria for PAF Full Depressive Syndrome). Fifty-two percent had Hostile Depressive features, 43% met PAF criteria for Anxious-Agitated Depressive Syndrome, and 42% had PAF Withdrawn Depressive features. The percentage of women who met PAF criteria for various categories is presented in Table 4.

It is noteworthy that even among the premenstrually depressed women, up to 21% also reported increased well-being premenstrually. Bipolar changes were also reported for some other dimensions and not only for mood; e.g., 50% of our sample reported increased *and* decreased activity, and 46% reported increased *and* decreased sleep during the premenstrual period. These seemingly contradictory reports are clarified in most cases when the reported PMC are monitored on a daily basis. Then it is apparent that there may be day-to-day swings in mood and behavior. This issue is of methodological importance for biological studies, as any biological determinant should be correlated with mood at the time of the test and not with general PMC. An example of bipolar changes in activity level during the premenstrual period is shown in Figure 4.

Table 1. Criteria of the Premenstrual Assessment Form Typological Categories Used to Select Subjects at Second Screening.*

FULL DEPRESSIVE SYNDROME

A. 1. Depressed or low mood — 1 of the following 5 items must be at least mild (3-6): Feel depressed (233) or Feel "empty" (263) or Feel sad or blue (265) or Feel lonely (271) or Pessimistic outlook (339)

OR 2. Loss of interest or pleasure — all of the following 4 items must be at least mild (3-6): Less sexual interest (323) and Avoid social activities (324) and Want to be alone (328) and Less leisure activities (343)

OR 3. Irritable — 1 of the following 2 items must be rated at least mild (3-6): Outbursts of irritability (264) or Feel "at war" (269)

B. If Depressed — at least 4 of the following 8 items, or item sets, must be rated at least mild (3-6). If Irritable or Loss of interest or pleasure only, at least 5 of the 8 items must be rated at least mild (3-6):

1. Appetite change — Loss of appetite (222) or Weight gain (273) or Increased appetite (331)
2. Sleep change — Hypersomnia (219) or Trouble sleeping (278)
3. Decreased energy (216)
4. Psychomotor change — Physical agitation (228) or Less desire to talk or move (237)
5. Less interest — Less sexual interest (323) or Avoid social activities (324) or Want to be alone (328) or Less leisure activities (343)
6. Self deprecation — Guilt feelings (262) or Decrease in self esteem (316)
7. Concentration difficulties (245)
8. Suicidal ideation (236)

ATYPICAL DEPRESSIVE FEATURES

A. Meets criteria for Full Depressive Syndrome

B. Rapid mood changes (215) or Mood swings (260)(rating of 3 or more)

C. At least 2 of the following 4 items rated 3 or more:

1. Hypersomnia (219)
2. Feel sleepy (241)
3. Crave specific foods (330)
4. Increased appetite (331)

ANXIOUS-AGITATED DEPRESSIVE FEATURES

A. Meets criteria for Full Depressive Syndrome

B. At least 2 of the following 4 items rated 4 or more:

1. Feel anxious (218)
2. Feel jittery or restless (221)
3. Physical agitation (228)
4. Pick skin/bite nails (259)

HOSTILE DEPRESSIVE FEATURES

A. Meets criteria for Full Depressive Syndrome

B. At least 3 of the following 6 items rated 3 or more:

1. Violent (240)
2. Outburst of irritability (264)
3. Feel "at war" (269)
4. Act spiteful (270)
5. Intolerant (274)
6. Blames others (317)

IMPAIRED SOCIAL FUNCTIONING

At least 3 of the following 11 items rated 3 or more:

1. Tend to nag (235)
2. Decreased judgment (247)
3. Family notes mood (268)
4. Stay at home (322)
5. Avoid social activities (324)
6. Lowered performance/efficiency (326)
7. Miss time at work (327)
8. Lack of inspiration (329)
9. Less attention to appearance (333)
10. Less housework (342)
11. Less leisure activities (343)

GENERAL DISCOMFORT SYNDROME

At least 1 of the following 3 items rated 3 or more:

1. Headaches or migraines (224)
2. Backaches/Joint/Muscle pains (267)
3. Abdominal discomfort/pain (276)

WATER RETENTION SYNDROME

At least 3 of the following 6 items rated 3 or more:

1. Breast pain or swelling (223)
2. Urinate less (272)
3. Weight gain (273)
4. Abdominal discomfort/pain (276)
5. Water retention signs (321)
6. Feel bloated (325)

AUTONOMIC PHYSICAL SYNDROME

At least 3 of the following 7 items rated 3 or more:

1. Nausea or vomiting (227)
2. Dizziness, faintness, vertigo (234)
3. Rapid heartbeat (243)
4. Urinate frequently (253)
5. Become constipated (254)
6. Urinate less (272)
7. Feel cold (334)

* Combination of certain of these Typological Categories are used in the Second Screening Phase (e.g., Full Depressive Syndrome, Atypical Depressive Features, and Impaired Social Functioning). See the accompanying "Flow Chart For Screening Process," which shows the sequential use of these criteria for the initial selection of subjects.

Table 2. Item Content of Unipolar Summary Scale Scores of the Premenstrual Assessment Form.*

Scale 1 — Low mood/loss of pleasure
233 Feel depressed
236 Suicidal ideation
252 Feel tearful
262 Guilty feeling
263 Feel "empty"
265 Feel sad or blue
271 Feel lonely
316 Decrease in self-esteem
328 Want to be alone
339 Pessimistic outlook

Scale 2 — "Endogenous" depressive features
222 Loss of appetite
237 Less desire to talk/move
254 Become constipated
314 Terminal insomnia; if true equals 6
332 Feel worse in A.M.

Scale 3 — Lability
215 Rapid mood changes
260 Mood swings
261 Hysterical if upset

Scale 4 — "Atypical" depressive features
215 Rapid mood changes
219 Hypersomnia
241 Feels sleepy
260 Mood swings
330 Crave specific foods
331 Increased appetite

Scale 5 — "Hysteroid" features
239 Dissatisfaction with appearance
251 More childlike
255 Self-indulgent
261 Hysterical if upset
336 Sensitive to rejection

Scale 6 — Hostility/anger
240 Violence
264 Outbursts of irritability
269 Feel "at war"
270 Act spiteful
274 Intolerant/impatient
317 Blames others

Scale 7 — Social withdrawal
237 Less desire to talk/move
322 Stay at home
324 Avoid social activities
328 Want to be alone

Scale 8 — Anxiety
218 Feel anxious
221 Feel jittery or restless
228 Physical agitation
258 Feel under stress

Scale 9 — Increased well-being
244 More enjoyment/excitement
249 Increased well-being
318 Increased activity/efficiency
335 Bursts of energy

Scale 10 — Impulsivity
240 Violence
250 Lack self control
256 Impulsive behavior
264 Outbursts of irritability

Scale 11 — "Organic" mental features
217 Poor motor coordination
225 Easily distracted
226 Tend to have accidents
238 More forgetful
245 Difficulty concentrating
246 Feel confused

Scale 12 — Signs of water retention
223 Breast pain or swelling
272 Urinate less
273 Weight gain
276 Abdominal discomfort/pain
321 Puffiness/edema
325 Feel bloated

Scale 13 —General physical discomfort
224 Headaches or migraines
267 Backaches, joint or muscle pains
276 Abdominal discomfort/pain

Scale 14 —Autonomic physical changes
227 Nausea or vomiting
234 Dizziness, faintness, vertigo
243 Rapid heartbeat
253 Urinate frequently
254 Become constipated
272 Urinate less
334 Feel cold

Scale 15 —Fatigue
216 Decreased energy
220 Feeling of malaise
229 Feelings of weakness
266 Tired legs

Scale 16 — Impaired social functioning
235 Tend to nag
247 Decreased judgment
268 Family notes mood
322 Stay at home
324 Avoid social activities
326 Lowered performance/efficiency
327 Miss time at work
329 Lack of inspiration
342 Less housework
343 Less leisure activities

Scale 17 — Miscellaneous mood/behavior changes
230 Feel overwhelmed
231 Feel insecure
242 Sense of unreality
248 Feel passive
257 Smoke/drink more
259 Pick skin/bite nails
275 Overtalkative
277 Increased sexual interest
278 Trouble sleeping
319 Brood over events
323 Less sexual interest
337 More affectionate
338 Seek advice
340 Drink more coffee/tea

Scale 18 — Miscellaneous physical changes
232 Flare-ups of allergy
315 Abdominal cramps
320 Skin problems
341 Pain during intercourse
344 Physical flare-ups
345 Eye problems

* Abbreviations are listed. The actual items are longer with examples, etc.

Table 3. Bipolar Continua of the PAF.

1.	Psychomotor activity	(Agitated-retarded)
2.	Appetite	(Increased-decreased)
3.	Sleep	(Increased-decreased)
4.	Goal-oriented activity	(Increased-decreased)
5.	Energy	(Increased-decreased)
6.	Sexual interest and activity	(Increased-decreased)
7.	Mood	(Depressed-increased well being)

Another interesting finding that is emphasized by the analysis of data along bipolar continua are reports of premenstrual increased sexual interest and/or activity, even among women who are depressed. This also distinguishes it from endogenous affective disorder, in which decreased sexual interest is the rule. Reports on the bipolar dimensions of some activities are presented in Figure 5.

Although the most prevalent subtypes of premenstrual dysphoric changes overlap with each other, they have been shown to have differential correlates with physical, organic, and behavioral PMC that are not part of the criteria for these subtypes. This finding emphasizes the value of differentiating among premenstrual dysphoric subtypes as opposed to the current prevalent practice of combining all negative changes into a single "premenstrual syndrome." For instance, premenstrual hostility was found to be differentially associated with suicidal ideation, pessimism, sensitivity to criticism, lack of judgment, wanting to be alone, and feeling guilty (Halbreich et al., 1983). This association resembles similar clusters of symptoms found among patients with depressive disorders. Differential association of premenstrual subtypes with other symptoms is also demonstrated in Table 5.

Such similarities between premenstrual subtypes of dysphoric changes and affective disorders further support the applicability of PMC as a model for depressions and the possible association between them.

The clinical distinction between various premenstrual subtypes may have implications for research and treatment (Halbreich, Endicott, & Lesser, 1985). Different pathophysiological mechanisms may contribute to the formation of different clinical features which may also call for more specific treatment for each subtype.

RELATIONSHIP BETWEEN PREMENSTRUAL DEPRESSION AND LIFETIME DIAGNOSIS OF MAJOR DEPRESSIVE DISORDER

So far, we have analyzed results for 194 women (patients and non-patient volunteers) on whom we have current and lifetime RDC diagnoses based on structured evaluations with the Schedule for Affective Disorders and Schizophrenia (SADS) and the PAF assessment (Halbreich & Endicott, 1985a). The structured psychiatric interview is described in Table 6.

```
AECOM STUDY  20 PAFS              APRIL 11, 1984                        PAGE  1
  ------PREMENSTRUAL ASSESSMENT FORM RECORD------

D:10232331, STUDY#20; DATE:09/17/83; AGE:37
            AV/MENS.CYCL:30 DAYS, REGULAR;
            AV.PREMENS.LEN:07 DAYS;AV.BLOOD FLOW:05DAYS;CURRENT STATUS: MNS.FLOW
            AGE 1ST MENS 12; 01 CHILD, NO ABORT/MISCARRY
            CONDITIONS (UNDERLINE=YES,STRICKEN=NO): MITTELSCHMERZ; DYSMENORREA;
                    ENDOMETRIOSIS; BIRTH-CONTROL-PILLS; IUD;
                    RX:PREMENS.CHANGE; RX:OTHER; OTHR-MEDICAL-DISORDER
            CURRENTLY:  NOT PREG.;        NOT POST MENOPAUS.
---------------------------------------------------------------------------------------
RAW  %MAX  UNIPOLAR SCALES    (RATING)ITEM NUMBER  ITEM ABBREVIATION
21    22.  LOW MOOD/PLEASUR   (3) 233.DEPRESSE     (2) 252.TEARFUL     (2) 262.GUILT
                              (2) 263.EMPTY        (2) 265.FEEL SAD    (2) 271.LONELY
                              (2) 316.NO EGO       (3) 328.BE ALONE    (2) 339.PESSIMIS
 7     8.  ENDOGEN DEP.FEAT   (2) 254.CONSTIPA     (2) 332.BAC MORN
 5    13.  LABILITY           (2) 260.MOODSWIN     (2) 261.HYSTERIA
20    47.  ATYPICAL DEP.FEA   (4) 219.HYPERSOM     (2) 241.SLEEPY      (2) 260.MOODSWIN
                              (5) 330.CRAVINGS     (6) 331.EAT MORE
13    32.  HYSTROID FEATURE   (6) 255.INDULGEN     (2) 261.HYSTERIA    (3) 336.SENSITIV
16    33.  HOSTIL/ANGER       (2) 240.VIOLENT      (2) 264.IRRITABL    (4) 269.AT WAR
                              (3) 270.SPITEFUL     (3) 274.IMPATIEN    (2) 317.BLAMES
 9    25.  SOCIAL WITHDRAWL   (3) 322.STAY HOM     (2) 324.ASOCIAL     (3) 328.BE ALONE
10    30.  ANXIETY            (4) 218.ANXIETY      (3) 221.JITTERY     (2) 258.STRESS
 6    10.  IMPULSIVITY        (2) 240.VIOLENT      (2) 264.IRRITABL
 9    25.  INC. WELLBEING     (2) 249.WELLBEIN     (2) 318.ACTIVITY    (4) 335.ENERGETI
31    24.  MISC.MOOD/BEHAVR   (3) 230.CAN'T CO     (3) 231.INSECURE    (2) 248.PASSIVE
                              (6) 257.UPS DRUG     (2) 259.PICK SKI    (2) 275.OVERTALK
                              (2) 319.BROODS       (2) 323.LESS SEX    (2) 337.KISSES
                              (2) 338.ADVICE       (2) 340.CAFFEINE
11    53.  GEN.PHYS.DISCOMF   (3) 224.HEADACHE     (6) 267.BACKACHE    (2) 276.ABDOMINA
14    27.  WATER RETENTION    (2) 223.BREASTS      (2) 273.+WEIGHT     (2) 276.ABDOMINA
                              (3) 321.OEDEMA       (4) 325.BLOATED
12    40.  FATIGUE            (4) 216.NO ENERG     (6) 266.TIRED LEG
12    14.  AUTONOMC PHYSCAL   (2) 254.CONSTIPA     (5) 334.FEEL COL
 9    10.  MISC.    PHYSICAL  (2) 315.CRAMPS       (2) 320.SKIN        (2) 341.SEX PAIN
31    36.  IMPAIR SOC.FUNC.   (4) 235.NAGS         (2) 247.JUDGMENT    (6) 268.IN A MOO
                              (3) 322.STAY HOM     (2) 324.ASOCIAL     (3) 326.LOW WORK
                              (3) 327.MISS WOR     (2) 329.UNINSPIR    (2) 333.SLOPPY
                              (2) 342.NO CLEAN     (2) 343.LESS TV
 9    10.  ORGANIC MENT.FEA   (3) 225.DISTRACT     (2) 238.FORGETFU
---------------------------------------------------------------------------------------
BIPOLAR CONTINUA
RAW (B=CHANGES IN BOTH DIRECTION, NO SCORE; 0=NO CHANGE; 1-5=MINIMAL-EXTREME CHANGE
 0         PSYCHOMOTOR
 5         APPETITE           (6) 331.EAT MORE
 3         SLEEP              (4) 219.HYPERSOM     (2) 241.SLEEPY
-1         SEX                (2) 323.LESS SEX
 B         ENERGY             (4) 216.NO ENERG     (4) 335.ENERGETI
 B         GOAL DIR ACTVITY   (2) 248.PASSIVE      (2) 318.ACTIVITY
 B         MOOD               (3) 233.DEPRESSE     (2) 265.FEEL SAD    (2) 249.WELLBEIN
---------------------------------------------------------------------------------------
       TYPOLOGICAL CLASSIFICATION:
    MAJOR DEPRESSION  (SUBTYPE IN PARENTHESIS):
                    (  HOSTILE            )
    GENERAL PAIN       IMPAIRED SOCIAL
```

Fig. 2. An example of computerized printout of analysis of the PAF. Shown are unipolar scale scores, scores of bipolar continua and the typologies for which the subject met criteria.

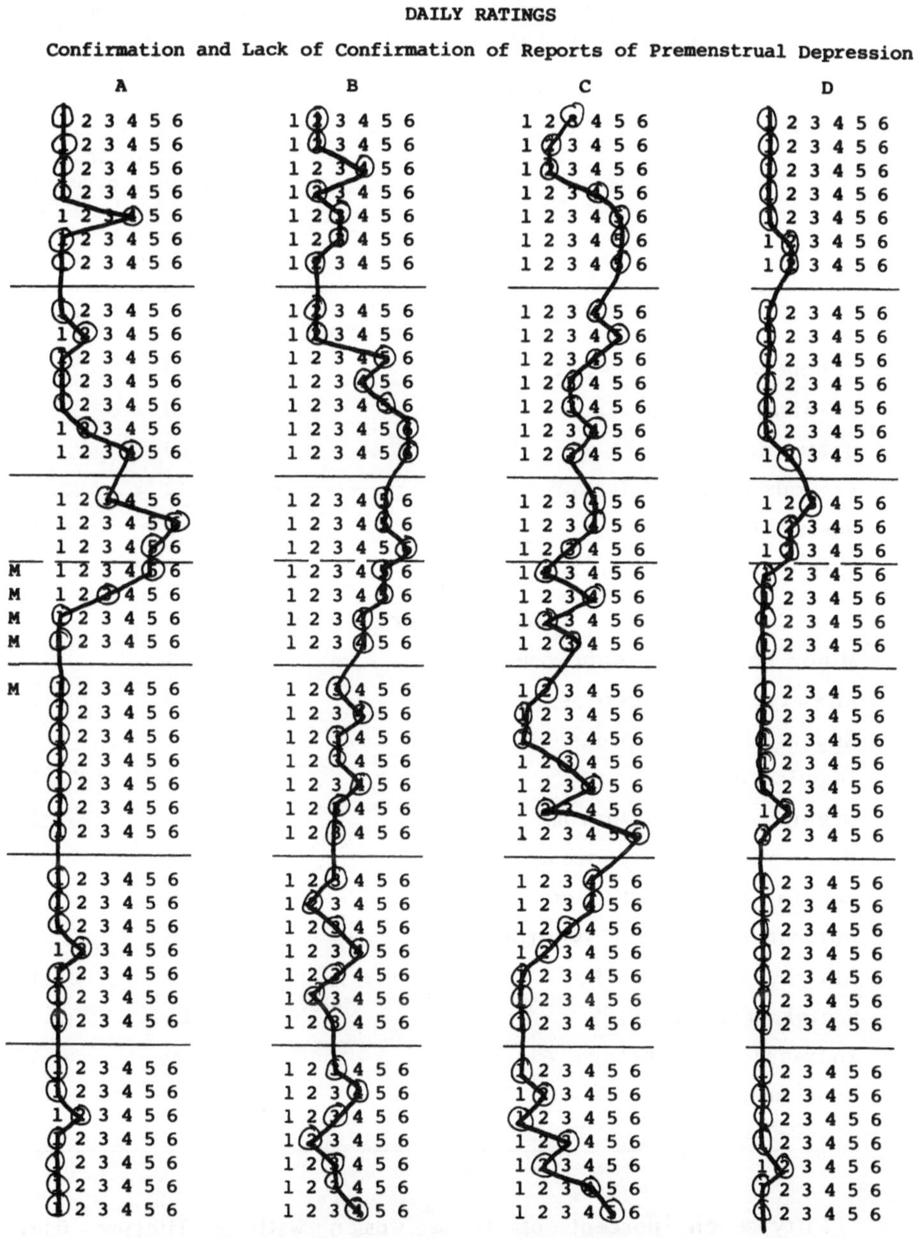

Fig. 3. *A*. Confirmation of Premenstrual Depression: There are changes in mood during the premenstrual period which return to baseline shortly after the beginning of menstrual blood flow. Except for very mild fluctuations, there are no such changes during other phases of the menstrual cycle. *B*. Lack of Confirmation: Chronic depression with some premenstrual worsening. Even though there is a severe premenstrual depression, the usual mood of the woman is low. *C*. Lack of Confirmation: Chronic depression, no connection to menstrual cycle. *D*. Lack of Confirmation: Severity of premenstrual depression is only minimal to mild. [From: Halbreich et al., 1985. Reprinted with permission of *Canadian Journal of Psychiatry*.]

Table 4. Categories of Premenstrual Changes in Women With and Without Premenstrual Assessment Form (PAF) Depressive Syndrome. [From: Halbreich et al., 1983. Reprinted With Permission of *Archives of General Psychiatry.*]

	Met Criteria for PAF Depressive Syndrome	
	No (N = 190)	Yes (N = 145)
Depressive Syndrome		
Endogenous features, %	0	0
Atypical features, %	0	63
Hysteroid features, %	0	17
Anxious-agitated features, %	0	43
Hostile features, %	0	52
Withdrawn features, %	0	42
Other Categories of Change		
Minor depressive syndrome, %	33	0
Anxiety without depression, %	3	0
Anger without depression, %	1	1
Impulsivity, %	9	52
Organic mental syndrome, %	1	27
Water retention syndrome, %	33	80
General discomfort syndrome, %	45	89
Autonomic physical syndrome, %	6	42
Fatigue syndrome, %	7	63
Social impairment, %	11	72
Increased well-being, %	9	21
None suitable, %	6	0

Fifty-seven percent of these women with a lifetime diagnosis of Major Depressive Disorder (MDD) also had Premenstrual Full Depressive Syndrome, while only 14% of the women who were "Never Mentally Ill" met these PAF criteria. The percentage of women meeting PAF criteria for Full Depressive Syndrome in the premenstruum was consistently higher in the subgroup of MDD women with recurrent Unipolar Depression. Eighty-four percent of the women who had PAF Full Depressive Syndrome had RDC Major Depressive Disorder and only 9% were "Never Mentally Ill."

The reported prevalence of PAF Full Depression, as well as that of other subtypes of PMC, depends on the recruitment and selection procedures used. It may be as high as 83% in women with current MDD and almost nonexistent in selected groups of women who were "Never Mentally Ill" (Halbreich & Endicott, 1985b).

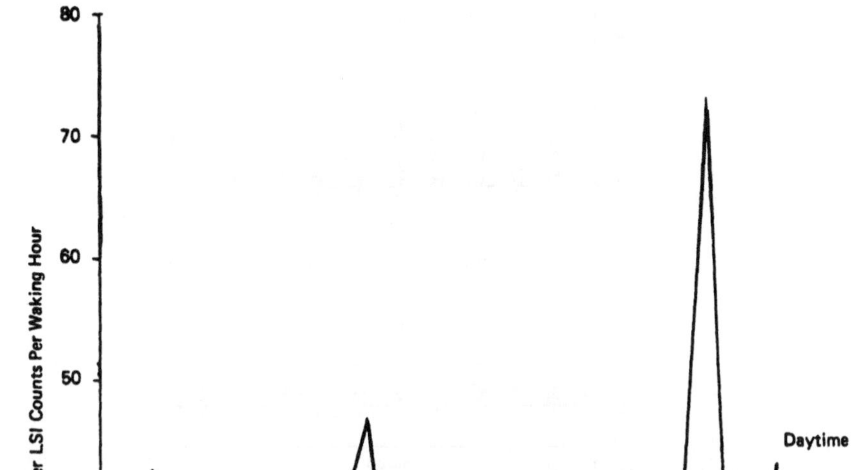

Fig. 4. Example of bipolar changes in activity level during the premenstrual period as measured with a wrist LSI activity monitor. [From: Halbreich et al., 1982. Reprinted with permission of *Acta Psychiatrica Scandinavica*.]

These differences may partially account for the great variability of rates reported in the literature. It is noteworthy that the few reports on the relationship between lifetime diagnosis of Affective Disorders and premenstrual "Affective Syndrome" are consistent despite major differences in definition and methodology.

Kashiwagi et al. (1976) reported that 65% of women who were diagnosed as having lifetime Affective Disorder [according to Feighner, Robin, & Guze's (1972) criteria] were also diagnosed as having a

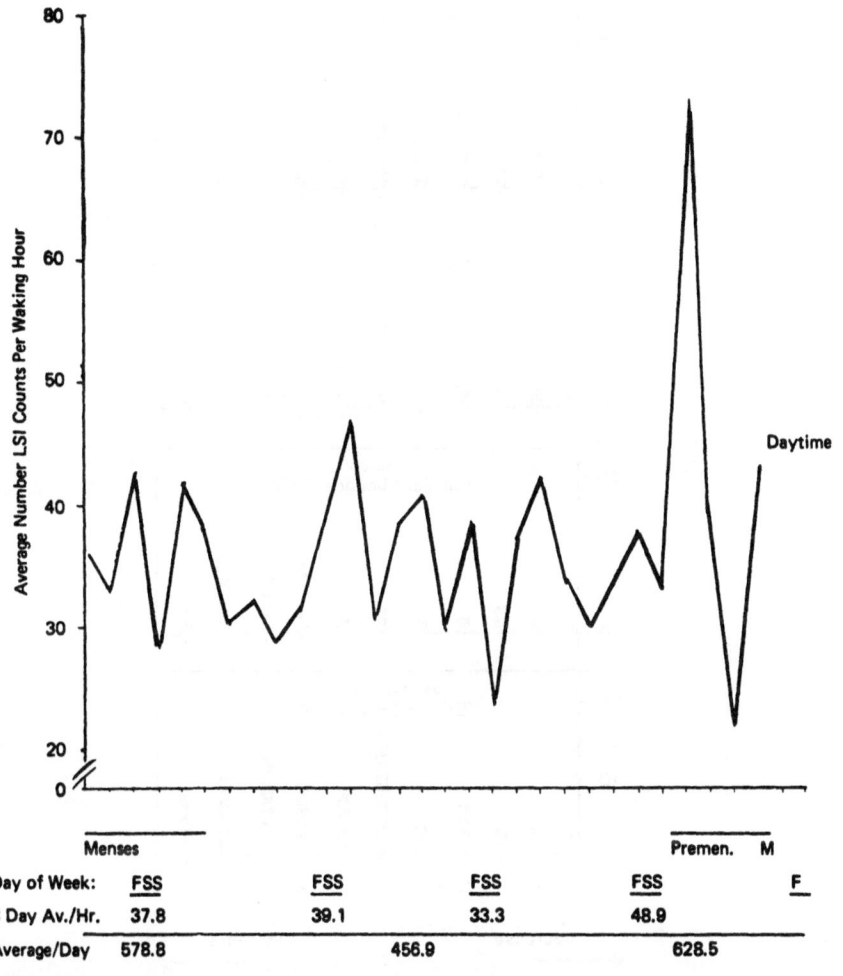

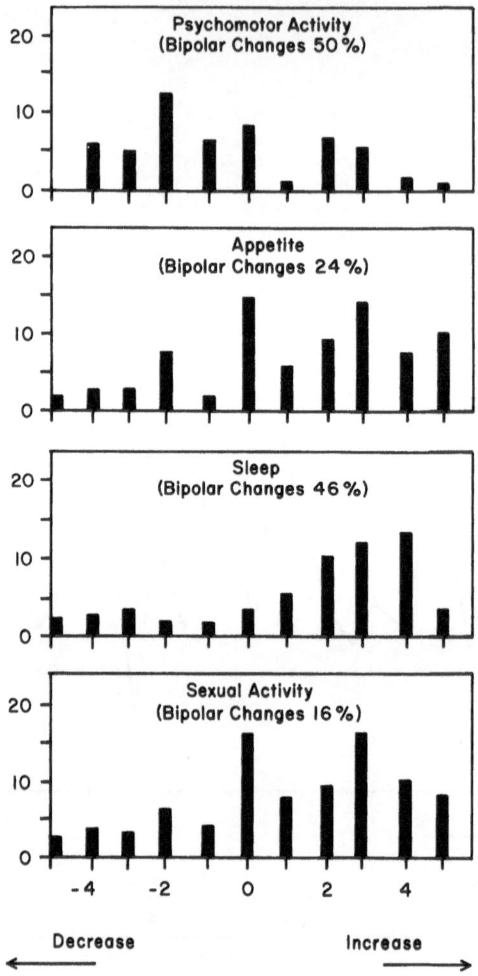

Fig. 5. Variability in severity and direction of Premenstrual Assessment Form, bipolar continua reported by women with premenstrual depression syndrome (N = 145). [From: Halbreich et al., 1982. Reprinted with permission of *Acta Psychiatrica Scandinavica.*]

premenstrual "affective syndrome," compared to only 14% of women with "other mental disorders." The same figure of 65% was reported by Diamond et al. (1976), who used the same Feighner criteria for the definition of Lifetime Affective Disorder. They also found that 57% of their "control groups" of social workers and patients' spouses had premenstrual depressive syndromes, but no lifetime diagnostic data were available for the "control groups."

Coppen (1965) reported that 72% of women in-patients with Affective Disorders also had a premenstrual disorder, about half of them to a moderate-to-severe degree. In a "Non-Affective Disorder" mixed group (lifetime diagnosis unknown), only 4-10% of the women had a severe premenstrual disorder, although many women had mild changes.

The predictive value of dysphoric PMC for the development of MDD in the future has been studied by two groups. Wetzel et al. (1975) reported that 18% of college students with Premenstrual Affective

Table 5. Differential Correlations of Physical and Organic Mental Changes With Subtypes of Depressive Features Among Women With Premenstrual Depression (N = 145).[a]

	Depressive Features		
	Atypical[b]	Hostile[b]	Anxious[b]
Physical Changes			
Have decreased energy or tend to fatigue easily	.36[c]	-.03	.12
Have feelings of weakness	.35[c]	-.14	.17
Have tired legs (weak, sore, tremble)	.35[c]	-.02	.02
Have relatively steady abdominal heaviness, discomfort or pain	.26[d]	.04	.07
Feel bloated	.31[c]	.07	.14
Tend to have backaches, joint and muscle pains, or stiffness	.35[c]	-.02	.20
Have skin problems, such as acne and pimples	.27[d]	-.02	.10
Have flare-up or appearance of cold sores, diarrhea, belching, spontaneous bruises, varicose veins, chest pain, hemorrhoids, numbing, tingling, epilepsy ("fits"), sensitivity of skin to sun	.28[d]	-.07	.14
Have flare-ups of allergy, breathing difficulties, stuffy feeling, or watery discharge from nose	.31[c]	-.26	.32[c]
Have nausea or vomiting	.16	-.04	.23[d]
Have periods of dizziness, faintness, vertigo (room spinning), ringing in the ears, numbness, tingling of skin, trembling, light-headedness	.16	-.17	.34[c]
Feel pounding of heart or have rapid heart beat	.15	-.07	.31[c]
Have a feeling of malaise (i.e., general, nonspecific bad feeling or vague sense of mental or physical ill health)	.09	.09	.33[c]
Have headaches or migraines	.19	-.15	.35[c]
Organic Mental Changes			
Be more easily distracted (i.e., attention shifts easily and rapidly)	.29[c]	-.03	.19
Have decreased ability to coordinate fine movements, poor motor coordination, or clumsiness	.10	-.05	.32[c]
Tend to have accidents, fall, cut self, or break things unintentionally	.19	.00	.39[c]
Have difficulty concentrating	.20	.03	.29[d]
Feel confused	.02	.18	.28[d]

[a] All 145 women met criteria for Premenstrual Assessment Form (PAF) depressive syndrome.

[b] The PAF scale score measuring the set of features noted was correlated with selected PAF items with the correlations of the other two sets of features partialed out. Items listed are those that were differentially related to the three sets of depressive features at at least the $p < .01$ level.

[c] Significant at the $p < .001$ level.

[d] Significant at the $p < .01$ level.

Syndrome developed Affective Disorders (according to Feighner et al.'s criteria) during a 4-year follow-up, compared with 10% of those without premenstrual affective syndrome. Similar results were reported by Schuckit et al. (1975), who found that 7% of those with a "premenstrual emotional syndrome" developed a depressive disorder within 12 months after entering into the study, compared to 0% of those without the "emotional syndrome."

Table 6. Structured Clinical Assessment: Psychiatric Patients *and* Normal Controls.

(A) Schedule for Affective Disorders and Schizophrenia (SADS) and Research Diagnostic Criteria (RDC)	Lifetime and current diagnosis of mental disorder using the Research Diagnostic Criteria. Number of episodes of various disorders. Hospitalizations, suicide attempts, social functioning, highest levels of occupation, etc. Summary scale scores and individual items of relevance for evaluation of severity of lifetime and current mental disorder.
(B) Family History-Research Diagnostic Criteria (FH-RDC)	Presence or absence of evidence of mental disorder in relatives. Cause of death of relatives.
(C) Demographic Form	Basic demographic information needed to describe the sample.
(D) SADS-Change Version (SADS-C)	Measurement of specific symptoms and their severity and degree of impairment due to them — during a specified period prior to the biological test.
(E) SCL-90	Initial screening of normals for presence of mental disorder.

The two latter studies are somewhat methodologically weak, especially in their clinical definitions and criteria for premenstrual changes. Nonetheless, they further confirm the possible relationship between premenstrual dysphoric changes and Affective Disorders.

POSSIBLE IMPLICATIONS OF AN ASSOCIATION BETWEEN DYSPHORIC PREMENSTRUAL CHANGES AND AFFECTIVE DISORDERS

The suggestion that premenstrual dysphoric changes in mood and behavior may be related to a lifetime history of Major Affective Disorder raises some practical and ethical issues that have not yet been solved.

The most important issue is whether the demonstration of a retrospective association between the two phenomena is also an indication that in younger women who do not have a lifetime history of MDD, the existence of dysphoric PMC may be a risk factor or a predictor for the development of MDD in the future. Two prospective studies (Schuckit et al., 1975; Wetzel et al., 1975) point in that direction. However, they should be confirmed by additional, well designed, prospective studies. If this is the case, and the predictive value of dysphoric PMC is established with reasonable sensitivity and specificity, then several ethical issues arise: (a) should a patient be informed of her higher risk of developing MDD? (b) should any preventive steps be taken? If so, what should these steps be and with what degree of rigorousness should they be undertaken?

At present, these issues are highly hypothetical because not only is the prospective confirmation of the association between dysphoric PMC and MDD far from being firm, but preventive measures for the development of MDD are virtually unknown. Assuming that the association between dysphoric PMC and MDD is confirmed, then the question of informing a woman with such changes of her being at higher risk is subject to a risk-benefit analysis. The situation would be further complicated by similar considerations regarding preventive interventions. Being assumptive and speculative where they stand alone, any discussion of the possible interrelationship between these intricate parameters can be compared to an elaborate speculation of how many angels can share an omelette prepared from an egg that has yet to be laid.

Another issue that may be raised, if an association between dysphoric PMC and depressive disorder is confirmed, is whether PMC can be studied as a model for affective disorders, especially for the study of possible biological correlates of changes in mood. This area may benefit from the currently developing processes of detailed diagnosis and subtyping of affective disorders and of PMC.

A further question raised by the association between premenstrual dysphoric changes and dysphoric symptomatology of a disorder's magnitude is when should the pattern of PMC be considered a "disorder" and at what level of severity is treatment warranted? This question should be addressed in this context because it seems that more women seek treatment due to dysphoric PMC than due to their physical PMC. The views that PMC constitutes a diversity of symptoms and changes, that not all of them are necessarily "negative," and that even the negative ones (those that are generally called "symptoms") constitute a continuum of severity — call for discussion on the decision of when to treat PMC. We believe that PMC should be treated any time the severity is such that there is an impairment of social or individual functioning to a degree that is clearly significant to the woman and/or those around her. Even in such a case, the risk-benefit ratio consideration should include the fact that we are dealing with a repetitive series of individually self-limited, usually short-lived situations. The assessment procedure devised by us (Halbreich et al., 1982, 1985) provides the necessary evaluation by including social impairment as a category of change (see Table 2), as well as unidimensional scores on other clusters of symptoms.

If treatment is warranted, then the question is posed of which treatment. At present, there is no treatment modality that has withstood the trial of well designed, double-blind, placebo-controlled tests to confirm its efficacy (Halbreich et al., 1985). However, the trial-and-error way in which most individual patients are treated for PMC at present does raise ethical issues; for instance, such concerns are raised when one evaluates the risk-benefit ratio of treatments for a condition whose severity varies from cycle to cycle and whose course probably depends upon sociopsychological and environmental influences while being essentially self-limited. Indeed, the observation that PMC are many times responsive to environmental influences provides support for treatments such as change of lifestyle or diet because, although unproven, they involve little risk of untoward side effects.

With our present understanding of PMC, the aforementioned issues constitute a matter for debate and speculation. Hopefully, they will become somewhat clearer with a better understanding of the background facts.

CONCLUSIONS

The diversity of premenstrual dysphoric changes has been demonstrated with the application of assessment procedures that are designed to measure these. However, retrospective reports, including the Premenstrual Assessment Form (PAF), should be confirmed by daily prospective ratings over at least one menstrual cycle.

The most prevalent PAF subtype of premenstrual dysphoric changes is the Atypical subtype, which is followed by the Hostile subtype, and then the subtype defined by Anxious-Agitated features. Premenstrual endogenous depression was not found. There is an overlap among the subtypes of premenstrual dysphoric changes. Moreover, there is some evidence that they are differentially related to other features of PMC.

In our sample, as well as in previous reports, about two-thirds of women with a lifetime diagnosis of Major Depressive Disorder (MDD) also had a premenstrual Full Depressive Syndrome, while very few women who were "Never Mentally Ill" met these criteria. Hence, it is suggested that there may be an association between Premenstrual Dysphoric Changes and MDD, and that this issue is well worth pursuing further.

ACKNOWLEDGMENTS

The research reported in this chapter was supported in part by the Albert Einstein College of Medicine, New York State Department of Mental Hygiene, NIMH grants MH30906 and MH36186, and the Ritter's Foundation.

REFERENCES

Abramowitz, E. S., A. H. Backer, and S. F. Freischer, 1982. Onset of depressive psychiatric crises and the menstrual cycle. *American Journal of Psychiatry 139:* 475-478.

Coppen, A., 1965. The prevalence of menstrual disorders in psychiatric patients. *British Journal of Psychiatry 3:* 155-167.

Diamond, S. B., A. A. Rubinstein, D. L. Dunner, and R. R. Fieve, 1976. Menstrual problems in women with primary affective illness. *Comprehensive Psychiatry 17:* 541-548.

Endicott, J., U. Halbreich, S. Schacht, and J. Nee, 1981. Premenstrual changes and affective disorders. *Psychosomatic Medicine 3:* 514-517.

Feighner, J. P., S. E. Robin, and S. B. Guze, 1972. Diagnostic criteria for use in psychiatric research. *Archives of General Psychiatry 26:* 57-63.

Halbreich, U. and J. Endicott, 1985a. The relationship of dysphoric premenstrual changes to depressive disorders. *Acta Psychiatrica Scandinavica 71:* 331-338.

Halbreich, U. and J. Endicott, 1985b. Methodological issues in studies of premenstrual changes. *Psychoneuroendocrinology 10:* 15-32.

Halbreich, U., J. Endicott, and J. Nee, 1982. The diversity of premenstrual changes as reflected in the Premenstrual Assessment Form. *Acta Psychiatrica Scandinavica 65:* 46-65.

Halbreich, U., J. Endicott, and J. Lesser, 1985. The clinical diagnosis and classification of premenstrual changes. *Canadian Journal of Psychiatry 30:* 489-497.

Halbreich, U., J. Endicott, and J. Nee, 1983. Premenstrual depressive changes: Value of differentiation. *Archives of General Psychiatry 40:* 535-542.

Kashiwagi, T., J. N. McClure, T. Reich, and R. D. Wetzel, 1976. Premenstrual affective syndrome and psychiatric disorder. *Diseases of the Nervous System 37:* 116-119.

Schuckit, M. A., V. Daly, G. Herrman, and S. Hineman, 1975. Premenstrual symptoms and depression in a university population. *Diseases of the Nervous System 36:* 516-517.

Wetzel, J. N., T. Reich, J. N. McClure, and I. Wald, 1975. Premenstrual affective syndrome and affective disorder. *British Journal of Psychiatry 127:* 219-221.

THE PSYCHOBIOLOGY OF PREMENSTRUAL SYNDROMES: THE MICHIGAN STUDIES

Meir Steiner,* M.D., Ph.D., F.R.C.P.(C) and
Roger F. Haskett,** M.B.B.S.

*Departments of Psychiatry and Neurosciences
McMaster University; and
Clinical Studies Program
McMaster Psychiatric Unit
St. Joseph's Hospital
Hamilton, Ontario, Canada

**Clinical Studies Unit
Department of Psychiatry
University of Michigan Medical School
Ann Arbor, Michigan

INTRODUCTION

Among adult women, the incidence and prevalence of depression, excessive anxiety, and related behavioral disturbances are disproportionately high. Sex differences and the epidemiology of depression have been reviewed to highlight this point (Weissman & Klerman, 1977). In every age group studied to date, at least a 2:1 female-to-male ratio of depression was found, and the incidence in community surveys is even more skewed toward women, with the ratio being as high as 4:1. These differences are conceptually and statistically significant and seem to be consistent between surveys (Robins, Helzer, Weissman, Orvaschel, Gruenberg, Burke, & Regier, 1984).

A variety of explanatory hypotheses have been proposed focusing mainly on psychosocial and/or biological predisposing gender differences (Norman, Johnson, & Miller, 1984). The psychosocial contributing factors are unclear. Community surveys have shown that women tend to report more affective symptoms than men, and some researchers believe that this could account for the increased incidence of depression in women. Employment and good social support seem to diminish the risk of depression in women (Clayton, 1983). To date, no conclusion can be reached as to whether women have a different psychobiological threshold for mental disorders.

A possible explanation for the higher incidence of mental illness in women would be a demonstrable relationship between these disorders and the female chromosome, the reproductive cyclicity, or any possible neuroendocrine changes. The data for a genetic linkage are inconclusive (Nurnberger & Gershon, 1982). The influence of hormones is not clear, although at puberty, depression ratings, depressive illness, and suicide attempts for females begin to exceed those of males.

Hormones are partial determinants of certain sexually dimorphic behaviors, interacting with psychologic, sociocultural, and other biologic factors. Areas of research which have focused on this interaction include the role of testosterone in aggression for men and mental disorders associated with child-bearing and climacteric changes for women, to name just a few (for reviews, see Rubin, Reinisch, & Haskett, 1981; Steiner, 1979, 1983).

Hormonal levels fluctuate over the menstrual cycle, and many women complain of menstrually-related symptoms which also fluctuate in a cyclical fashion. Thus, it is not surprising that many researchers, including ourselves, were tempted to study the cyclical biological changes along the menstrual cycle and their possible relevance to premenstrual syndromes (PMS).

This chapter will briefly review some of the earlier theories of possible hormonal influences on premenstrual dysphoria, but will be primarily devoted to the summary and discussion of our own studies.

BACKGROUND TO THE STUDIES

In our reviews of the literature (Carroll & Steiner, 1978; Steiner & Carroll, 1977), we stated that various psycho-socio-biological theories of PMS have been suggested, but without convincing evidence, and that this difficulty was reflected in the enormous number of suggested treatments.

In an attempt to provide a better understanding of the syndromes and their potential treatments, we initially identified what we considered to be the central issues. These could be summarized as follows:

(1) The clinical dimensions of PMS were too broad, and the only available rating scale at that time, the Menstrual Distress Questionnaire (MDQ; Moos, 1969), covers many non-specific phenomena.

(2) The obvious possibility that episodic mood shifts which occur premenstrually might be related to manic-depressive illness remained almost unexplored. None of the studies have detailed the phenomenology of PMS in a way which made comparison with primary affective disorders possible.

(3) No menstrually-related hormonal changes, which might distinguish women with PMS from unaffected women, have been conclusively identified.

(4) The timing of premenstrual symptoms coinciding with late luteal elevation of plasma prolactin (PRL), as well as some indirect evidence from human and animal studies, suggested a role for PRL in PMS which warranted further investigation (Carroll & Steiner, 1978).

(5) Suppression of PRL secretion with bromocriptine, the interaction of PRL with lithium, and other reported treatments which may suppress PRL secretion or antagonize its peripheral effects have all been suggested as treatments for PMS, but the rationale for using them has not been established and their effectiveness has not been substantiated (Carroll & Steiner, 1978).

On the basis of these questions, we decided to: (a) reassess the specificity of symptoms included in PMS; (b) re-examine psychoneuroendocrine mechanisms possibly involved in these conditions; and (c) establish the therapeutic efficacy of lithium and bromocriptine in women with severe premenstrual dysphoria.

DELINEATION OF THE SYNDROME AND THE DEVELOPMENT OF RESEARCH DIAGNOSTIC CRITERIA AND NEW RATING SCALES

Our first task was to define which clinical features of the syndrome are most prominent in the premenstruum. We decided to study a group of severely affected women who were free of physical or psychological pathology at all other times. Since no single rating scale has been designed to measure specifically the changes in *severe* PMS, we chose to use a group of existing instruments. These included the:

(1) Menstrual Distress Questionnaire (MDQ; Moos, 1969).

(2) Visual Analogue Scale (VAS; Aitken, 1969; Maxwell, 1978).

(3) Multiple Affect Adjective Check List (MAACL; Zuckerman & Lubin, 1965).

(4) State-Trait Anxiety Inventory (STAI; Spielberger, Gorsuch, & Lushene, 1979).

(5) Hamilton Depression Scale (HDS; Hamilton, 1960).

(6) Carroll Depression Scale (CDS; Carroll, Feinberg, Smouse, Rawson, & Greden, 1981a).

Women who met our strict inclusion criteria (Haskett, Steiner, Osmun, & Carroll, 1980) went through an evaluation phase which lasted for at least two complete menstrual cycles. Visits to the clinic were scheduled to coincide as closely as possible with two specific points in the menstrual cycle. These were a follicular phase visit on Day 9 (where Day 1 was the onset of menses) and a luteal phase visit on, or around, Day 26 but always 2-6 days premenstrual. The evaluation was considered complete when all measures had been obtained for these two points in a single menstrual cycle. This extended evaluation permitted confirmation of the major inclusion criteria: all women suffered a severe premenstrual dysphoria, and the disturbance was an ON-OFF phenomenon.

All the rating scale measurements indicated that we were studying a group of women with a severe disturbance in the premenstruum which was not present in the follicular phase. The change in group means between the two visits was highly significant for all current state ratings. The range of scores obtained at the follicular phase visits was also consistent with normative data published for most instruments. The specific anxiety, depression, and hostility scales produced results which did not indicate that any of these dimensions alone constitute the core syndrome in PMS.

In addition to considering total scores, we performed an individual item analysis of the MDQ, examining the change in scores between follicular and premenstrual visits and the distribution of items which were recorded at the follicular visit.

The analyses sought to rank order the items according to degree of change between visits and frequency of response. First, any of the 47 MDQ items for which more than half of the subjects recorded a score change of less than two were excluded. A severity index score was derived for the remaining items by summing for each, the product of score change and the number of subjects recording that value, where the minimum score change considered was three. To permit comparison between the total group and sub-groups, the severity index scores were expressed as a percentage of the maximum possible in each group (for details, see Haskett et al., 1980).

Analysis of the changes for individual items on the MDQ between follicular and late luteal visits revealed that only 27 of 47 MDQ items qualified (e.g., were different in the two phases). The emotional descriptors which appear in the most highly ranked items (in a sub-group of women with low follicular scores) were Irritability, Mood Swings, Restlessness, and Tension. This describes an aroused, brittle individual who is liable to become hostile or dysphoric with or without provocation. These responses are reflected in the next two items: Depression and Anxiety. Down the list were additional items which refer specifically to impaired functioning as well as physical symptoms (Haskett et al., 1980).

Based on a comprehensive review of the literature, our own clinical observations, and the rank-ordered lists of items from the MDQ and the other rating scales used, we compiled a list of the major symptoms and signs of severe PMS. Using the patients' own words where possible, descriptors of the most characteristic aspects of this disorder were then incorporated into a list of operational criteria for PMS. The format used was intentionally similar to that used by Spitzer, Endicott, and Robins (1978) in the Research Diagnostic Criteria (RDC) and is shown in Figure 1.

Subcategory "A" contains descriptors which have been shown in this study to define the core changes which occur with PMS. "B" is a severity factor to ensure that only women who are severely affected will be included in this category. To obtain homogeneity in populations to be studied, it is necessary to distinguish minor variants of this disorder from the severe disabling condition. This is analogous to the need to separate individuals with minor mood fluctuations from those suffering from a major affective disorder in studies of that condition (see also Haskett & Steiner, 1986).

Many of the women in this study indicated that their PMS symptoms were not of identical severity in each menstrual cycle. Subcategory "C" is included to ensure that subjects are suffering from an essentially recurrent condition. Subcategory "D" describes one of the major inclusion criteria used for this study. It emphasizes our suggestion that research into this condition must clearly define the particular time period under discussion. We do not believe that these symptoms are seen only in the premenstrual phase. There are many reports in the literature which suggest that variations of this complex are present at other phases of the menstrual cycle (Smith, 1975; Sutherland & Stewart, 1965). We stress, however, the need to define this disturbance when it is confined to the premenstruum before considering other syndromes which differ either in specific symptom configuration or temporal relationship.

The Primary/Secondary distinction is proposed for reasons similar to those justifying its inclusion in the criteria for Major Depressive Disorder. To facilitate research, it is necessary to separate subjects who suffer from PMS alone from those who manifest an interaction between other psychopathology and PMS.

PRIMARY RECURRENT PREMENSTRUAL TENSION DISORDER

This category is applied to female subjects in their fertile years who do not currently meet the criteria for any other psychiatric disorder.

The psychological and behavioral symptoms included in this disorder frequently occur in association with physical premenstrual symptoms; e.g., painful or tender breasts, headaches, swelling of abdomen, breasts or ankles, with water retention, weight gain, etc. These are not necessary for the psychiatric diagnosis.

A through D are required.

A. At least 5 of the following are required for definite diagnosis and 4 for probable diagnosis as part of a current episode.

1. Irritable, hostile, angry, short-fused.
2. Tense, restless, jittery, upset, high-strung, unable to relax.
3. Decreased efficiency, fatigue.
4. Dysphoric, marked spontaneous emotional lability, crying.
5. Lowered motor coordination, clumsy, prone to accidents (cut finger, break dish, etc.).
6. Distractable, confused, forgetful, difficulty in concentration, lowered judgement.
7. Change in eating habits (cravings, overeating, etc.).
8. Marked change in libido.

B. Overall disturbance is so severe that at least one of the following is present:

1. Serious impairment socially, with family, at home, at school or work.
2. Sought or was referred for help from someone or took medication (especially tranquilizers and/or diuretics) at least once during a premenstrual period.

C. Premenstrual dysphoric symptoms for at least six of the nine preceding menstrual cycles.

D. Symptoms only during the premenstrual period with relief soon after onset of menses.

SECONDARY RECURRENT PREMENSTRUAL TENSION DISORDER

This category is applied for subjects who meet the criteria A through D for Primary Recurrent Premenstrual Tension Disorder but at the same time meet the criteria for another psychiatric disorder.

N.B. Some women previously given the diagnoses Intermittent Depressive Disorder, Minor Depressive Disorder and/or Labile Personality may now be more accurately classified as having Primary Recurrent Premenstrual Tension Disorder.

Fig. 1. Research Diagnostic Criteria for PMS.

Using the same composite list of descriptors for this syndrome, self-report and observer-rating questionnaires were constructed. These are shown in the appendix to this chapter. It is intended that these scales should be complementary. The questionnaires are designed to monitor changes in the same specific PMS phenomenology, and the relationship between items is described in the original publication (Steiner, Haskett, & Carroll, 1980a).

The most pertinent clinical items are presented in terms designed to be meaningful for women suffering from PMS and therapists working with them. We have tried to avoid linguistic pitfalls which have confused the issues in the past. For example, we found that the MDQ items "anxiety" and "depression" were interpreted by many women as "tension" and "dysphoria," respectively. The same two items have been repeatedly used by clinicians to designate the syndrome as "Premenstrual Anxiety" and "Premenstrual Depression," when it is highly likely that women were using these emotional descriptors for quite different meanings. We believe that these terms are very misleading. PMS does not appear to be an abbreviated form of an Anxiety Disorder, nor is it a mini-episode of Endogenous Depression. The core symptomatology of PMS includes irritability, dysphoria, restlessness, tension, and emotional lability. Additional features include fatigue, avoidance of social activity, decreased efficiency, difficulty concentrating, and occasional impairment of motor coordination. Symptoms of anxiety or depression, when present, seem to be reactive to the unexplained irritability and dysphoria.

To date, at least 15 researchers around the world are using our rating scales and diagnostic criteria. It is our expectation that the use of the same instruments will enable investigators of PMS to more effectively compare data with each other.

PSYCHONEUROENDOCRINE MECHANISMS

Prolactin

The pattern of circulating sex steroid hormones and gonadotrophins in the course of the normal menstrual cycle has been well described in recent years (Kaulhausen, Leyendecker, Benker, & Breuer, 1978; Punnonen, Nummi, Ylikorkala, Alapiessa, Karvonen, & Viinikka, 1976). Studies which have attempted to demonstrate a link between PMS and a relative imbalance of hormones, including not only estrogens and progesterone but also aldosterone, have produced inconsistent results (Backstrom & Mattsson, 1975; Janowsky, Berens, & Davis, 1973; Smith, 1975).

Earlier reports of elevated prolactin (PRL) levels during the late luteal phase in women with PMS (Halbreich, Assael, Ben-David, & Bornstein, 1976; Horrobin, Karmali, Mtabaji, Manku, & Nassar, 1976), together with the claim that symptoms of PMS have been markedly ameliorated by bromocriptine, a PRL suppressant (Benedek-Jaszmann & Hearn-Sturtevant, 1976), have led us to further investigate whether a late luteal hyperprolactinemia, in fact, coincides with the timing of PMS.

We studied 37 adult women (ages 22-42 years) who complained of a severe dysphoric syndrome in the premenstruum, but who showed no evidence of emotional disorder at other times. Single PRL levels were obtained from all 37 women at 4 p.m. during both the follicular (Day 9) and late luteal (Day 26) phases. In 21 of the subjects, a 10 a.m. PRL sample was also taken (Steiner, Haskett, Carroll, Hays, & Rubin, 1984a).

All mean PRL values in this study were within the normal range (12.8-17.3 nanograms per milliliter). There was no significant difference between morning (10 a.m.) and afternoon (4 p.m.) samples during either phase of the cycle. No significant difference was found between follicular and late luteal mean PRL levels at 10 a.m. There was, however, a significant increase in mean PRL levels at 4 p.m. from follicular to late luteal phase ($p < 0.05$; two-tailed t-test). Although statistically significant, the implications of this finding are unclear. One-third of the subjects (12 of the 37 women sampled at 4 p.m. and six of the 21 sampled at 10 a.m.) showed lower PRL levels during the late luteal (premenstrual) phase than during the follicular phase. There was no obvious clinical difference between women who had increased and those who had decreased late luteal phase PRL levels.

In addition, two subjects with extremely severe PMS and two asymptomatic healthy female controls participated in a study of circadian hormone secretory profiles. These women were admitted to the Clinical Research Center on Days 9 and 26 of their menstrual cycles. The follicular phase (Day 9) studies preceded the luteal phase (Day 26) studies in all subjects. Blood samples for PRL, growth hormone (GH), and cortisol were collected every 30 minutes for 26 hours from an in-dwelling catheter in the antecubital vein (Steiner, Haskett, Carroll, Hays, & Rubin, 1984b).

The cortisol and GH results in our study did not indicate a major neuroendocrine stress or arousal response associated with PMS. The elevated PRL levels in one woman with PMS and in one of the control subjects are also unlikely to be the result of non-specific stress of PMS. Markedly elevated PRL levels were seen in the absence of PMS.

It is clear from our data that measurement of circadian profiles is superior to plasma level estimation in single samples. The pulsatile secretion pattern of these hormones clearly demonstrates the difficulties of interpreting values obtained from single samples. We have also demonstrated that the comparison of mean daily hormone levels with behavioral observations that are scored once a day does not appear to be meaningful.

Our data failed to show any specific relationship between serum PRL levels and PMS. Even though there was a slight premenstrual increase of PRL, neither the PRL measurements from single blood samples nor the circadian PRL secretion profiles support the hypothesis that PMS is associated with an elevation in serum PRL levels. Similar results have been reported by Backstrom and Aakvaag (1981) and O'Brien and Symonds (1982).

We also estimated serum PRL levels in 10 women participating in a bromocriptine treatment trial who received doses ranging from 2.5 to 7.5 mg daily. They received medication from day 10 until the onset of menses for three consecutive cycles. The blood samples were drawn around 10 a.m. on Days 9 and 26 of a pretreatment cycle and for each of the three cycles of the trial.

Our data confirmed that bromocriptine suppressed PRL on Days 26, but PRL levels on Days 9 were significantly elevated. Despite this marked "rebound" hyperprolactinemia following the cessation of bromocriptine, all subjects remained free of symptoms, with no observable effects on mood, behavior, or menstrual regularity. The lack of emotional or behavioral changes during a "rebound" hyperprolactinemia has not been reported before.

The 24-hour PRL profiles from the subjects in this study showed great variation and no obvious relationship to PMS or menstrual cycle phase. One other study of 24-hour PRL profiles in an asymptomatic subject, measuring episodic release and diurnal variation, showed an increase in nocturnal PRL release at midcycle or the time of ovulation (Ehara, Siler, Vandenberg, Sinha, & Yen, 1973). Other stimuli of PRL secretion include meal ingestion and changes in ambient temperature (Mills & Robertshaw, 1981; Quigley, Ropert, & Yen, 1981). Previous studies have not controlled for these variables, and it is obvious that future studies should.

Finally, even if PRL secretion can be shown to be associated with the clinical features of PMS, this hormone may be serving as an endocrine reflection of central neurotransmitter activity rather than as a direct etiological agent for these symptoms. Many of the transmitters which influence the activity of the hypothalamic-pituitary-gonadal (HPG) axis during the normal menstrual cycle are also believed to alter the secretion of PRL; e.g., dopamine and endogenous opiates (Fritz & Speroff, 1982). The timing of PMS symptoms makes it a reasonable hypothesis that they are related to the cyclical neuroendocrine changes in the HPG axis, so that it is possible that changes in PRL, estrogens, or progesterone, which are an important part of the menstrual cycle, have an indirect but unclear relationship to PMS (Vaitukaitis, 1984).

The Hypothalamic-Pituitary-Adrenocortical (HPA) Axis

The measurement of various hormone plasma levels associated with PMS has not yielded particularly reliable or informative results (Abplanalp, Haskett, & Rose, 1980). An alternative strategy would be a search for those endocrine abnormalities that have been noted to be associated with specific forms of psychopathology. The presence of such phenomena might suggest some similarity between the pathophysiology of PMS and other psychiatric disorders.

The hypothalamic-pituitary-adrenocortical (HPA) axis is the most intensively studied endocrine system in situations of altered psychological state, and some specific associations have been described. Adrenocortical activity is noted to increase in response to various stressful stimuli and is persistently elevated in many patients during an episode of endogenous depression (ED) (see Carroll, 1972 for review). The clinical similarities between PMS and some depressive disorders would be of greater heuristic significance if these women also demonstrated disinhibition of the HPA axis, similar to that seen in patients with ED. Although estrogen or progesterone treatment, or pregnancy, can alter adrenocortical function (Bulbrook, Herian, Tong, Hayward, Swain, & Wang, 1973; Hellman, Yoshida, Zumoff, Levin, Kream, & Fukushima, 1976; Lindholm & Schultz-Moller, 1973), evaluation of this system in PMS is facilitated by the apparent absence of cyclic fluctuations in baseline cortisol secretion in medication-free women with normal menstrual cycles (Aubert, Lemarchand-Beraud, Deguillaume, & Desaulles, 1971; Carr, Parker, Madden, MacDonald, & Porter, 1979; Saxena, Dusitsin, & Lazarus, 1974).

Urinary measures of cortisol excretion during a 24-hour period provide an integrated measure of adrenocortical functioning over time. This is preferred to the measurement of plasma cortisol levels, since the pulsatile release pattern of cortisol limits the amount of information provided by the latter method unless frequent blood samples are obtained. Urinary-free cortisol (UFC) is reported to reflect the effective level of free plasma cortisol better than any other urinary parameter

(Beisel, Cos, Horton, Chao, & Forham, 1964; Burke & Beardwell, 1973; Greaves & West, 1960; Rosner, Cos, Bigliera, Hane & Forsham, 1963).

This study compared the clinical features of severe PMS with the syndrome of ED. Indices of adrenocortical function that are abnormal in many patients with ED, such as 24-hour UFC (Carroll, Curtis, Davies, Mendels, & Sugerman, 1976a) and the 1 mg Dexamethasone Suppression Test (DST) (Carroll, Feinberg, Greden, Tarika, Albala, Haskett, James, Kronfol, Lohr, Steiner, de Vigne, & Young, 1981b), were also assessed in these women. In addition, to evaluate the possible contribution of a non-specific stress response to HPA axis activation, we examined the relationship between cortisol excretion and reported levels of psychological distress. Forty-two women participated in this study (Haskett, Steiner, & Carroll, 1984). Clinical interviews, self-report scales, and endocrine measurements were performed for each subject at each of two visits during the menstrual cycle. In addition, information was obtained on the symptoms and signs necessary for psychiatric syndromal categorization according to the RDC (Spitzer et al., 1978).

Thirty-eight women completed the DST at the time of the follicular and premenstrual phase visits. UFC was measured in urine collected during the 24-hour periods immediately before and after the administration of the dexamethasone. Total plasma cortisol was estimated from a blood sample drawn at 4 p.m. on the following day according to the standard DST procedure for outpatients (Carroll et al., 1981b). Cortisol was measured in plasma and urine by the competitive protein-binding methods of Murphy (1967, 1968) with modifications described by Carroll, Curtis, and Mendels (1976b).

All 42 subjects complained of a prominent dysphoric mood when interviewed during the premenstrual visit. The clinical disturbance reported by each woman at that time only met the RDC for Major Depressive Disorder (MDD) if the duration of symptoms criterion in this diagnostic category was reduced from 2 weeks to 2 days. None, however, met criteria for the endogenous subtype. At the follicular visit, psychopathology was either absent or minimal, and no subject met RDC for any category of psychiatric illness.

Twenty-four-hour UFC values obtained during the DST showed no evidence of cortisol hypersecretion before dexamethasone. The mean baseline UFC excretion values of 46.7 and 47.9 micrograms/24 hours were no different than those found by Murphy (1968) in normal subjects. Despite the definitive premenstrual increase in symptoms, UFC values obtained in the premenstrual and follicular phases were not significantly different.

Four women showed an abnormal DST result in the follicular phase, and three women in the premenstrual phase. No woman had an abnormal result on both occasions.

The typical HPA axis dysfunction reported in many patients with ED was only occasionally seen in these subjects. There was no association between the premenstrual disorder and hypercortisolemia or resistance of cortisol secretion to suppression by dexamethasone. The rate of abnormal DST result was much lower than that reported in patients with ED and did not significantly change between follicular and premenstrual phases of the menstrual cycle. Thus, in these women with no other psychiatric disorder, PMS did not appear to be a model for ED. We concluded that the HPA axis functioning does not appear to be a useful neuroendocrine marker of the distress that is reported by women suffering from severe PMS.

THE THERAPEUTIC RELEVANCE OF LITHIUM AND BROMOCRIPTINE

Lithium

Given the cyclic nature of the PMS and the very few scanty reports on the effects of lithium in women with premenstrual dysphoria, we decided to investigate the possible utility of this drug in our clinic. Fifteen women suffering severe premenstrual symptoms were selected for this study (Steiner, Haskett, Osmun, & Carroll, 1980b). They received 600-900 mg lithium carbonate daily, and the plasma lithium levels ranged between 0.3 and 0.85 milliequivalent per liter (mEq/1)(average 0.54). Six patients were unable to complete the 3-month study, three because of drug-related side effects and three for other reasons. Six patients reported significant side effects but were willing to complete the 3-month schedule. Five patients seemed to benefit from the treatment, but only three requested to be maintained on lithium past the study period. None of the patients experienced any beneficial effects on the physical premenstrual symptoms, and in five patients lithium seemed to have aggravated the symptoms.

In contrast to anecdotal clinical studies, we have studied only women who have not experienced major psychiatric disorders in the past. Most of the women experienced severe side effects even on low dose lithium, reminiscent of observations in normal volunteers (Judd, Hubbard, Janowsky, Huey, & Attewell, 1977). The three women who clearly benefited from the treatment would probably qualify as having "subsyndromic" affective disorders (Akiskal, Djenderedjian, Rosenthal, & Khani, 1977). Two of them had first-degree relatives with diagnosed affective illness. We believe that these women comprise a specific subgroup. Lithium seems to help some cyclothymic features without directly affecting their premenstrual tension. Consequently, while on lithium they seem to be able to better cope with the PMS symptoms. We believe that the non-specific emotional symptoms which disappeared in some of the women while on lithium cannot be completely attributed to a specific effect of medication. A general placebo effect seems to play a major role in PMS treatments (Smith, Cleghorn, Streiner, & Younglai, 1975), the full meaning of which needs further clarification.

Unlike some previously reported studies, we were unable to show that lithium carbonate is indicated in premenstrual syndromes.

Bromocriptine

We were in part responsible for the vogue and enthusiasm for bromocriptine (Carroll & Steiner, 1978). Some reports on dysphoric women having higher prolactin levels throughout the cycle, as well as a higher premenstrual increase when compared to controls, have contributed to the increased attention devoted to the use of bromocriptine in PMS.

Bromocriptine (2-bromo-alpha-ergocryptine, CB-154, Parlodel) is a specific long-acting dopaminergic agonist which is known to be very effective in suppressing prolactin secretion (Del Pozo, Del Re, Varga, & Friesen, 1972; Fluckiger, 1978). Bromocriptine has been claimed to be of some merit in the treatment of PMS. According to Benedek-Jaszmann and Hearn-Sturtevant (1976), when prolactin secretion was suppressed by bromocriptine, more than 90 percent of their subjects obtained complete relief from premenstrual symptoms for up to 11 months. An extensive single-case study reported by Horrobin et al. (1976) also suggested that bromocriptine is effective against both the physical and behavioral components of PMS. Several additional groups have reported the beneficial effect of bromocriptine in the treatment of severe cyclical mastalgia (pain in the breasts), but without clearly differentiating between this condition and PMS (Blichert-Toft, Andersen, Hendriksen, & Mygind, 1979; Schulz, Del Pozo, Lose, Kunzig, & Geiger, 1975). Controlled studies have demonstrated that mastalgia and possibly peripheral edema are the only symptoms of PMS that would be improved by the use of bromocriptine (Andersch, Hahn, Wendestam, Ohman, & Abrahamsson, 1978; Andersen, Larsen, Steenstrup, Svendstrup, & Nielsen, 1977; Ghose & Coppen, 1977; Graham, Harding, Wise, & Berriman, 1978).

The purpose of our double-blind, parallel group study was to evaluate the safety and efficacy of three strengths of bromocriptine in comparison with placebo in the treatment of severe emotional premenstrual dysphoria. Thirty women suffering from severe premenstrual symptoms were carefully selected for this study (Steiner, Haskett, Osmun, Starkman, Peterson, Metski, & Carroll, 1983). Each of the 30 patients was randomly assigned under double-blind, parallel design conditions to one of four treatment groups. Six patients received placebo treatment. Eight patients in each of the other three groups received bromocriptine 2.5, 5.0, or 7.5 milligrams per day, respectively.

There was no significant difference in premenstrual baseline scores among the different groups. There was also no difference in the degree of severity of physical symptoms (especially breast tenderness) among the various groups. The mean scores for all groups showed an improvement in emotional symptoms with treatment. There was no significant difference between the group given placebo and the groups receiving bromocriptine.

Comparison of score changes in individual rating scales revealed no noticeable difference between the effect of placebo and that of bromocriptine 2.5, 5.0, or 7.5 milligrams per day on any particular item. Score changes failed to show any significant difference between the four treatment groups. Bromocriptine did not appear to be superior to placebo in its capacity to ameliorate severe premenstrual syndrome.

As already stated, a general placebo response seems to be prominent in trials of PMS treatments (see also chapters by Reid and Sampson, this volume). We concluded that in order to establish or refute the efficacy of an allegedly specific treatment such as bromocriptine, a double-blind cross-over, rather than parallel, study design is mandatory.

More recently, Andersch (1983) surveyed 14 placebo-controlled studies regarding the treatment of PMS with bromocriptine. He also concluded that there is no substantial support that bromocriptine is an effective drug in PMS as an entity.

CONCLUSIONS

Despite our persistent ignorance about the pathogenesis of PMS, identification of this disorder has important treatment implications (Haskett & Steiner, 1986). As noted earlier (Haskett & Abplanalp, 1983; Haskett et al., 1980), some women suffer from severe PMS in the absence of any other emotional disorder. Various substances have been enthusiastically recommended for the treatment of this condition (for details, see chapter by Reid, this volume). Unfortunately, we still believe that well controlled studies have been unable to reliably demonstrate the specific efficacy of any intervention (Rubinow & Roy-Byrne, 1984). It has also been noted repeatedly that the disturbance often responded favorably to placebo (Smith et al., 1975).

Women suffering from PMS, either alone or accompanied by situational or interpersonal problems, frequently report improvement, at least in the short term, when provided with non-specific support and an increased understanding of the disturbance. Conversely, PMS may combine with other sources of psychological distress and exacerbate symptoms when both are present. To recommend the use of "medical ovariectomy" (Muse, Cetel, Futterman, & Yen, 1984) for women with PMS seems premature. Our observations suggest that, with the possible exception of "periodic premenstrual psychosis" where complete suppression of ovulation may be useful (Dennerstein, Judd, & Davis, 1983), the decision to treat PMS pharmacologicaly should be greatly influenced by the likelihood of significant side effects.

Finally, there has been some controversy about the psychosocial implications of diagnosing PMS. Several investigators have questioned whether there is sufficient evidence to support the hypothesis that PMS is a discrete diagnostic category (Parlee, 1973; Ruble, 1977). They have suggested that flawed research methods and negative social attitudes towards women and menstruation have been partly responsible for the findings of premenstrual dysfunction in large numbers of women (for further discussion, see chapters by Parlee, and Ruble & Brooks-Gunn, this volume; see also those by Bell and Ericksen, this volume). Many of these methodological criticisms are still valid, although their comments may be more relevant to studies of asymptomatic volunteers. Despite this, a small percentage of adult women continue to seek help for distressing and unwelcome changes that affect them regularly during the premenstruum. Attempts to improve our understanding of this disturbance and to alleviate the associated discomfort in affected women should be clearly differentiated from unwarranted generalizations about the emotional stability of women in general.

Through our endocrine studies and our close contact with a large population of women visiting a special clinic for PMS, we developed diagnostic tools and established research diagnostic criteria for the syndrome (Haskett et al., 1980; Steiner et al., 1980a). We strongly suggest that definite criteria of severity and disability be applied in selecting patients for future research. The presence of PMS should be considered during the clinical assessment of any adult woman with intermittent or fluctuating psychological symptoms (Haskett & Steiner, 1986). Women suffering from severe episodic PMS do differ from other women (Osmun, Steiner, & Haskett, 1983), and this difference probably has a physiological basis yet to be determined. The main difficulty in the evaluation of publicized psychobiologic explanations and therapeutic successes in PMS resides in major methodological problems (Halbreich & Endicott, 1985; see also their chapter in this volume).

The clinician must carefully ascertain the relationship between the clinical features and the menstrual cycle; evaluation must include several phases of the cycle and may need to extend over more than one menstrual cycle. Although severe "pure" PMS is probably biological in origin, the relative contributions of biological and psychosocial influences to psychopathology related to the menstrual cycle are still unclear.

ACKNOWLEDGMENTS

The authors thank Dr. Bernard J. Carroll for his active participation in and support of the studies described in this chapter.

The authors also thank Drs. R.T. Rubin, S.E. Hays, M.N. Starkman, and E. Peterson for their assistance with these studies; J.N. Osmun, J. Ritchie, and R. Metski for their important contributions to the clinical and laboratory aspects; and Barbara Roszel for her excellent assistance in preparing the manuscript.

This work was supported by USPHS Grant MH28294, by the Mental Health Research Institute, the Upjohn Centre for Clinical Pharmacology, University of Michigan, and by Sandoz, Inc.

REFERENCES

Abplanalp, J. M., R. F. Haskett, and R. M. Rose, 1980. The premenstrual syndrome. *Psychiatric Clinics of North America 3:* 327-347.

Aitken, R., 1969. Measurement of feelings using Visual Analogue Scales. *Proceedings of the Royal Society of Medicine 62:* 989-993.

Akiskal, H., A. Djenderedjian, R. Rosenthal, and M. Khani, 1977. Cyclothymic disorder: Validating criteria for inclusion in the bipolar affective group. *American Journal of Psychiatry 134:* 1227-1233.

Andersch, B., 1983. Bromocriptine and premenstrual symptoms: A survey of double blind trials. *Obstetrics and Gynecology Survey 38:* 643-646.

Andersch, B., L. Hahn, C. Wendestam, R. Ohman, and L. Abrahamsson, 1978. Treatment of premenstrual tension syndrome with bromocriptine. *Acta Endocrinologica Supplement 216:* 165-174.

Andersen, A. N., J. F. Larsen, O. R. Steenstrup, B. Svendstrup, and J. Nielsen, 1977. Effect of bromocriptine on the premenstrual syndrome: A double blind clinical trial. *British Journal of Obstetrics and Gynaecology 84:* 370-374.

Aubert, M. L., T. Lemarchand-Beraud, R. Deguillaume, and P. Desaulles, 1971. Cortisol secretion during the normal menstrual cycle. *Acta Endocrinologica Supplement 155:* 78.

Backstrom, T. and A. Aakvaag, 1981. Plasma prolactin and testosterone during the luteal phase in women with premenstrual tension syndrome. *Psychoneuroendocrinology 6:* 245-251.

Backstrom, T. and B. Mattsson, 1975. Correlation of symptoms in premenstrual tension to estrogen and progesterone concentrations in blood plasma: A preliminary study. *Neuropsychobiology 1:* 80-86.

Beisel, W., J. Cos, R. Horton, P. Chao, and P. Forsham, 1964. Physiology of urinary cortisol excretion. *Journal of Clinical Endocrinology 24:* 887-893.

Benedek-Jaszmann, L. J. and M. D. Hearn-Sturtevant, 1976. Premenstrual tension and functional infertility. *The Lancet 1:* 1095-1098.

Blichert-Toft, M., A. Andersen, O. Hendriksen, and T. Mygind, 1979. Treatment of mastalgia with bromocriptine: A double blind cross-over study. *British Medical Journal 1:* 237.

Bulbrook, R., J. Herian, D. Tong, J. Hayward, M. Swain, and D. Wang, 1973. Effect of steroidal contraceptives on levels of plasma androgen sulphates and cortisol. *The Lancet 1:* 628-631.

Burke, C. and C. Beardwell, 1973. Cushing's syndrome — An evaluation of the clinical usefulness of urinary free cortisol and other urinary steroid measures in diagnosis. *Quarterly Journal of Medicine 42:* 175-204.

Carr, B. R., C. R. Parker, Jr., J. D. Madden, P. C. MacDonald, and J. C. Porter, 1979. Plasma levels of adrenocrticotropin and cortisol in women receiving oral contraceptive steroid treatment. *Journal of Clinical Endocrinology and Metabolism 49:* 346-349.

Carroll, B. J., 1972. The hypothalamic-pituitary-adrenal axis in depression. In: B. Davies, B. J. Carroll, and R. M. Mowbray (Eds.), *Depressive Illness: Some Research Studies.* Charles C. Thomas, Springfield, IL, pp. 23-68.

Carroll, B. J., G. C. Curtis, B. M. Davies, J. Mendels, and A. Sugerman, 1976a. Urinary free cortisol excretion in depression. *Psychological Medicine 6:* 43-50.

Carroll, B. J., G. C. Curtis, and J. Mendels, 1976b. Neuroendocrine regulation in depression: 1. Limbic system-adrenocortical dysfunction. *Archives of General Psychiatry 33:* 1039-1044.

Carroll, B. J., M. Feinberg, P. E. Smouse, S. G. Rawson, and J. F. Greden, 1981a. The Carroll Rating Scale for Depression: 1. Development, reliability and validation. *British Journal of Psychiatry 138:* 194-200.

Carroll, B. J., M. Feinberg, J. F. Greden, J. Tarika, A. A. Albala, R. F. Haskett, N. M. James, Z. Kronfol, N. Lohr, M. Steiner, J. P. de Vigne, and E. Young, 1981b. A specific laboratory test for the diagnosis of melancholia: Standardization, validation, and clinical utility. *Archives of General Psychiatry 38:* 15-22.

Carroll, B. J. and M. Steiner, 1978. The psychobiology of premenstrual dysphoria: The role of prolactin. *Psychoneuroendocrinology 3:* 171-180.

Clayton, P. J., 1983. Gender and depression. In: J. Angst (Ed.), *The Origins of Depression: Current Concepts and Approaches.* Springer-Verlag, Berlin, pp. 77-89.

Del Pozo, E., R. B. Del Re, L. Varga, and H. Friesen, 1972. The inhibition of prolactin secretion in man by CB 154 (2-Br.-alpha-ergocryptine). *Journal of Clinical Endocrinology and Metabolism 35:* 768-771.

Dennerstein, L., F. Judd, and B. Davies, 1983. Psychosis and the menstrual cycle. *Medical Journal of Australia 28:* 524-526.

Ehara, Y., T. Siler, G. Vandenberg, Y. N. Sinha, and S.S.C. Yen, 1973. Circulating prolactin levels during the menstrual cycle: Episodic release and diurnal variations. *American Journal of Obstetrics and Gynecology 117:* 962-970.

Fluckiger, E., 1978. Effects of bromocriptine on the hypothalamo-pituitary axis. *Acta Endocrinologica Supplement 216:* 111-117.

Fritz, M. A. and L. Speroff, 1982. The endocrinology of the menstrual cycle: the interaction of folliculogenesis and neuroendocrine mechanisms. *Fertility and Sterility 38:* 509-529.

Ghose, K. and A. Coppen, 1977. Bromocriptine and premenstrual syndrome: Controlled study. *British Medical Journal 1:* 147-148.

Graham, J. J., P. E. Harding, P. H. Wise, and H. Berriman, 1978. Prolactin suppression in the treatment of premenstrual syndrome. *Medical Journal of Australia Supplement 3:* 18-20.

Greaves, A. R. and H. F. West, 1960. Relation of free corticosteroids in urine to steroid dosage. *The Lancet 1:* 368.

Halbreich, U., M. Assael, M. Ben-David, and R. Bornstein, 1976. Serum prolactin in women with premenstrual syndrome. *The Lancet 2:* 654-656.

Halbreich, U. and J. Endicott, 1985. Methodological issues in studies of premenstrual changes. *Psychoneuroendocrinology 10:* 15-32.

Hamilton, M., 1960. A rating scale for depression. *Journal of Neurology, Neurosurgery, and Psychiatry 23:* 56-62.

Haskett, R. F. and J. M. Abplanalp, 1983. Premenstrual tension syndrome: Diagnostic criteria and selection of research subjects. *Psychiatry Research 9:* 125-138.

Haskett, R. F. and M. Steiner, 1986. The diagnosis of premenstrual tension syndrome in psychiatric practice. *Hospital and Community Psychiatry 37:* 33-36.

Haskett, R. F., M. Steiner, and B. Carroll, 1984. A psychoendocrine study of premenstrual tension syndrome: A model for endogenous depression? *Journal of Affective Disorders 6:* 191-199.

Haskett, R. F., M. Steiner, J. N. Osmun, and B. J. Carroll, 1980. Severe premenstrual tension: Delineation of the syndrome. *Biological Psychiatry 15:* 121-139.

Hellman, L., K. Yoshida, B. Zumoff, J. Levin, J. Kream, and D. Fukushima, 1976. The effect of medroxyprogesterone acetate on the pituitary-adrenal axis. *Journal of Clinical Endocrinology and Metabolism 42:* 912-917.

Horrobin, D. F., R. A. Karmali, J. P. Mtabaji, M. S. Manku, and B. A. Nassar, 1976. Prolactin and mental illness. *Postgraduate Medical Journal Supplement 3:* 79-85.

Janowsky, D. S., S. C. Berens, and J. M. Davis, 1973. Correlations between mood, weight, and electrolytes during the menstrual cycle: A renin-angiotensin-aldosterone hypothesis of premenstrual tension. *Psychosomatic Medicine 35:* 143-154.

Judd, L., B. Hubbard, D. Janowsky, L. Huey, and P. Attewell, 1977. The effect of lithium carbonate on affect, mood, and personality of normal subjects. *Archives of General Psychiatry 34:* 346-351.

Kaulhausen, J., G. Leyendecker, G. Benker, and H. Breuer, 1978. The relationship of the renin-angiotensin-aldosterone system to plasma gonadotropin, prolactin and ovarian steroid patterns during the menstrual cycle. *Archives of Gynaekologie 225:* 179-200.

Lindholm, J. and N. Schultz-Moller, 1973. Plasma and urinary cortisol in pregnancy and during estrogen gestagen treatment. *Scandinavian Journal of Clinical Laboratory Investigations 31:* 119-122.

Maxwell, C., 1978. Sensitivity and accuracy of the visual analogue scale: A psychophysical classroom experiment. *British Journal of Clinical Pharmacology 6:* 15-24.

Mills, D. E. and D. Robershaw, 1981. Response of plasma prolactin to changes in ambient temperature and humidity in man. *Journal of Clinical Endocrinology and Metabolism 52:* 279-283.

Moos, R. H., 1969. *Menstrual Distress Questionnaire. Preliminary Manual.* Social Ecology Laboratory, Stanford, CA.

Murphy, B., 1967. Some studies of the protein-binding of steroids and their application to the routine micro and ultramicro measurement of various steroids in body fluids by competitive protein-binding radioassay. *Journal of Clinical Endocrinology and Metabolism 27:* 973-990.

Murphy, B., 1968. Clinical evaluation of urinary cortisol determinations by competitive protein-binding radioassay. *Journal of Clinical Endocrinology and Metabolism 28:* 343-348.

Muse, K. N., N. S. Cetel, L. A. Futterman, and S.S.C. Yen, 1984. The premenstrual syndrome. *New England Journal of Medicine 311:* 1345-1349.

Norman, W. H., B. A. Johnson, and I. W. Miller III, 1984. Depression: A behavioral-cognitive approach. In: E. A. Blechman (Ed.), *Behavior Modification with Women.* Guilford Press, New York, NY, pp. 275-307.

Nurnberger, F. I. and E. S. Gershon, 1982. Genetics. In: E. S. Paykel (Ed.), *Handbook of Affective Disorders.* Guilford Press, New York, NY, pp. 126-145.

O'Brien, P.M.S. and E. M. Symonds, 1982. Prolactin levels in the premenstrual syndrome. *British Journal of Obstetrics and Gynaecology 89:* 306-308.

Osmun, J. N., M. Steiner, and R. F. Haskett, 1983. Psychosocial aspects of severe premenstrual tension. *International Journal of Women's Studies 6:* 65-70.

Parlee, M. B., 1973. The premenstrual syndrome. *Psychopharmacological Bulletin 80:* 454-465.

Punnonen, R., S. Nummi, O. Ylikorkala, U. Alapiessa, P. Karvonen, and L. Viinikka, 1976. A composite picture of the normal menstrual cycle. *Acta Obstetrica and Gynecologica Scandinavica Supplement 51:* 63-70.

Quigley, M. E., J. F. Ropert, and S.S.C. Yen, 1981. Acute prolactin release triggered by feeding. *Journal of Clinical Endocrinology and Metabolism 52:* 1043-1045.

Robins, L. N., J. E. Helzer, M. M. Weissman, H. Orvaschel, E. Gruenberg, J. D. Burke, Jr., and D. A. Regier, 1984. Lifetime prevalence of specific psychiatric disorders in three sites. *Archives of General Psychiatry 41:* 949-958.

Rosner, J., J. Cos, E. Biglieri, S. Hane, and P. Forsham, 1963. Determination of urinary unconjugated cortisol by glass fiber chromatography in the diagnosis of Cushing's Syndrome. *Journal of Clinical Endocrinology and Metabolism 23:* 820-827.

Rubin, R. T., J. M. Reinisch, and R. F. Haskett, 1981. Postnatal gonadal steroid effects on human behavior. *Science 211:* 1318-1324.

Rubinow, D. R. and P. Roy-Byrne, 1984. Premenstrual syndromes: Overview from a methodologic perspective. *American Journal of Psychiatry 141:* 163-172.

Ruble, D. N., 1977. Premenstrual symptoms: A reinterpretation. *Science 197:* 291-292.

Saxena, B. N., J. Dusitsin, and L. Lazarus, 1974. Human growth hormone (HGH), thyroid stimulating hormone (TSH) and cortisol levels in the serum of menstruating Thai women. *Journal of Obstetrics and Gynaecology of the British Commonwealth 81:* 563-567.

Schulz, K., E. Del Pozo, K. Lose, H. Kunzig, and W. Geiger, 1975. Successful treatment of mastodynia with the prolactin inhibitor bromocriptine (CB-154). *Archives Gynaekologie 220:* 83-87.

Smith, S. L., 1975. Mood and the menstrual cycle. In: E. J. Sachar (Ed.), *Topics in Psychoendocrinology.* Grune and Stratton, New York, NY, pp. 19-58.

Smith, S. L., J. M. Cleghorn, D. L. Streiner, and E. V. Younglai, 1975. A study of estrogens and progesterone in premenstrual depression. In: H. Hirsch (Ed.), *The Family.* Karger, Basel, pp. 538-542.

Spielberger, C. D., R. L. Gorsuch, and R. E. Lushene, 1970. *STAI Manual.* Consulting Psychologist Press, Palo Alto, CA.

Spitzer, R. L., J. Endicott, and E. Robins, 1978. Research diagnostic criteria: rationale and reliability. *Archives of General Psychiatry 35:* 773-782.

Steiner, M., 1979. Psychobiology of mental disorders associated with childbearing: An overview. *Acta Psychiatrica Scandinavica 60:* 449-464.

Steiner, M., 1983. Psychobiologic aspects of the Menopausal Syndrome. In: H. J. Buchsbaum (Ed.), *The Menopause.* Springer-Verlag, New York, NY, pp. 151-160.

Steiner, M. and B. J. Carroll, 1977. The psychobiology of premenstrual dysphoria: Review of theories and treatments. *Psychoneuroendocrinology 2:* 321-335.

Steiner, M., R. F. Haskett, and B. J. Carroll, 1980a. Premenstrual tension syndrome: The development of research diagnostic criteria and new rating scales. *Acta Psychiatrica Scandinavica 62:* 177-190.

Steiner, M., R. F. Haskett, J. N. Osmun, and B. J. Carroll, 1980b. Treatment of premenstrual tension with lithium carbonate: A pilot study. *Acta Psychiatrica Scandinavica 61:* 96-102.

Steiner, M., R. F. Haskett, J. N. Osmun, M. N. Starkman, E. Peterson, R. Metski, and B. J. Carroll, 1983. The treatment of severe premenstrual dysphoria with bromocriptine. *Journal of Psychosomatic Obstetrics and Gynecology 2:* 223-227.

Steiner, M., R. F. Haskett, B. J. Carroll, S. E. Hays, and R. T. Rubin, 1984a. Plasma prolactin and severe premenstrual tension. *Psychoneuroendocrinology 9:* 29-35.

Steiner, M., R. F. Haskett, B. J. Carroll, S. E. Hays, and R. T. Rubin, 1984b. Circadian hormone secretory profiles in women with severe premenstrual tension syndrome. *British Journal of Obstetrics and Gynaecology 91:* 466-471.

Sutherland, H. and L. Stewart, 1965. A critical analysis of the premenstrual syndrome. *The Lancet 1:* 1180.

Vaitukaitis, J. L., 1984. Premenstrual syndrome. *The New England Journal of Medicine 311:* 1371-1373.

Weissman, M. M. and G. L. Klerman, 1977. Sex differences and the epidemiology of depression. *Archives of General Psychiatry 34:* 98-111.

Zuckerman, M. and B. Lubin, 1965. *Manual for Multiple Affect Adjective Check List*. Educational and Industrial Testing Service, San Diego, CA.

APPENDIX

SELF-RATING SCALE FOR PREMENSTRUAL TENSION SYNDROME

Name: Date:
Identification No.:

Instructions: The following questions are concerned with the way you feel or act today (or the way you felt or acted during the week).

Please answer all questions by circling YES or NO as indicated.

1.	Do you find your self avoiding some of your social commitments?	YES NO
2.	Have you gained 5 or more pounds during the past week?	YES NO
3.	Is your coordination so poor that you are unable to use kitchen utensils, garden tools, or unable to drive?	YES NO
4.	Do you feel more angry than usual?	YES NO
5.	Do you avoid family activities and prefer to be left alone?	YES NO
6.	Do you doubt your judgment or feel that you are prone to hasty decisions?	YES NO
7.	Do you feel more irritable than usual?	YES NO
8.	Is your efficiency diminished?	YES NO
9.	Do you feel tense and restless?	YES NO
10.	Do you feel a marked change in your sexual drive or desire during the last week?	YES NO
	If YES, is it increased or decreased?	
11.	Are your present physical symptoms causing so much pain and discomfort that you are unable to function?	YES NO
12.	Have you recently cancelled previously scheduled social activities?	YES NO
13.	Do you feel as if you were unable to relax at all?	YES NO
14.	Do you feel confused?	YES NO
15.	Do you suffer from painful or tender breasts?	YES NO
16.	Do you have an increased desire for specific kinds of food (e.g., cravings for candy, chocolate, etc.)?	YES NO
17.	Do you scream/yell at family members (friends, colleagues) more than usual? Are you "short-fused"?	YES NO
18.	Do you feel sad, gloomy, and hopeless most of the time?	YES NO
19.	Do you feel like crying?	YES NO
20.	Do you have difficulty completing your daily household/job routine?	YES NO
21.	Was there a marked change in your sexual drive with definite change in your sexual behavior during the last week?	YES NO
22.	Do you find yourself being more forgetful than usual or unable to concentrate?	YES NO
23.	Do you happen to have more "accidents" with your daily housework/job (cut fingers, break dishes, etc.)?	YES NO
24.	Have you noticed significant swelling of your breasts and/or ankles and/or bloating of your abdomen?	YES NO
25.	Does your mood change suddenly without obvious reason?	YES NO
26.	Are you easily distracted?	YES NO
27.	Do you think that your restless behavior is noticeable by others?	YES NO
28.	Are you clumsier than usual?	YES NO
29.	Are you obviously negative and hostile towards other people?	YES NO
30.	Are you so fatigued that it interferes with your usual level of functioning?	YES NO
31.	Do you tend to eat more than usual or at odd irregular hours (sweets, snacks, etc.)?	YES NO
32.	Do you become more easily fatigued than usual?	YES NO
33.	Is your handwriting different (less neat than usual)?	YES NO
34.	Do you feel jittery or upset?	YES NO
35.	Do you feel sad or blue?	YES NO
36.	Have you stopped calling or visiting some of your best friends?	YES NO

RATING SCALE FOR PREMENSTRUAL TENSION SYNDROME

Name: Rater:
Identification No.: Date:

Circle the most appropriate score for each item:

1. *Irritability -- Hostility (0-4)*
   (Irritable, hostile, negative attitude, angry, short-fused, yelling and screaming at others)
   0. Not irritable.
   1. Doubtful, trivial. Not reported without direct questioning.
   2. Mild. Occasional outbursts of anger and hostile behavior. Spontaneously reported.
   3. Moderate. Irritable behavior evident. Frequent outbursts.
   4. Severe. Affects most interactions between patient and significant others.

2. *Tension (0-4)*
   (Tense, restless, jittery, upset, high-strung, unable to relax)
   0. Not tense.
   1. Doubtful, trivial.
   2. Mild. Reports occasional tension.
   3. Moderate. Tense, jittery, unable to relax. Restless behavior evident.
   4. Severe. Constantly tense and upset.

3. *Efficiency (0-4)*
   (Decreased efficiency, easily fatigued)
   0. No disturbance.
   1. Doubtful, trivial.
   2. Mild. Somewhat reduced efficiency.
   3. Moderate. Easily fatigued, gets much less done than usual.
   4. Severe. Fatigue causes serious interference with functioning.

4. *Dysphoria (0-4)*
   (Dysphoric mood, distinguish from depression)
   0. Not dysphoric.
   1. Somewhat blue, sad. Elicited only on direct questioning.
   2. Mild dysphoric and labile mood,, spontaneously reported.
   3. Marked spontaneous emotional lability; occasional crying; feelings of loneliness.
   4. Severe, obvious and persistent.

5. *Motor coordination (0-4)*
   (Clumsy, prone to accidents, lowered motor coordination)
   0. No disturbance.
   1. Doubtful, trivial.
   2. Mild clumsiness, feels awkward.
   3. Moderate. Frequent "accidents" while doing simple housework or on the job.
   4. Severe impairment in motor co-ordination, e.g. unable to write properly, sew, or unable to drive.

6. *Mental -- cognitive functioning (0-4)*
   (Forgetful, poor concentration, distractable, confused, lowered judgement)
   0. No disturbance.
   1. Doubtful, trivial.
   2. Mild. Slight forgetfulness and distractability.
   3. Moderate. Performance impaired by poor concentration, cognitive disorganization, forgetfullness, etc.
   4. Severe. Marked deterioration in cognitive capacity, poor judgement, leading to regrettable decisions.

7. *Eating habits (0-2)*
   0. No change.
   1. Mild increase in food intake, eating at odd, irregular hours, mostly snacks and sweets.
   2. Obvious, marked increase. Uncontrollable cravings for sweets, chocolate, etc.

8. *Sexual drive and activity (0-2)*
   0. No change.
   1. Mild but consistent increase or decrease in sexual drive, desire, libido.
   2. Marked change in sexual drive with definite change in sexual behavior.

9. *Physical symptoms (0-4)*
   (Painful or tender breasts; swelling of abdomen, breasts, ankles, or fingers; water retention; weight gain; headaches; low-back pain, etc.)
   0. No physical symptoms.
   1. Doubtful or trivial.
   2. Mild. Some symptoms, increased awareness of bodily changes.
   3. Moderate. Obvious changes and complaints.
   4. Severe. Physical symptoms are incapacitating. Pain and discomfort. Marked water retention and edema. Weight gain more than 5 lbs.

10. *Social impairment (0-4)*
    (Avoidance of social activities and interactions with family, at home, at work, at school, etc.)
    0. No social impairment.
    1. Doubtful, trivial.
    2. Mild avoidance of social activity.
    3. Moderate but obvious impairment of social activity, mainly noticeable at home and with family.
    4. Severe. Marked impairment of most social interactions including at work or school. Withdrawal, isolation.

Total score: ....

CONCLUSIONS

THE MULTIPLE FACETS OF EVE: THE PLACE OF PREMENSTRUAL SYNDROME IN THE TAXONOMY OF AFFECTIVE BEHAVIOR

Benson E. Ginsburg, Ph.D.

Biobehavioral Sciences Graduate Degree Program
Department of Psychology
The University of Connecticut
Storrs, Connecticut; and
Department of Psychiatry
The University of Connecticut Health Center
Farmington, Connecticut

INTRODUCTION

What is Premenstrual Syndrome?

My interest in premenstrual syndrome (PMS) was, like Virginia Cassara's (see her chapter, this volume), personally motivated. Where hers was a response to subjectively felt distress associated with the premenstrual phase of her cycle, mine, while also a reaction to such experiences, was necessarily observational. I have known a young woman undergoing troublesome periodic changes of mood who, once she had related these to her menstrual cycle, sought medical help and information with only limited success. One has only to see and know such a person, let alone to be one, in order to be convinced that the phenomenon we are here calling PMS is real, and that whatever psychological manifestations are involved, that it is also biologically based by virtue of its tight correlation with the hormonal events associated with the menstrual cycle. It would seem, therefore, a reasonable expectation to find clinical studies in which hormonal differences between women experiencing premenstrual psychological stress and women not seriously affected in this way would have been described, and, further, to find clinical practice taking advantage of these findings and providing diagnostic tests to identify the particular imbalance involved in each case, as well as the means to achieve a normal equilibrium with the expected amelioration of symptoms. Given the complexity of the hormonal systems involved in the menstrual cycle, it was also my expectation that there would be multiple etiologies, and that these would not necessarily be confined to the hormonal changes associated with the cycle, but would include neural and psychological events as well. It was my further expectation that the neural and psychological events could be controlling the moods and acts which characterize PMS, since these moods and acts can also be found in depressions and other conditions not associated with the menstrual cycle and can be experienced by men as well as by women. Moreover, many normally menstruating women do not experience cyclically disruptive psychological episodes. Together with some others whose works are represented in this volume (e.g., chapter by Halbreich & Endicott), I entertained the hypothesis that where the psychological manifestations were severe, they might represent an underlying vulnerability that crossed a threshold from latent to manifest under a particular set of hormonal conditions arising during the premenstruum. As a geneticist, I further entertained the idea that the underlying psychological vulnerability and/or any physiological disharmonies could have a genetic basis.

Our Attempt to Clarify the Status of Premenstrual Syndrome

At this point, the search for a treatment to help a particular person identified not only a widening complexity of issues, but disparities in the conclusions of various experts, such that an exchange of evidence and opinions in a "think-tank" environment leading to a possible re-evaluation of the field in its various ramifications seemed the only way to identify where there was scientific knowledge, where there was disagreement, and how the now widening problems could be addressed. It is hoped that this volume, resulting from such a series of scholarly exchanges, will provide a comprehensive picture of the state of our knowledge concerning PMS — and may help those who suffer from its symptoms and the professionals to whom they come for help to more realistically evaluate their options.

CAN ADAM UNDERSTAND EVE? — SUBJECTIVE ASPECTS OF PREMENSTRUAL SYNDROME

There is an internal as well as an external aspect to every behavioral event. As seen from the outside, it consists of an act or a verbalization that can be described or elicited in its own terms as well as in its social or interactive context. As experienced subjectively, the act may or may not directly reflect the affect. I have never been Eve, but like every Adam, I have seen and known many variations of her, just as I have seen and known aspects of myself in others. Thinking first introspectively, I can best relate to observed, measured, reported, or shared behaviors in terms of projecting my own affect and cognition on them and, where these limits are too circumscribed, extending the range of my personal capacities by extrapolating from them — but I am still bound by them. My bonds are the range of my own experience, the social and genetic factors that have made me what I am, and the scientific traditions that direct and limit my hypotheses. At the same time, I am at least a partial resonator to any behaviors and emotions exhibited by others, since I, too, am capable of feeling what they feel, and potentially of acting out, at least in my mind, whatever it is that they do. I therefore have four complementary approaches to the understanding and evaluation of theories regarding behaviors that I have not and cannot directly experience:

(1) *Subjective Resonance:* I am essentially capable of feeling whatever emotions are involved in PMS or any other presumably biologically-based behavior, even though I have not experienced these emotions in the same context or from the same causes. Although PMS, by definition, can affect only females, I would maintain that the affective experiences involved, whatever their range, are not the exclusive property of one sex. Besides, where would we draw the line? Must a psychiatrist have experienced a psychotic break in order to understand and treat a patient who has had one, let alone to infer from his or her personal experience what the patient must be feeling?

(2) *Descriptive Analysis:* I have available to me a variety of "objective" studies, some based on rating scales such as those reported in this volume (see chapters by Halbreich & Endicott; Ruble & Brooks-Gunn; and Steiner & Haskett) that characterize the behavioral stigmata attributed to PMS and that present reasoned arguments drawing on psychological, anthropological, sociological, and biomedical research. There are also self reports and psychiatric interviews that overlap and supplement the questionnaires, as well as reports and observations of behaviors that are taken as signs of depression: irritability, impaired judgment, hostility, memory lapses, and automatism. Because these can arise in contexts other than PMS and are exaggerated during the premenstruum in some instances, a distinction has to be made between PMS-exacerbated symptomatology and PMS-initiated changes in affect and behavior (see Foreword by P. J. Fink, this volume). Some investigators regard only the changes that occur on a normal baseline as PMS related, while others consider that even these constitute instances of latent psychopathy that become manifest only during the premenstruum. While these two views have different implications with respect to etiology and treatment, the subjective, affective components could be the same. Again, the inner feelings associated with PMS would be much more broadly shared if they were qualitatively different for PMS than when experienced in other contexts.

(3) *Clinical Intervention:* Therapy (including behavior modification, the use of hormones, diet, placebos, and neuroleptic drugs) has been tried with varying degrees of success. In some instances, the success depends on the particular therapy matching the particular etiology. In others, it involves matching the treatment to symptoms, as in the use of neuroleptic drugs or in the use of behavior modification. There is also the problem of evaluating therapy on a statistical basis, since what may work in the main for one sample (assuming multiple etiologies converging on a syndrome) may not for another. This is because the etiological spectrum can be different across individuals. Hypotheses regarding appropriate therapies range from those that treat the symptoms (for example, antidepressants for depression) to those that treat the condition (for example, progesterone for PMS, whatever the acts or the affect). Comparing these approaches, both leave open the possibility that a given affective attribute is much the same whatever its basis, but one approach holds that treatment must be matched to etiology, while the other emphasizes convergent symptoms as amenable to similar treatment and, therefore, very likely based on similarities in essential links in chains of mechanisms, although other links may differ.

(4) *Studies of Underlying Mechanisms:* These range from social and psychological conditioning to neuroendocrine factors and include interactions among these variables. Here, the search for identifiable mechanisms carries with it the implied promise of preventive intervention appropriate to each case. Both the literature and clinical evidence indicate that a single variable approach is too simplistic, and that so far no one has hit upon a final common path or trajectory that might be intercepted by a magic missile. Still, attempts continue to find a universal treatment, or at least one that will work for a particular characterization of PMS, as, for example, in the use of progesterone therapy by Dr. Katharina Dalton for those cases conforming to her criteria.

WHAT IS THE PREMENSTRUAL SYNDROME?

The term "premenstrual sydnrome" has been used, in the broad sense, to include any and all physical, physiological, and behavioral deviations associated with the menstrual cycle. While many of these are entirely benign, our concern is with those that are not. The premenstrual syndrome, as I view it here, is not simply a recurrent transitory condition associated with episodic psychological and physical discomfort in some women, but for many, it is a source of acute anguish that is disruptive of family and other interpersonal relations; and for some, it results in apparently biologically-driven behavior that, in extreme instances, places the person at legal risk. Thus, we have not only those cases reported by some investigators as medically treatable, where aggression against persons or property may be involved, but a spectrum of less troublesome behaviors that nevertheless corrode family ties, including marital relationships, and often result in severe depressions and persistent feelings of inadequacy. The significance of this problem for some women — including their families — and for society at-large is attested to by the formation of self-help networks (see chapter by Cassara, this volume) that attempt to disseminate information and advice to the many women who seek it. Far from being a women's problem, it is a societal problem. To retreat from it because women are the primary actors, although not the only victims, is to discriminate against women on the erroneous premise that letting the problem out of the closet may be prejudicial to them. That this is a problem involving ethics and values within our society cannot be in doubt. The current handbook on *Obstetrics and Gynecology*, edited by Danforth and Scott (1986), lists and describes PMS as a clinical entity and reviews the literature dealing with its causes and treatments (see Goldsmith, 1986, pp. 160-161). Psychiatrists are now confronting the existence of PMS as a diagnostic entity for inclusion in the proposed revision of the *Diagnostic and Statistical Manual of Mental Disorders*, third edition (DSM-III, The American Psychiatric Association, 1980), the ostensibly rare psychiatric condition to be called "Periluteal Phase Dysphoric Disorder."

PREMENSTRUAL SYNDROME: A MULTIDISCIPLINARY ISSUE

The scientific and ethical issues are inexorably intertwined. Without the benefit of the best scientific knowledge in this area and an effort to disseminate it, we can accomplish little of social value. Where is an affected family or individual to turn for help? Most medical practitioners can treat the problem symptomatically at best, if at all. The networks assembling and disseminating information are only as good as their sources, and cannot help diagnose or prescribe for the individual case. Feminist theorists are divided into those who want help for their sex and those who treat the problem pejoratively because they are afraid that addressing it publicly will be prejudicial to women on the job and elsewhere. This is neither an idle fear nor a trivial issue. It does not, however, warrant evading the problem.

Legal scholars, practicing attorneys, bioethicists, and other criminal justice practitioners who must deal with the severe cases have no reliable way of knowing whether effective remediation is available or of evaluating the conflicting claims in this area. Even were those responsible for judicial decisions disposed to prescribe biomedical solutions where these are available, we cannot intelligently discuss ethical, social, or philosophical issues or those of culpability and remediation where the criminal justice system becomes involved without the type of synthesis and evaluation being sought by us collectively in this volume (see especially chapters by Boorse and by Jeffery). Our major scientific and ethical goals converge in the effort to collate and disseminate the best knowledge available to those who should have it, and, at the same time, to examine the underlying issues relating to the pursuit and application of such knowledge. Presently, this requires a tolerance of uncertainty that many find difficult to entertain (see chapter by Carter, this volume). In planning this volume as a multidisciplinary approach to legal and ethical implications of the biobehavioral sciences and focusing on the premenstrual syndrome as a particular example, Dr. Carter and I sought also to emphasize the broader ethical issues involving research on biological factors affecting the capacity for responsible behavior, of which, as mentioned, PMS is one example.

PREMENSTRUAL SYNDROME IN A BIOLOGICAL CONTEXT

As a biologist, and particularly as a geneticist concerned with the biological bases of behavior, I should like to describe and justify my theoretical position before applying it to the evidence on PMS. One important principle that has emerged from our researches (and those of others in behavioral genetics) is that there are multiple biological mechanisms underlying the propensity to any particular type of behavior in virtually any studied population, be it human or animal. For example, Reid (this volume) points out that with respect to PMS, some medications are effective for some cases but not for others. O'Brien (this volume) similarly summarizes the diversities of selectively effective treatments.

In studies of aggressive behavior under well controlled conditions with dogs and mice, precisely the same behavioral manifestations could be obtained on a variety of genetic bases (Fisher, 1955; Ginsburg, 1966). In one genetic condition, increased aggression is associated with a prepubertal surge in testosterone in males. By the time the aggression is displayed in the postpubertal animal, the hormone level is normal. Other genotypes that converge in their behavioral manifestations of aggressive behavior do not show the same hormonal developmental profile and, in one instance at least, the behavior appears to be related to the capacity for normal amounts of steroid hormones to exert disproportionate effects on brain centers associated with these behaviors rather than to variations in hormone levels. There is no behavioral clue that reflects these differences in mechanism. Yet, if one were developing strategies of ameliorative intervention, they would be different in the two cases (Selmanoff & Ginsburg, 1981).

We have published a number of studies using extreme aggressive behavior as an endpoint in which, depending on the particular genetic predisposition, different regimens of early rearing would either exacerbate, attenuate, or have no effect on the later behavior, again depending on the biological substratum (Ginsburg, 1966, 1979, 1981; Ginsburg, Vigue, Larson, & Maxson, 1981; Selmanoff & Ginsburg, 1981). Similar situations have been described for dogs (Fisher, 1955). Clearly, no formula approach for the reduction of aggressive behavior is possible with these species, let alone for our own. What, then, can we say regarding the aggressive behaviors encountered in rare instances of PMS (see chapters by Boorse and by Dalton, this volume)?

In recent studies of familial affective behaviors, particularly those involving bipolar depression, at least two genetic modes of transmission have been reported. In one, the condition is associated with the X-chromosome. In another, there is father-to-son transmission, thus eliminating involvement of the X. On the pharmacological side, an entire science of pharmacogenetics is developing. Since differences in the biological basis of a condition are associated with differences in response to treatments with drugs and bioactive agents, we are currently, with the help of clinical collaborators, developing a genetic taxonomy of a number of these conditions. This taxonomy will not homogenize such biological differences, but, rather, will take account of them in order to study biological variations within a syndrome, each in their own right. Since there will not be an infinite number of these for each condition, we should eventually arrive at appropriate diagnostic criteria for a taxonomy of such syndromes, which would, in turn, aid in unravelling their diverse and possibly related underlying biological mechanisms and in developing appropriate treatments for each substituent biological type.

Two further findings from such researches deserve mention before attempting a further application of these concepts to PMS. One finding is that of the behavioral priming of gene expression. In monozygotic twins vulnerable to the same familially-based psychiatric disorder, there are a number of instances in which, despite similar environments, one twin has expressed the vulnerability and the other has not (Nicol & Gottesman, 1983). Where such studies have been carried forward for several generations, the ability to transmit the condition is not affected by whether or not it has been manifested. The second significant finding derives from animal models. We have been able to demonstrate in a series of collaborative experiments that genetic vulnerability for a behavioral syndrome involving an ability to sustain a learned inhibitory act will not be expressed unless a separation syndrome has previously been induced (Corson, Corson, Becker, Ginsburg, Trattner, Connor, Lucas, Panksepp, & Scott, 1980; Ginsburg, Becker, Trattner, & Bareggi, 1984). In some of these instances, we are accumulating evidence that particular regulatory genes are affected by internal hormonal and other changes induced by environmental events, and that these, in turn, can trigger the expression of encoded genetic systems which otherwise would remain latent. Additionally, studies of extreme temperamental variants, particularly in dogs, support the idea of genetic set-points or equilibrium points, towards which the individual will tend (Mac Donald & Ginsburg, 1981). In order to effect lasting changes, it is necessary to separate and differentiate those factors that will affect variations in behavioral expression around the equilibrium points from those that are involved in the setting of the equilibrium points themselves.

What emerges from these researches is a somewhat different picture of the relationship between biological mechanisms, experiential history, and behavior. Biology must not only be seen as an interactive system embracing external (environmental) and internal events, but also as one that produces diverse interactions converging on common phenotypic expressions (that is, syndromes). When extreme enough to warrant intervention, these syndromes must be diagnosed and treated in the light of this biological variability, which, to be understood, must be differentiated and separately studied. In order to pursue such research endeavors in the case of PMS and to channel the results into clinical practice, it must first be recognized that these variations do occur and must be differentiated. Perhaps such a subtyping of PMS will best be accomplished by pharmacogenetic means. If, then, PMS represents a multiplicity of underlying conditions, these will have to be separately identified and researched in order for the multiple mechanisms to be discovered and appropriate treatments for each to be developed.

LEGAL IMPLICATIONS OF THE BIOLOGICAL MODEL

Turning next to those extreme cases, such as the ones described by Dr. Katharina Dalton and into which the case of Shirley Santos may also fit (see chapters by Dalton and by Boorse, this volume), what are the ethical and legal implications of the application of imperfect and scientifically uncertain knowledge to clinical practice; of the use of such tentative knowledge as a basis for legal defenses; and of the remanding for treatment using a medical model of women with histories of antisocial and violent acts that appear to be associated with their menstrual cycle? On ethical grounds, it would seem that no person should be denied the opportunity to alter their behavior in a socially constructive way and to adjust their lives in ways more satisfying for themselves and more constructive for society (see chapter by Jeffery, this volume). This is an issue that warrants separation from culpability for acts society defines as criminal — yet the separation cannot be complete.

PREMENSTRUAL SYNDROME: ETHICAL CONSIDERATIONS BASED ON OTHER BIOBEHAVIORAL MODELS

Macklin (this volume) has drawn the analogy between the present status of PMS and the XYY controversy. Males with an extra Y-chromosome (the determining chromosome for maleness) were at first thought to be biologically predisposed to violence and to be actually driven beyond voluntary control. Later, they were found to constitute a heterogeneous group for whom the simple presence of the extra Y-chromosome was not an indicator of potential aggressive behavior. We have established in mice that the effect of the Y-chromosome on aggressive behavior depends upon the particular Y-chromosome itself, as well as the autosomal complement with which it is associated (Maxson, Ginsburg, & Trattner, 1979). Even where a predisposing complement exists, the analogy from animal experiments to humans cannot be made directly. With the exception of the higher primates, other mammals do not interpose a cerebral cortical screen between incoming stimuli and hypothalamic structures; and even for the higher primates, the intervening cortical mechanisms have not been conditioned to any moral imperatives.

The question of where the boundary exists between biologically-driven behavior that escapes conscious control and biological predisposing factors that can, nevertheless, be resisted is a difficult one to answer. Given that PMS arises from diverse etiologies — biological and social — there can be no generic answer. Also, given that in many instances the condition responds to treatments by multiple agents, including psychotherapy, and that there are evidently "different strokes for different folks," PMS must be seen as a spectrum disorder that is potentially amenable to amelioration but is not yet sufficiently understood to enable the "expert" to prescribe any universally effective treatment.

Jeffery (this volume) views PMS as an example of a more general problem. He argues that aberrant and criminal behavior must be researched in a biobehavioral perspective. If some forms of unacceptable social behaviors are biologically driven, then research into these conditions becomes socially and economically important by offering hope of rehabilitation through medical intervention. Although we have seen serious abuses of the medical model (e.g., prefrontal lobotomies, sterilization of sex offenders, inappropriate use of electroconvulsive shock, and other simplistic applications of premature and inadequately researched techniques with punitive aspects), Jeffery has argued that the biomedical model is potentially appropriate and applicable to many conditions (including PMS) that can result in legally culpable behavior. He has further argued that research in these areas could be astonishingly effective in reducing crime and changing our philosophic focus from retribution to rehabilitation. In its emphasis on investigating biological mechanisms as a medium for responsible change, this view constitutes the other side of the coin of biological determinism.

MEDICALIZATION OF PREMENSTRUAL SYNDROME

While the criminal cases are dramatic, we should not lose sight of situations that do not involve infractions of the law, but are nonetheless due to serious disruptions of personal and family life. In both sets of circumstances, the same desiderata apply. There is the presumably driven person who has established a history of disruptive acts directed against self, friends, family, and/or society; and there is the possibility of using the medical model to affect changes in her behavior and to affect changes in her milieu, which may also warrant involvement in the therapeutic process. (It would be interesting to find out more about the environmental aspects in the case histories cited by Dalton.) To stay with the more extreme criminal cases a moment longer, there is an interesting difference in the approach exemplified by Dalton (see her chapter, this volume) versus that used in the Santos case (see chapters by Boorse and by Jeffery, this volume). For Dalton, the relationship of PMS to the criminal justice system is on the basis of diminished capacity. For the legal profession in general, it is in the commitment of an unconscious act. This raises an interesting question: To what extent is such behavior (including less extreme versions) biologically driven? Is it a condition over which the person can exercise no conscious control unless the intervening biological mechanism is changed by using progesterone or other biological interventions? Is it a condition that can be made accessible to control by methods involving primarily behavior modification techniques (see chapter by Blechman & Clay, this volume)? Do both situations exist? Is it possible to judge in an individual instance whether the act was performed consciously or unconsciously, as developed in the Santos case?

Various PMS therapies have been claimed and evaluated, but with no clear consensus. Do progesterone therapies, vitamin and other dietary therapies, and placebos differentially succeed depending on the particular underlying biological mechanisms (see chapters by Halbreich & Endicott; O'Brien; Reid; Rubinow; and Steiner & Haskett, this volume)? From my own theoretical perspective, these interventions, wherever effective, appear to simply augment the potential for acceptable behavior, but do not change the genetic set-point; they do not constitute a cure, but instead rely on the continuing correction of a biological deviation that expresses itself in behavioral and affective manifestations. The same is true in those instances where the behavior is treated symptomatically, as if there were an underlying sub-threshold condition of, for example, depression, which breaks through episodically during the menstrual cycle, but which should be treated as an affective disorder like any other.

GENETICS

Given that PMS is difficult to characterize as a syndrome, and that biological, social, and psychological factors are all involved, it is legitimate to ask whether there is a genetic predisposition to this condition in its more extreme forms. It should be noted that evidence suggesting genetic involvement in some cases does not indicate that other instances must also be genetically based, or even that those cases that presumably have a genetic component all share a common genetic mechanism. Norris and Sullivan (1983), in their book, *PMS: Premenstrual Syndrome*, and Dalton (see her chapter, this volume) cite instances of familial occurrence and of concordance in monozygotic twins, both suggestive of a genetic etiology. Others report co-variation across twin pairs for menstrual symptoms, as well as for state anxiety and depression (the latter two being personality variables as well as premenstrual symptoms), and, further, that trait neuroticism was due almost entirely to pleiotropic gene action (Silberg, Martin, & Heath, personal communication, 1986). Twin data have also been reported with respect to psychiatric side effects of oral contraceptives (primarily depression and irritability). Martin, Kendler, Heath, Handelsman, and Eaves (1986) concluded that genetic factors are involved and are separable from those affecting basic levels of psychiatric symptomatology. Such studies are compatible with the findings that emotional distress experienced in PMS is not associated with hormonal differences between affected and unaffected women. These studies do not resolve the issue of whether the affective disturbances in PMS are independent of an underlying vulnerability to these symptoms. While suggesting such independence in some cases, associations found between underlying psychopathologies and premenstrual psychiatric distress (Kinch & Robinson, 1985; MacKenzie, Wilcox, & Baron, 1986) remain unexplained. Where women are clearly evaluated as exhibiting premenstrual distress but not underlying psychopathology, this may be taken as evidence that the two are not necessarily related — at least not in all cases — or it may indicate that an underlying vulnerability to psychosis is essential, but only becomes manifest during the premenstruum.

CONCLUSIONS

We are left with an ethical dilemma that can best be served by continued research and exchange of knowledge since we do not know at present how to diagnose and prescribe for each individual case. This remains true whether intervention involves changing societal attitudes, on the one hand, or pharmacological treatment, on the other. The research strategies, for biology and for environment, appear to be dictated by our present knowledge of how these factors interact within the context I have described in this chapter. As noted in my initial subjective comments, the menstrual cycle is certainly associated with changes in affect (and to a greater or lesser degree in different women), but these same variations in affect are also experienced by men, even if not in the same biological context. To attempt to find the best ameliorative strategies at the individual and societal level need not be taken as pejorative to women. Centering on PMS as one example of the relationship between responsible behavior and biosocial factors represents a segment of a taxonomy that is also needed in the further analysis of other syndromes.

Standard double-blind, crossover studies will not, in my opinion, by themselves provide the ultimate answers. While such studies can distinguish placebo effects from treatment effects, the veracity of the conclusions is dependent either on an assumption of etiologic homogeneity or statistical averaging across a sufficiently large sample. If the study sample is sufficiently heterogeneous with respect to the diversity of underlying mechanism, an effective treatment for one segment of the sample will not necessarily be effective for others. Such distinctions are likely to be submerged in the static of the placebo. If, however, cases were also followed on an individual basis, a crossover design could reveal differential treatment effectiveness. Usually statistically-oriented techniques pool data and homogenize incommensurables, and this creates a loss of significant information. The inclusion of individual case analysis avoids this pitfall and, further, provides a means of identifying true responders versus non-responders to a particular agent. These (non-responding) individuals could then be separately investigated and potentially treated. Either group might well represent a number of etiologies, and each of these could ultimately respond differently from the others. Individual data analysis is crucial if research is to have direct clinical applicability.

As with the six blind men and the elephant, a number of seemingly very different conceptions may all be correct. We need each individual view and the whole integrated reality to fully understand PMS.

REFERENCES

Corson, S. A., E. O'L. Corson, R. E. Becker, B. E. Ginsburg, A. Trattner, R. L. Connor, L. A. Lucas, J. Panksepp, and J. P. Scott, 1980. Interaction of genetics and separation in canine hyperkinesis and in differential responses to amphetamine. *Pavlovian Journal of Biological Sciences 15:* 5-11.

Danforth, D. N. and J. R. Scott (Eds.), 1986. *Obstetrics and Gynecology* (fifth edition). J. B. Lippincott, Philadelphia, PA.

Fisher, A. E., 1955. The effects of differential early treatment on the social and exploratory behavior of puppies. Ph.D. dissertation, Department of Psychology, Pennsylvania State University, University Park, PA.

Ginsburg, B. E., 1966. All mice are not created equal: Recent findings on genes and behavior. *Social Service Review 40:* 121-134.

Ginsburg, B. E., 1979. The violent brain: Is it everyone's brain? In: C. R. Jeffery (Ed.), *Biology and Crime. Sage Research Progress Series in Criminology, Volume 10.* Sage Publications (in cooperation with the American Society of Criminology), Beverly Hills, CA, pp. 47-64.

Ginsburg, B. E., 1983. Genetic factors in aggressive behavior. *Psychoanalytic Inquiry 2:* 49-71.

Ginsburg, B. E., R. E. Becker, A. Trattner, and S. R. Bareggi, 1984. A genetic taxonomy of hyperkinesis in the dog. *International Journal of Developmental Neuroscience 2:* 313-322.

Ginsburg, B. E., L. C. Vigue, W. A. Larson, and S. C. Maxson, 1981. Y-Chromosome length in sublines of two mouse strains. *Behavior Genetics 11:* 359-368.

Goldsmith, L. T., 1986. Puberty, adolescence and the clinical aspects of normal menstruation. In: D. N. Danforth and J. R. Scott (Eds.), *Obstetrics and Gynecology* (fifth edition). J. B. Lippincott, Philadelphia, PA, Chapter 8.

Kinch, R. A. and G. E. Robinson, 1985. Symposium: Premenstrual syndrome — Current knowledge and new directions. *Canadian Journal of Psychiatry 30:* 467-468.

Mac Donald, K. B. and B. E. Ginsburg, 1981. Induction of normal prepubertal behavior in wolves with restricted rearing. *Behavioral and Neural Biology 33:* 133-162.

MacKenzie, T. B., K. Wilcox, and H. Baron, 1986. Lifetime prevalence of psychiatric disorders in women with perimenstrual difficulties. *Journal of Affective Disorders 10:* 15-19.

Martin, N. G., K. S. Kendler, A. C. Heath, D. Handelsman, and L. J. Eaves, 1986. Genetic factors in use and side effects of oral contraceptives. Paper presented at the 16th annual meeting of the Behavior Genetics Association, Honolulu, HI, June.

Maxson, S. C., B. E. Ginsburg, and A. Trattner, 1979. Interaction of Y-chromosomal and autosomal gene(s) in the development of intermale aggression in mice. *Behavior Genetics 9:* 219-226.

Nicol, S. E. and I. I. Gottesman, 1983. Clues to the genetics and neurobiology of schizophrenia. *American Scientist 71:* 398-404.

Norris, R. V. and C. Sullivan, 1983. *PMS: Premenstrual Syndrome.* Rawson Associates, New York, NY.

Selmanoff, M. K. and B. E. Ginsburg, 1981. Genetic variability in aggression and endocrine function in inbred strains of mice. In: P. F. Brain and D. Benton (Eds.), *Multidisciplinary Approaches to Aggression Research.* Elsevier/North-Holland Biomedical Press, Amsterdam, pp. 247-268.

APPENDIX

SUMMATION OF CONFERENCE ON
ETHICAL ISSUES FOR RESEARCH ON BIOLOGICAL FACTORS AFFECTING
THE CAPACITY FOR RESPONSIBLE BEHAVIOR

Albert Greenfield Center at SugarLoaf
Philadelphia, PA
September 17-21, 1984

Conference Organizers and Committee Coordinators:

Bonnie Frank Carter, Ph.D.
Clinical Psychologist/Behavior Geneticist
Department of Psychiatry
Albert Einstein Medical Center
Northern Division
Philadelphia, PA 19141

Benson E. Ginsburg, Ph.D.
Behavior Geneticist
Department of Biobehavioral Sciences
The University of Connecticut
Storrs, CT 06268

This Conference, focusing on premenstrual syndrome (PMS) as an example of issues in biobehavioral sciences, has been jointly organized by Bonnie Frank Carter, of the Department of Psychiatry at Albert Einstein Medical Center, Northern Division in Philadelphia, PA, and by Benson E. Ginsburg, of the Department of Biobehavioral Sciences at The University of Connecticut, Storrs, CT.

Human behavior is complex. While it is better understood now than it has been in the past, there remain enormous areas of uncertainty. Such is the nature of the complexity of the behaviors we seek to understand and the questions we seek to answer. The express purpose of the present Conference was to consider ways of utilizing and applying as yet uncertain data arising from the diverse behavioral sciences. This is not unique to premenstrual syndrome, but includes many areas of medicine and behavior, where we do the best we can with what we have. Toward the end of being able to understand how to proceed most effectively with uncertain information, we functioned this week as a think-tank.

The 22 participants met as a group for a very full week, and we worked toward educating one another. This multidisciplinary interaction covered our various professional efforts, as we perceived these to have

---

This Conference was supported by grant RII-840935 from the Ethics and Values in Science and Technology (EVIST) section of the National Science Foundation, and by a grant from the Humanities, Science and Technology (HST) program of the National Endowment for the Humanities.

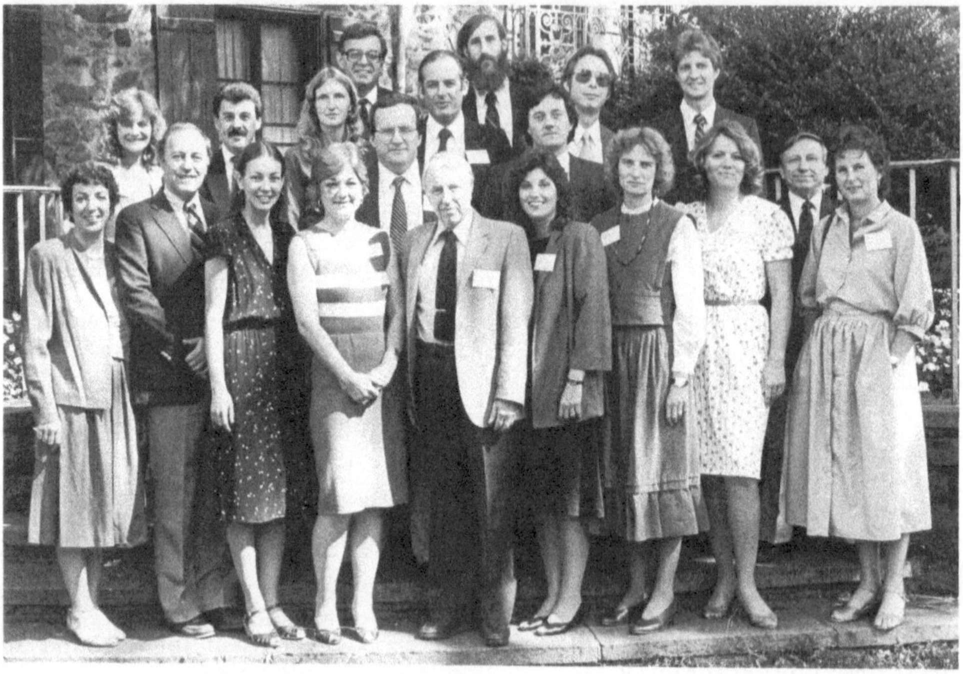

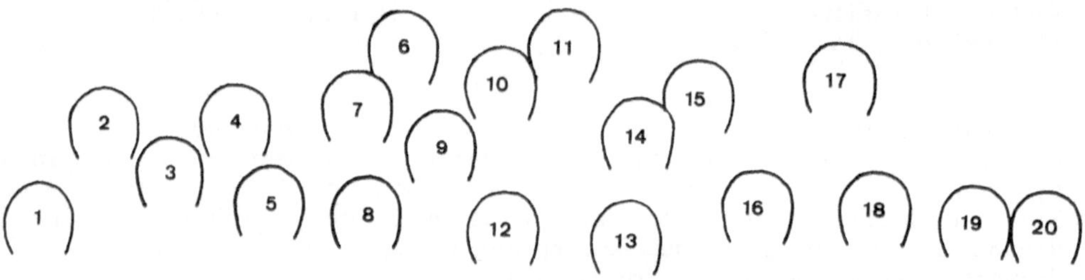

Conference Participants

1. Virginia Cassara
2. Jeanne Brooks-Gunn
3. Michael J. Vergare
4. Meir Steiner
5. Stephanie L. Benson
6. Robert L. Sadoff
7. S. Louise Carter
8. Karen Paige Ericksen
9. Ronald V. Norris
10. Uriel Halbreich
11. David R. Rubinow
12. Benson E. Ginsburg
13. Bonnie Frank Carter
14. P.M.S. O'Brien
15. Christopher Boorse
16. Susan E. Bell
17. Robert L. Reid
18. Stephanie J. Bird
19. C.R. Jeffery
20. Gwyneth A. Sampson

Absent for photograph: Katharina Dalton, Laurence D. Houlgate, Ruth Macklin, and Diane N. Ruble relevance to premenstrual syndrome and the scientific, legal, and ethical issues raised by the attention being given to the syndrome. Even more importantly, we struggled with the difficult task of educating one another about our diverse professional viewpoints; viewpoints that sometimes come into direct conflict, but all of which are valid. As clinicians, physicians, philosophers, lawyers, ethicists, and researchers, we utilize a variety of methods and priorities to accomplish different, but equally important tasks. The compilation of our pre-Conference manuscripts constituted a workbook for the week.

Our final sessions were devoted to synthesizing our week-long efforts. This task was addressed by dividing into three sub-groups: Social Science Research and Public Policy; Biomedical Issues; and Legal Ethics. The summary statements of these three sub-groups follow. These summary statements represent an enormous amount of effort and a significant accomplishment in terms of synthesizing diverse bodies of information.

PARTICIPANTS

The participants, occupational fields, institutional affiliations, and titles of the papers presented at this Conference were:

Susan E. Bell, Ph.D., Sociologist; Bowdoin College, Brunswick, ME; "Premenstrual Syndrome and the Medicalization of Menopause: Sociological Perspectives."

Stephanie L. Benson, J.D.; Attorney; New York City, NY; "Utilization of Premenstrual Stress Syndrome as a Criminal Defense."

Stephanie J. Bird, Ph.D.; Physiologist/Pharmacologist; Massachusetts Institute of Technology, Cambridge, MA; "Neuroscience Research and PMS: Scientific and Ethical Concerns."

Christopher Boorse, Ph.D.; Philosopher; University of Delaware, Newark, DE; "The Relevance of PMS to Criminal Responsibility."

Bonnie Frank Carter, Ph.D.; Clinical Psychologist/Behavior Geneticist; Albert Einstein Medical Center, Northern Division, Philadelphia, PA; "Interdisciplinary Problem Solving: The Premenstrual Syndrome."

S. Louise Carter, Ph.D.; Psychologist and Science Writer; Seattle, WA.

Virginia Cassara, M.A., M.S.S.W.; Social Worker/Educator; PMS Action, Irvine, CA; "Premenstrual Syndrome (PMS): View From the Top of a Consumer Organization."

Katharina Dalton, F.R.C.G.P.; Physician; University College Hospital, London (paper read in Dr. Dalton's absence); "Should Premenstrual Syndrome Be a Legal Defense?"

Karen Paige Ericksen, Ph.D.; Psychologist; University of California at Davis, CA; "Menstrual Symptoms and Menstrual Beliefs: National and Cross-National Patterns."

Benson E. Ginsburg, Ph.D.; Behavior Geneticist; The University of Connecticut, Storrs, CT; "The Multiple Facets of Eve."

Uriel Halbreich, M.D.; Psychiatrist; Albert Einstein College of Medicine, Bronx, NY; "Dysphoric Premenstrual Changes: Are They Related to Affective Disorders?"

Laurence D. Houlgate, Ph.D.; Philosopher; California Polytechnic State University, San Luis Obispo, CA; "Mental Abnormality and Responsibility."

C.R. Jeffery, Ph.D.; Criminologist; Florida State University, Tallahassee, FL; "Criminal Law and Biological Psychiatry: Conflicting Perspectives."

Ruth Macklin, Ph.D.; Philosopher/Bioethicist; Albert Einstein College of Medicine, Bronx, NY; "Implications of Labeling a Biological Phenomenon as a 'Disease' Versus Normal Variation."

Ronald V. Norris, M.D.; Psychiatrist; The Premenstrual Syndrome Program, Inc., Lynnfield, MA; "Historical Development of Progesterone Therapy."

P.M.S. O'Brien, M.D., M.R.C.O.G.; Obstetrician/Gynaecologist; University of Nottingham, England; "Controversial Aspects of Endocrine, Physical Factors and Treatment of Premenstrual Syndrome."

Robert L. Reid, M.D.; Obstetrician/Gynecologist, Reproductive Endocrinologist; Queen's University, Kingston, Ontario; "Premenstrual Syndrome as a Psychoendocrine Disorder."

David R. Rubinow, M.D.; Psychiatrist; National Institutes of Health, Bethesda, MD; "Practical and Ethical Aspects of Pharmacotherapeutic Evaluation of PMS."

Diane N. Ruble, Ph.D.; Psychologist; New York University, New York City, NY; "Perceptions of Menstrual and Premenstrual Symptoms: Self Definitional Processes at Menarche" (Jeanne Brooks-Gunn, Ph.D., co-author).

Robert L. Sadoff, M.D.; Clinical/Forensic Psychiatrist; University of Pennsylvania, Philadelphia; and Villanova University School of Law, Villanova, PA; "The Insanity Defense in Criminal Law."

Gwyneth A. Sampson, D.P.M., M.R.C.Psych.; Psychiatrist; Middlewood Hospital and University of Sheffield, England; "Premenstrual Syndrome: Characterization, Therapies, and the Law."

Meir Steiner, M.D., Ph.D.; Psychiatrist/Neuroscientist; St. Joseph's Hospital, Hamilton, Ontario; "Multiple Etiologies of Premenstrual Syndrome."

Michael J. Vergare, M.D.; Psychiatrist; Albert Einstein Medical Center, Northern Division, Philadelphia, Pa; "Premenstrual Syndrome: Implications for Psychiatric Practice."

COMMITTEE ON SOCIAL SCIENCE RESEARCH AND PUBLIC POLICY

The menstrual cycle is a normal event in the lives of most women of reproductive age. It does not disrupt their behavior and it does not disrupt their lives. A small percentage of women experience recurring menstrual-related problems, and some of these women find that those problems seriously affect their lives. Despite cases claiming an association between violent acts and the menstrual cycle, there are no studies confirming this. It is a violation of the dignity of all women to perpetuate stereotypes about the effect of menstruation on behavior.

Regardless of etiology, the experience of cyclic symptoms is an important and sometimes a serious one. We need to recognize women's experiences of these recurring symptoms and not dismiss them as figments of their imagination. At the same time, we need to distinguish these problems from other problems that have been mistakenly called PMS.

Unfortunately, the nature of the phenomenon called PMS remains ill-defined. Various aspects of the menstrual cycle need further interdisciplinary investigation. Psychological research shows clearly that using self-reports results in biases of various sorts. Social and cultural factors influence women's reported experiences and memories of them. This conclusion is shown by the research indicating that women's reported experiences vary as a function of culture, religion, social class, socialization at menarche, and current life events. (For this reason, we encourage the careful development and use of instruments that are sensitive to these factors and, when possible, verification with other measures.)

The attempts to study the phenomenon as a purely biological entity are inconclusive. We recommend: (1) further basic research on cycle physiology and the psychology of emotion; (2) the formation of interdisciplinary research teams to study menstrual-related experiences collaboratively; (3) cooperation between researchers and the organizations/groups composed of women with first-hand experience of PMS; (4) development of well-designed experimental approaches; (5) giving top priority to funding interdisciplinary research; and (6) funding an abstracting and referencing service that can make available the current research from all disciplinary fields to researchers, clinicians, and interested consumers.

Because the etiology of this phenomenon is unknown, all treatments are experimental. No treatment is risk-free. We urge caution and consideration of risks and benefits on the part of both health care professionals and people seeking treatment. We are concerned about the commercialization of treatments based upon limited and inconclusive evidence.

To correct the widespread misunderstanding of menstrual cycle-related experience, education should be top priority. We recommend creative education programs directed toward the general public, including both children and adults. In addition, special attention should be paid to the training and continuing education of members of the biomedical community. Because of their perspective, women's groups should be centrally involved in these programs.

Committee Members

Susan E. Bell, Ph.D. (Chair)
Sociologist
Bowdoin College
Brunswick, ME

Stephanie J. Bird, Ph.D.
Physiologist/Pharmacologist
Massachusetts Institute of Technology
Cambridge, MA

Virginia Cassara, M.A., M.S.S.W.
Social Worker/Educator
Premenstrual Syndrome Action, Inc.
Irvine, CA

Karen Paige Ericksen, Ph.D.
Psychologist
University of California
Davis, CA

Ruth Macklin, Ph.D.
Philosopher/Bioethicist
Albert Einstein College of Medicine
Bronx, NY

Diane N. Ruble, Ph.D.
Psychologist
New York University
New York, NY

Michael J. Vergare, M.D.
Psychiatrist
Albert Einstein Medical Center
Northern Division
Philadelphia, PA

COMMITTEE ON BIOMEDICAL ISSUES

Many women report a variety of physical and behavioral changes that occur in temporal relation to the menses, but there is, at present, no universally accepted definition of PMS. Although a number of symptoms such as irritability, abdominal bloating, mood lability, breast tenderness, hostility, and tension are frequently reported in relation to the premenstruum, diagnosis of PMS cannot be made solely on the basis of symptomatology. Most experts agree that a precise definition of PMS must incorporate information about severity and timing of symptoms. The importance of obtaining this information *prospectively* cannot be overemphasized. Prospective records have, in fact, revealed the existence of a group of women in whom symptoms cyclically reappear in the premenstrual phase of the cycle, with relief following the onset of menstruation. At times, premenstrual symptoms are sufficiently distressing to result in reports of significant impairment of function. However, it is not yet known if PMS is an extreme form of normal premenstrual symptoms, or if it is a distinctive clinical entity.

The current uncertainty arises in part from the differences that can be expected when separate disciplines examine a subject and from the inherent difficulty in comparing work that uses widely disparate constructs. It is even questionable whether various investigators have been examining the same basic phenomenon. Much of the confusion may result from the tendency to generalize findings from restricted samples of women.

Many modalities have been reported to be effective in the treatment of PMS. However, evidence at present does not support any current etiological model, nor does it support the therapeutic superiority of any prescribed treatment. The cornerstone of the treatment of PMS at present should be careful, comprehensive, longitudinal evaluation with attention paid to the severity and pattern of appearance of symptoms, as well as to medical, social, and psychological factors that may affect symptom appearance. Treatment may include such modalities as social support, education, counseling, life-style changes, and pharmacotherapy tailored to the patient's individual needs.

Much of the present difficulty in assessing treatments results from methodology that omits necessary control and placebo conditions, as well as the failure to select patients/subjects on the basis of multiple prospective ratings throughout the menstrual cycle and over the course of several cycles. Further conclusions concerning the efficacy of treatment modalities must await the results of rigorously designed studies that include the following: utilization of clear and consistent definitions of PMS; prospective diagnostic confirmation; double-blind placebo control trials; utilization of treatment cells that are long enough to avoid the obfuscating effects of intercycle symptomatic variation; and consideration of sociocultural variables. In addition, collateral objective assessment of symptoms is recommended to evaluate the reliability of subjective ratings.

It appears that the least ambiguous results will be obtained by studies of women who are severely affected premenstrually yet have no clinical evidence of emotional or behavioral disturbance at other phases of their menstrual cycle. If PMS could be defined in these women and the data used to construct operationally-defined criteria and specific symptom-rating tools, it should be possible to more reliably compare future studies of the etiology and treatment of this disabling condition.

Currently available data do not permit reliable estimates of the prevalence and impact of this disorder, highlighting the importance of the need for well-designed, prospective, epidemiological studies. Future research should consider the interactions of psychosocial, cultural, and biological factors in the development and expression of menstrually-related symptoms and should take advantage of interdisciplinary methods and expertise.

Increasing social pressures and demands for treatment have led to a heightened awareness of PMS in clinical practice, and constitute a mandate for careful research on the incidence, etiology, and treatment of PMS. The public should be fully educated in order to avoid exploitation inherent in the marketing of untested, ineffective, and often expensive therapies. Equally important is the need to establish educational programs for health care providers. Development and implementation of such educational programs will enable health professionals to deal more effectively with the needs of affected women and their families. Finally, a broad-based, multidisciplinary understanding of PMS and its relation to other menstrual symptoms may provide an important model for studying interactions of biological, cultural, and social concomitants of biobehavioral changes.

Committee Members

David R. Rubinow, M.D. (Chair)
Psychiatrist
National Institutes of Health
Bethesda, MD

Christopher Boorse, Ph.D.
Philosopher
University of Delaware
Newark, DE

S. Louise Carter, Ph.D.
Psychologist and Science Writer
Seattle, WA

Uriel Halbreich, M.D.
Psychiatrist
Albert Einstein College of Medicine
Bronx, NY

Ronald V. Norris, M.D.
Psychiatrist
The Premenstrual Syndrome Program, Inc.
Lynnfield, MA

P.M. Shaughn O'Brien, M.D., M.R.C.O.G.
Obstetrician/Gynaecologist
University of Nottingham
Nottingham, England

Robert L. Reid, M.D.
Obstetrician/Gynecologist, Reproductive Endocrinologist
Queen's University
Kingston, Ontario, Canada

Gwyneth A. Sampson, D.P.M., M.R.C.Psych.
Psychiatrist
Middlewood Hospital, and
University of Sheffield
Sheffield, England

Meir Steiner, M.D., Ph.D.
Psychiatrist/Neuroscientist
St. Joseph's Hospital
Hamilton, Ontario, Canada

A crime consists of two parts: *actus reus* and *mens rea*. "*Actus reus*" is a Latin term meaning "guilty act;" that is, the act must be voluntary and the product of free will. "*Mens rea*" is a Latin term referring to the mental state of the actor. Examples of legally recognized mental states are: purposely, knowingly, recklessly, and negligently. In order for a defendant to be found guilty of a crime, the prosecution must prove beyond a reasonable doubt both elements of the crime, the *actus reus* and the *mens rea*.

Premenstrual syndrome — whatever the definition or etiology — while not a defense *per se*, can be relevant to the determination of the the requisite criminal intent *(mens rea)* and/or the voluntariness of the defendant's act *(actus reus)*. For example, automatism *is* a complete defense, based on a lack of *actus reus* (that is, it is behavior that is not part of any conscious plan of action). It is possible that a woman suffering from PMS may be excused from criminal liability by utilizing a defense of automatism. Moreover, there is the possibility that a woman suffering from PMS may have a mental, emotional, and/or physiological condition or disorder that interferes with her ability to form the requisite criminal intent *(mens rea)*.

Medical science and law approach their objectives from different perspectives. Medicine demands a scientific basis of proof and validity with a high degree of reliability and certainty. At present, there are no scientific studies to show that PMS causes violent behavior, although cases have surfaced suggesting such an association. Scientific evidence is usually not admissible without consensus of the scientific community. On the other hand, the criminal defense attorney is obligated by the ethics of the legal profession to zealously defend his or her client, and to this end, to raise all possible and reasonable defenses. This could require courtroom presentation of PMS in order to highlight any reasonable doubt regarding *actus reus* (voluntariness) or *mens rea* (criminal intent).

We do not anticipate a large number of criminal cases utilizing PMS inasmuch as the defendant must have been suffering from PMS at the time of the offense, and PMS must have caused or contributed to the behavior at issue. It is anticipated that PMS will be introduced into various areas of civil law. In 1983, PMS was considered a factor, but ultimately rejected as insufficient to discharge a debt in bankruptcy court. It may also surface in domestic relations cases, including child custody matters, and suits involving personal injury and property damage. Inasmuch as the definition and etiology of PMS are still uncertain, we would caution against its misuse or abuse in these cases. PMS may be a relevant factor in these cases, and like all other cases, each should be judged on its own merits. Finally, interdisciplinary research and education may modify our current concepts and recommendations.

Committee Members

Robert L. Sadoff, M.D. (Chair)
Clinical/Forensic Psychiatrist
University of Pennsylvania
Philadelphia, PA; and
Villanova University School of Law
Villanova, PA

Stephanie L. Benson, J.D.
Attorney
New York, NY

Laurence D. Houlgate, Ph.D.
Philosopher
California Polytechnic State University
San Luis Obispo, CA

C. Ray Jeffery, Ph.D.
Criminologist
Florida State University
Tallahassee, FL

AUTHOR INDEX

INDEX